PLANS OF CARE FOR
SPECIALTY PRACTICE

*Obstetric and Gynecologic
Nursing*

PLANS OF CARE FOR
SPECIALTY PRACTICE

Obstetric and Gynecologic Nursing

MEG GULANICK, RN, PhD
Assistant Professor
Niehoff School of Nursing
Loyola University of Chicago
Chicago, Illinois

MICHELE KNOLL PUZAS, RNC, MHPE
Pediatric Nurse Clinician
Michael Reese Hospital and Medical Center
Chicago, Illinois

DEIDRA GRADISHAR, RNC, BS
Obstetric Outreach Educator
University of Chicago Perinatal Network
Assistant Clinical Manager, Birth Rooms
University of Chicago Hospitals
Chicago, Illinois

KATHY V. GETTRUST, RN, BSN ~ *Series Editor*
Case Manager
Midwest Medical Home Care
Milwaukee, Wisconsin

Delmar Publishers Inc.™
ITP

NOTICE TO THE READER

Publisher does not warrant or guarantee any of the products described herein or perform any independent analysis in connection with any of the product information contained herein. Publisher does not assume, and expressly disclaims, any obligation to obtain and include information other than that provided to it by the manufacturer.

The reader is expressly warned to consider and adopt all safety precautions that might be indicated by the activities described herein and to avoid all potential hazards. By following the instructions contained herein, the reader willingly assumes all risks in connection with such instructions.

The publisher makes no representations or warranties of any kind, including but not limited to, the warranties of fitness for particular purpose or merchantability, nor are any such representations implied with respect to the material set forth herein, and the publisher takes no responsibility with respect to such material. The publisher shall not be liable for any special, consequential or exemplary damages resulting, in whole or in part, from the readers' use of, or reliance upon, this material.

Delmar publishing team:
Publisher: David C. Gordon
Administrative Editor: Patricia Casey
Associate Editor: Elisabeth F. Williams
Project Editor: Danya M. Plotsky
Production Coordinator: Mary Ellen Black
Art and Design Coordinator: Megan K. DeSantis
Timothy J. Conners

For information, address

Delmar Publishers Inc.
3 Columbia Circle, Box 15015
Albany, NY 12212-5015

COPYRIGHT © 1994 BY DELMAR PUBLISHERS INC.

The trademark ITP is used under license.

Printed in the United States of America
Published simultaneously in Canada
by Nelson Canada,
a division of The Thomson Corporation

1 2 3 4 5 6 7 8 9 10 XXX 00 99 98 97 96 95 94

Library of Congress Cataloging-in-Publication Data

Obstetric and gynecologic nursing / [edited by] Meg Gulanick, Deidra
    Gradishar, Michele Knoll Puzas
        p. cm.—(Plans of care for specialty practice.)
    Includes index.
    ISBN 0-8273-5468-1
    1. Gynecologic nursing.   2. Maternity nursing.   3. Nursing care
plans.   I. Gulanick, Meg.   II. Gradishar, Deidra.   III. Puzas,
Michele Knoll.   IV. Series.
    [DNLM: 1. Obstetrical Nursing—methods.   2. Gynecology—nurses'
instruction.   3. Patient Care Planning.   4. Genital Diseases,
Female—nursing.   5. Pregnancy—nurses' instruction.   6. Labor—
nurses' instruction.   WY 157 O122 1994]
RG105.O27 1994
610.73'678—dc20
DNLM/DLC
    for Library of Congress   93-5045
                                                                              CIP

TABLE OF CONTENTS

CONTRIBUTORS

Sharon Broderick, RN, MS
Clinic Manager, Perinatal Services
University of Chicago Hospitals,
Chicago
Lying-in Hospital, Chicago, Illinois
• Chemical Addiction During
  Pregnancy

Monalisa S. Bron, RN, BSN
Staff Nurse, Obstetrics and
Gynecology
Michael Reese Hospital and Medical
Center
Chicago, Illinois
• Anemia: Iron Deficiency
  Postpartum

Ursula Brozek, RN, MS
Clinical Consultant
Horizon Mental Health Services, Inc.
Chicago, Illinois
• Eating Disorders: Anorexia
  Nervosa and Bulemia Nervosa
• Rape—Trauma Syndrome

Reneau A. Buckner, RNC, MS
Assistant Clinical Manager, Labor
and Delivery
Rush-Presbyterian-St. Luke's Hospital
Chicago, Illinois
• Preterm Premature Rupture of
  Membranes

Connie J. Campbell, RN, MSN, MJ
Nurse Manager, Family Centered
Maternity/Gynecology Unit
St. Joseph's Hospital & Health Care
Center
Chicago, Illinois
• Vaginal Delivery: Post Partum
  Care

Elicita A. Chavez, RN
Assistant Nurse Manager, Labor and
Delivery
Michael Reese Hospital and Medical
Center
Chicago, Illinois
• Prolapsed Cord/Emergency
  Cesarean Section

Sarah Cohen, RN
Staff Nurse, Labor and Delivery
Michael Reese Hospital and Medical
Center
Chicago, Illinois
• Epidural Anesthesia During Labor
  and Delivery
• Hypertension, Pregnancy-Induced/
  HELLP Syndrome

Joanne Coleman, RN, BSN
Staff Nurse, Labor and Delivery
Michael Reese Hospital and Medical
Center
Chicago, Illinois
• Placenta Previa

Peggy Cowling, RNC, MSN
Clinical Nurse Specialist, Obstetrics
and Gynecology
South Suburban Hospital
Hazel Crest, Illinois
• Urinary Tract Infections

Patricia Douglas, RN
Staff Nurse, Labor and Delivery
Michael Reese Hospital and Medical
Center
Chicago, Illinois
• Amnioinfusion, Intrapartum Care
  of Patient Receiving

Janet L. Engstrom, RN, PhD, CNM
Assistant Professor, Maternal and
  Child
Nursing, College of Nursing
University of Illinois at Chicago
Chicago, Illinois
- Infertility
- Pelvic Inflammatory Disease
- Vulvovaginitis

Linda Escobar, RN, BSN
Clinical Supervisor
Obstetrics and Gynecology
Humana-Michael Reese Health Plan
Chicago, Illinois
- Intrauterine Fetal Demise
  (Stillbirth)

Imelda Fahy, RN
Staff Nurse, Labor and Delivery
Michael Reese Hospital and Medical
  Center
Chicago, Illinois
- Fourth Stage of Labor

Ann Filipski, RN, MS
Assistant Professor, School of
  Nursing
St. Xavier University
Chicago, Illinois
- Depression
- Loss

Catherine Folker-Maglaya, RN,
  MSN, IBCLC
Lactation Consultant/Clinical Nurse
  Specialist
Lutheran General Hospital
Park Ridge, Illinois
- Breast Self-Examination (BSE)
- Facilitating Breast Feeding
- Newborn Assessment From First
  Two Hours of Life Through Three
  Days
- Promoting Parent-Infant
  Attachment

Deidra Gradishar, RNC, BS
Obstetric Outreach Educator
University of Chicago Perinatal
  Network;
Assistant Clinical Manager, Birth
  Rooms
University of Chicago Hospitals
Chicago, Illinois
- Abruptio Placentae
- Battered Woman
- Breast Biopsy
- Ectopic/Tubal Pregnancy
- Hyperemesis Gravidarum
- Mammogram
- Pelvic Examination and the
  Papanicolaou Test (PAP Smear)
- Pregnant Patient in First Trimester
- Pregnant Patient in Third
  Trimester

Joy C. Grohar, RNC, MS
President, Comprehensive Perinatal
  Consultants
Chicago, Illinois
- Pain Management During Labor

Meg Gulanick, RN, PhD
Assistant Professor
Niehoff School of Nursing
Loyala University of Chicago
Chicago, Illinois
- Menopause
- Osteoporosis: Prophylaxis and
  Treatment

Lisa Hauser, RN, BSN
Women's Health Resources
Illinois Masonic Medical Center
Chicago, Illinois
- Lesbian Health Concerns

Margaret Hixson, RN, BSN
Staff Nurse, Labor and Delivery
Michael Reese Hospital and Medical
  Center
Chicago, Illinois
- Cesarean Birth: Postpartum
- Infertility as Emotional Crisis

Bernadette Keller, RNC, BSN
Staff Nurse, Labor and Delivery
Michael Reese Hospital and Medical
    Center
Chicago, Illinois
• Colposcopy
• Intrapartum Patient
• Newborn Assessment From Birth
    to 2 Hours of Life

Cheryl A. King, RN, BSN
Assistant Nurse Manager, Labor and
    Delivery
Michael Reese Hospital and Medical
    Center
Chicago, Illinois
• Prolapsed Cord/Emergency
    Cesarean Section

Joan Klein, RN, MS
Associate Professor, School of
    Nursing
St. Xavier University
Chicago, Illinois
• Substance Abuse

Jill Kollman, RN, BSN
Nurse Manager of Labor and
    Delivery/OB-GYNE
Riverside Medical Center
Kankakee, Illinois
• Pregnant Patient in First Trimester

Mary Ann Krol, RN, MSN
Clinical Nurse Specialist, Surgery
Loyola University Medical Center
Maywood, Illinois
• Mastectomy

Margo Elizabeth Lewis-Brown, RN,
    MS
Research Nurse, OB/Gyne Units
University of Chicago Hospitals
Chicago, Illinois
• Contraception Methods

Daria Lieber, RN
Staff Nurse, Obstetrics and
    Gynecology
Michael Reese Hospital and Medical
    Center
Chicago, Illinois
• Cesarean Birth: Postpartum

Mary Christine McCarthy, RN, BSN
Staff Nurse, Obstetrics and
    Gynecology
Michael Reese Hospital and Medical
    Center
Chicago, Illinois
• Oxytocin Induction/Augmentation
    of Labor
• Premature Labor (Tocolysis)

Lou Ellen McElmurray, BSN, RN
Nurse Manager
St. Mary's Hospital
Kankakee, Illinois
• Battered Woman

Christine Potaczak McFadden, RN,
    BSN
Staff Nurse, Birth Rooms
University of Chicago Hospitals
Chicago, Illinois
• Pregnant Patient in Second
    Trimester

Mary McGoldrick-Charliza, RN,
    MPH
Perinatal Outreach Educator
University of Illinois Perinatal Center
Chicago, Illinois
• Condyloma Acuminata (Genital
    Warts)
• Dilatation and Curretage (D&C)

Pat Moss, RN, MSN
AIDS Clinical Nurse Specialist
Michael Reese Hospital and Medical
    Center
Chicago, Illinois
• Human Immunodeficiency Virus
    Disease

Marleen Mrozek, RN, BSN
Staff Nurse, Labor and Delivery
Michael Reese Hospital and Medical
    Center
Chicago, Illinois
• Chemical Addiction during
    Pregnancy

Mary Mullee, RN, BSN
Staff Nurse, Labor and Delivery
Michael Reese Hospital and Medical
  Center
Chicago, Illinois
- Oxytocin Induction/Augmentation
  of Labor
- Postpartum Hemorrhage

Charlotte Niznik, RN, MS, CDE
Diabetes Clinical Nurse Specialist
Northwestern Memorial Hospital
Chicago, Illinois
- Gestational Diabetes Mellitus

Manie Omsin, RN, BSN
Staff Nurse, Obstetrics
Michael Reese Hospital and Medical
  Center
Chicago, Illinois
- Anemia: Iron Deficiency
  Postpartum

Denise Pang-Hong, RNC, MS
Clinical Supervisor
Edgewater Medical Center
Chicago, Illinois
- Ectopic/Tubal Pregnancy

Patrice Perez, RN, MSN
School Nurse, Hinsdale Community
  School
District 181, Hinsdale, Illinois
- Breast Biopsy
- Mammogram
- Pelvic Examination and the
  Papanicolaou Test (PAP Smear)

Charlotte Razvi, RN, PhD, MSN
Clinical Nurse Specialist
Obstetrics and Gynecology/Lactation
Specialist, Michael Reese Hospital
  and Medical Center
Chicago, Illinois
- Newborn Assessment From First
  Two Hours of Life to Three Days

Caroline Reich, RN, MS
Nurse Manager, Obstetrics/Nursery
  and Special Care Nursery
Riverside Hospital
Kankakee, Illinois
- Circumcision Care

Mary Therese Rinzel, RN, MS
Nurse Manager, Mother-Baby Unit
Lutheran General Hospital
Park Ridge, Illinois
- Promoting Parent-Infant
  Attachment

Mary Sandelski, RN, MSN
Nurse Manager & Clinical Nurse
  Specialist Obstetrics
St. Mary's Medical Center
Hobart, Indiana
- Intrapartum Patient
- Newborn Assessment From Birth
  to 2 Hours of Life
- Perinatal Loss
- Spontaneous Abortion (First
  Trimester)

Paula Schipiour, RN, MS
Nurse Manager/Nurse Clinician
Antenatal Unit
Michael Reese Hospital and Medical
  Center
Chicago, Illinois
- Fetal Well-being/Fetal Stress

Deborah Schy, RNC, MSN
Obstetric Outreach Educator
Lutheran General Hospital
Park Ridge, Illinois
- High-Risk Pregnant Patient
- Premenstrual Syndrome

Kathy Stewart, RN
Staff Nurse, Labor and Delivery
Michael Reese Hospital and Medical
  Center
Chicago, Illinois
- Promoting Parent-Infant
  Attachment

Denise Talley-Lacy, RN, MSN
Staff Nurse, Labor and Delivery
Michael Reese Hospital and Medical
  Center
Chicago, Illinois
- Premature Labor (Tocolysis)

Maripat Tomaszkiewicz, RN, MSN
Staff Nurse, Labor and Delivery
Michael Reese Hospital and Medical
    Center
Chicago, Illinois
* Intrauterine Fetal Demise
    (Stillbirth)

Theresa Vanderhei, RN
Staff Nurse, Labor and Delivery
Michael Reese Hospital and Medical
    Center
Chicago, Illinois
* Postpartum Hemorrhage

Denise Wheeler, RN, MS, CNM
Certified Nurse Midwife
Broadlawns Medical Center
Des Moines, Iowa
* Bartholin Cyst/Abscess
* Hysterectomy
* Uterine Fibroids

Janet Williams, RN, BSN
Staff Nurse, Labor and Delivery
Michael Reese Hospital and Medical
    Center
Chicago, Illinois
* Prostaglandin-Induced Abortion
    (Second Trimester)

Valerie Wolf, RN, BSN
Staff Nurse, Labor and Delivery
Michael Reese Hospital and Medical
    Center
Chicago, Illinois
* Hypertension, Pregnancy-Induced/
    HELLP Syndrome

Jeffrey Zurlinden, RN, MS
Director Community Program for
    Clinical Research on AIDS
Chicago, Illinois
* Chlamydia
* Gonorrhea
* Herpes
* Syphilis

PREFACE

This book is about women's health. This project was born out of an interest to produce a book addressing women's health needs across their life cycle. We believe that this approach provides a more holistic framework than the fragmented systems approach. While we make no claims to being all inclusive in the selection of our topics, we direct your attention to the care plan guides on loss, lesbian health, rape-trauma syndrome, HIV disease, battered woman, facilitating breast feeding, eating disorders, abortion, and many obstetrical topics. Some of these titles have appeared in specialty books, but others are quite unique. What is special is that they have never before been published in a single reference specifically designed for the individual interested in women's health.

The planning guides selected for this publication represent the work of 52 authors whose special interests and life's work and study are directed toward enhancing the nursing care for the women they serve. These contributors developed their care guides for the practicing nurse. We imagined nurse practitioners, midwives, and perinatal nurses, as well as ambulatory care nurses, using this text as a reference, a template for planning the care they would give their patients. We did not include obvious information or principles commonly understood by the mature practitioner or facts contained in more basic texts. There are already many texts that do this admirably. Instead, this book focuses on the "clinical pearls."

For the novice and the student nurse we integrated very specific teaching guidelines and rationale that explain the complex rather than the obvious. This book supports the process of nursing practice while presuming that where and when nurses provide care, the nursing process is in operation. We articulate for nurses the things they do every day in the care of their patients.

This book is testimony to the fact that the nurse expert lives and works in rural as well as urban areas, ambulatory as well as inpatient settings, the community hospital as well as the medical center, for the contributors of this book come from all of these areas. The authors integrated professional and regional standards into the care guides that they developed. Most of all, they recorded what they see, what they assess, what they do, why they do it that way, and what outcomes they want to see for their patients.

We invite you to use this book to bring added dimension to the care you render and better understanding of the women you serve.

Meg Gulanick
Deidra Gradishar
Michele Knoll Puzas

ACKNOWLEDGMENTS

We are very grateful to our colleagues who have helped with this book: Barbara Norwitz for her vision and support of this project in its earliest stages. Patricia E. Casey, Elisabeth F. Williams, and the Delmar staff for their expertise and guidance through the publishing process. Emma Glover and Rosalie Clay for their quality work in preparing the manuscript. The nurse authors for their willingness to share their knowledge. To the many patients who served as our "teachers" in the clinical setting.

SERIES INTRODUCTION

Scientific and technological developments over the past several decades have revolutionized health care and care of the sick. These rapid and extensive advancements of knowledge have occurred in all fields, necessitating an ever-increasing specialization of practice. For nurses to be effective and meet the challenge in today's specialty settings, the body of clinical knowledge and skill needs to continually expand. *Plans of Care for Specialty Practice* has been written to aid the practicing nurse in meeting this challenge. The purpose of this series is to provide comprehensive, state-of-the-art plans of care and associated resource information for patient situations most commonly seen within a specialty that will serve as a standard from which care can be individualized. These plans of care are based on the profession's scientific approach to problem solving—the nursing process. Though the books are written primarily as a guide for frontline staff nurses and clinical nurse specialists practicing in specialty settings, they have application for student nurses as well.

DOCUMENTATION OF CARE

The Joint Commission on Accreditation of Healthcare Organizations (JCAHO) assumes authority for evaluating the quality and effectiveness of the practice of nursing. In 1991, the JCAHO developed its first new nursing care standards in more than a decade. One of the changes brought about by these new standards was the elimination of need for every patient to have a handwritten or computer-generated care plan in his or her chart detailing all or most of the care to be provided. The Joint Commission's standard that describes the documentation requirements stipulates that nursing assessments, identification of nursing diagnoses and/or patient care needs, interventions, outcomes of care, and discharge planning be permanently integrated into the clinical record. In other words, the nursing process needs to be documented. A separate care plan is no longer needed; however, planning and implementing care must continue as always, but using whatever form of documentation that has been approved by an institution. *Plans of Care for Specialty Practice* can be easily used with a wide variety of approaches to documentation of care.

ELEMENTS OF THE PLANS OF CARE

The chapter title is the presenting situation, which represents the most commonly seen conditions/disorders treated within the specialty setting. It may be a medical diagnosis (e.g., diabetes mellitus), a syndrome (e.g., acquired immunodeficiency syndrome), a surgical procedure (e.g., mastectomy), or a diagnostic/therapeutic procedure (e.g., thrombolytic therapy).

An opening paragraph provides a definition or concise overview of the presenting situation. It describes the condition and may contain pertinent physiological/psychological bases for the disorder. It is brief and not intended to replace further investigation for comprehensive understanding of the condition.

Etiologies

A listing of causative factors responsible for or contributing to the presenting situation is provided. This may include predisposing diseases, injuries or trauma, surgeries, microorganisms, genetic factors, environmental hazards, drugs, or psychosocial disorders. In presenting situations where no clear causal relationship can be established, current theories regarding the etiology may be included. For those chapters pertaining to clinical procedures, indications for the procedure are listed instead of etiologies and clinical manifestations.

Clinical Manifestations

Objective and subjective signs and symptoms which describe the particular presenting situation are included. This information is revealed as a result of a health history and physical assessment and becomes part of the data base.

Clinical/Diagnostic Findings

This component contains possible diagnostic tests and procedures which might be done to determine abnormalities associated with a particular presenting situation. The name of the diagnostic procedure and the usual abnormal findings are listed.

Nursing Diagnosis

The nursing management of the health problem commences with the planning care phase of the nursing process. This includes obtaining a comprehensive history and physical assessment, identification of the nursing diagnoses, expected outcomes, interventions, and discharge planning needs.

Diagnostic labels identified by NANDA through the Tenth National Conference in April 1992 are being used throughout this series. (Based on North American Nursing Diagnosis Association, 1992. *NANDA Nursing Diagnoses: Definitions and Classification 1992.*) We have also identified new diagnoses not yet on the official NANDA list. We endorse NANDA's recommendation for nurses to develop new nursing diagnoses as the need arises and we encourage nurses using this series to do the same.

"Related to" Statements

Related to statements suggest a link or connection to the nursing diagnosis and provide direction for identifying appropriate nursing interventions. They are termed contributing factors, causes, or etiologies. There is frequently more than one related to statement for a given diagnosis. For example, change in job, marital difficulties, and impending surgery may all be "related to" the patient's nursing diagnosis of anxiety.

There is disagreement at present regarding inclusion of pathophysiological/medical diagnoses in the list of related to statements. Frequently, a medical diagnosis does not provide adequate direction for nursing care. For example, the nursing diagnosis of chronic pain related to rheumatoid arthritis does not readily suggest specific nursing interventions. It is more useful for the nurse to identify specific causes of the chronic pain such as inflammation, swelling, and fatigue; these in turn suggest more specific interventions. In cases where the medical diagnosis provides the best available information, as occurs with the more medically oriented diagnoses such as decreased cardiac output or impaired gas exchange, the medical terminology is included.

Defining Characteristics

Data collection is frequently the source for identifying defining characteristics, sometimes called signs and symptoms or patient behaviors. These data, both subjective and objective, are organized into meaningful patterns and used to verify the nursing diagnosis. The most commonly seen defining characteristics for a given diagnosis are included and should not be viewed as an all-inclusive listing.

Risk Factors

Nursing diagnoses designated as high risk are supported by risk factors that direct nursing actions to reduce or prevent the problem from developing. Since these nursing diagnoses have not yet occurred, risk factors replace the listing of actual defining characteristics and related to statements.

Patient Outcomes

Patient outcomes, sometimes termed patient goals, are observable behaviors or data which measure changes in the condition of the patient after nursing treatment. They are objective indicators of progress toward prevention of the development of high-risk nursing diagnoses or resolution/modification of actual diagnoses. Like other elements of the plan of care, patient outcome statements are dynamic and must be reviewed and modified periodically as the patient progresses. Assigning realistic "target or evaluation dates" for evaluation of progress toward outcome achievement is crucial. Since there are so many considerations involved in when the outcome could be achieved (e.g., varying lengths of stay, individual patient condition), these plans of care do not include evaluation dates; the date needs to be individualized and assigned using the professional judgment and discretion of the nurse caring for the patient.

Nursing Interventions

Nursing interventions are the treatment options/actions the nurse employs to prevent, modify, or resolve the nursing diagnosis. They are driven by the related to statements and risk factors and are selected based on the outcomes to be achieved. Treatment options should be chosen only if they apply realistically to a specific patient condition. The nurse also needs to determine frequencies for each intervention based on professional judgment and individual patient need.

We have included independent, interdependent, and dependent nursing interventions as they reflect current practice. We have not made a distinction between these kinds of interventions because of institutional differences and increasing independence in nursing practice. The interventions that are interdependent or dependent will require collaboration with other professionals. The nurse will need to determine when this is necessary and take appropriate action. The interventions include assessment, therapeutic, and teaching actions.

Rationales
The rationales provide scientific explanation or theoretical bases for the interventions; interventions can then be selected more intelligently and actions can be tailored to each individual's needs.

The rationales provided may be used as a quick reference for the nurse unfamiliar with the reason for a given intervention and as a tool for patient education. These rationales may include principles, theory, and/or research findings from current literature. The rationales are intended as reference information and, as such, should not be transcribed into the permanent patient record. A rationale is not provided when the intervention is self-explanatory.

Discharge Planning/Continuity of Care
Because stays in acute care hospitals are becoming shorter due to cost containment efforts, patients are frequently discharged still needing care; discharge planning is the process of anticipating and planning for needs after discharge. Effective discharge planning begins with admission and continues with ongoing assessment of the patient and family needs. Included in the discharge planning/continuity of care section are suggestions for follow-up measures, such as skilled nursing care; physical, occupational, speech, or psychiatric therapy; spiritual counseling, social service assistence; follow-up appointments, and equipment/supplies.

References
A listing of references appears at the conclusion of each plan of care or related group of plans. The purpose of the references is to cite specific work used and to specify background information or suggestions for further reading. Citings provided represent the most current nursing theory and/or research bases for inclusion in the plans of care.

Health Teaching Guides
These comprehensive teaching guides highlight the relevant information necessary for comprehensive patient education.

A Word About Family
The authors and editors of this series recognize the vital role that family and/or other significant people play in the recovery of a patient. Isolation from the family unit during hospitalization may disrupt self-concept and feelings of security. Family members, or persons involved in the patient's care, must be included in the teaching to ensure that it is appropriate and will be followed. In an effort to constrain the books' size, the patient outcome, nursing intervention, and discharge planning sections usually do not include reference to the family or other significant people; however, the reader can assume that they are to be included along with the patient whenever appropriate.

Any undertaking of the magnitude of this series becomes the concern of many people. I specifically thank all of the very capable nursing specialists who authored or edited the individual books. Their attention to providing state-of-the-art information in a quick, usable form will provide the reader with current reference information for providing excellent patient care.

The editorial staff, particularly Patricia E. Casey and Elisabeth F. Williams, and production people at Delmar Publishers have been outstanding. Their frank criticism, comments, and encouragement have improved the quality of the series.

Finally, but most importantly, I thank my husband, John, and children, Katrina and Allison, for their sacrifices and patience during yet another publishing project.

Kathy V. Gettrust
Series Editor

LIST OF TABLES

LIST OF FIGURES

Psychosocial Concerns

▼

ℬATTERED WOMAN

Lou Ellen McElmurray, RN, BSN
Deidra Gradishar, RNC, BS

Battering is marked by psychological or physical abuse; the perpetrator attempts to coerce the victim in defiance of her personal rights. This care plan addresses nursing management in the acute phase of treatment. Battering includes four types of interpersonal violence:

1. Sexual: forced sexual activity of any kind
2. Physical: including choking, slapping, kicking, biting, pushing, use of weapons, punching
3. Social: including degradation, threats to children, isolation, excessive jealousy
4. Threatened or actual destruction of property

Every socioeconomic group is represented among battered women.

ETIOLOGIES

The cycle of violence may have begun for both abuser and victim when they were children:

- Abuser and victim may have
  − observed abuse of the women in their families.
  − suffered physical or sexual abuse.
  Abused women characteristically
- have low self-esteem
- have difficulty in protecting themselves
- feel they are to blame for the abuse

CLINICAL MANIFESTATIONS

- Injuries at different stages of healing
- Inconsistent description of how injuries occurred
- Reports of battering
- Injuries to the head, face, neck, or trunk

3

▼

NURSING DIAGNOSIS: DECISIONAL CONFLICT REGARDING RELATIONSHIP WITH ABUSER

Related To
- Lack of experience with decision-making
- Lack of relevant information
- Support system deficit
- Multiple sources of information

Defining Characteristics
Uncertainty about choices
Vacillation between alternative choices
Delayed decision-making
Physical signs of distress/tension
Rationalization of partner's behavior
Return to abusive environment
Lack of confidence in ability to manage alone and make independent
    decisions

Patient Outcome
Patient will receive the information and support she needs to make an effective decision about continuing/changing her relationship with her abuser.

Nursing Interventions	Rationales

Provide information about the cycle of violence. The perpetrator's cyclic pattern is three-phased:
1. Phase I
   • experiences increased tension
   • gets increasingly angry
   • blames victim for untoward circumstances in his life
   • provokes violent arguments
2. Phase II
   • engages in battery: physical, sexual, emotional
3. Phase III
   • feels remorse over what he has done
   • denies, minimizes, or blames the victim for his violence
   • promises never to hurt the victim again
4. Phase III becomes progressively shorter over time.
5. Eventually Phase I is reentered.
	Information about cyclic pattern provides understanding of role of perpetrator vs. victim.

Assess for behaviors suggestive of abuse: 1. comments about emotional abuse 2. attempts to minimize injuries 3. anxiety about being away from partner too long 4. anger, defensiveness 5. change in routine appointment patterns 6. vague somatic complaints 7. expression of suicidal ideation or gestures, depression, substance abuse 8. complaints of a jealous partner 9. reports of sleep, performance disturbances 10. degree of clinical depression	Some of the symptoms of abuse are subtle. The presence of these symptoms may, upon exploration with the patient, reveal domestic violence as a contributing factor.
Assess the woman's strengths and coping mechanisms and the effect to which the abuse is resulting in other dysfunctional behaviors.	Victims of domestic violence are at risk for other emotional problems, including substance abuse and suicide.

Nursing Interventions	**Rationales**
Provide the patient with information about the symptoms of escalating physical danger: 1. a weapon brought into the home 2. extreme jealousy/increased jealousy 3. rape 4. assaults extending to other vulnerable family members (children, elderly parents, pets) 5. stalking or surveillance of the victim 6. remorse for violence no longer expressed after abuse 7. weapons used during assaults	Battering must be seen as potentially lethal. Individuals immersed in the cycle of violence may not be aware of the subtle changes in behaviors that signal imminent deadly danger.
Help patient identify and explore her options. Indicate that hope exists.	Hopelessness and social isolation are frequent experiences of these patients. They may require enormous amounts of support to break the cycle.
Provide information about options: 1. immediate access to shelter 2. information about shelter should she choose to access it later 3. referral to legal or police agencies to pursue legal recourse 4. return to abusive partner with follow-up appointment.	Fear may prevent the victim from seeing all the options open to her.
Assist the patient in devising an exit plan, including a safe place to go. Suggest she have important papers and some money and clothes in a safe place in case she decides to leave in a hurry.	Having a plan of escape aids the woman in seeing change as an option to the abuse.

Nursing Interventions	Rationales
Inform patient of legal statutes in resident state: 1. Many states allow victims to make a police report without signing a criminal complaint. 2. Illinois law provides that victims of domestic violence have the right to press charges against the abuser. 3. The court may enter an order of protection on the victim's behalf, the victim may petition for an order of protection, or an order of protection can be requested on a victim's behalf if the victim is a child or incapacitated.	Patient must be given information about her rights under the law and her options. Illinois and many other states require health care providers to give patients suspected of battering adequate information regarding services available.
Respect a battered woman's decision to return home.	The victim's fear and anxiety may prevent her from terminating the abusive relationship. The professional needs to be aware of her personal response to the patient's ambivalence and to remain nonjudgmental. The patient has a right to beliefs/activities that conflict with those of the nurse.
Assess patient's support system.	

▼

NURSING DIAGNOSIS: HIGH RISK FOR TRAUMA

Risk Factors
Physical abuse

Patient Outcomes
- The victim of battering is identified.
- The trauma is identified and treated.

Nursing Interventions	Rationales
Separate the woman from any partner who may have accompanied her for treatment. Provide a quiet, private environment for the interview.	The patient may not feel safe verbalizing concerns in the presence of her partner.
Interview the patient using open-ended questions. Encourage—but do not force—responses.	The patient may not choose disclosure at this time.
Assess for signs of abuse. 1. Multiple emergency room visits 2. Injuries at various stages of healing 3. Inconsistent description of how injuries occurred 4. Poor healing of old injuries 5. A pattern of injuries about the head, face, neck, or trunk	If a pregnant woman presents with physical injuries, suspect battering; 25% to 45% of all battered women report battering during pregnancy.
Complete a head-to-toe physical assessment, including a neurological examination. Use a body map to identify the site and extent of any old and new injuries.	This examination serves as documentation of the extent of injuries.
Obtain required diagnostic tests to confirm injuries.	Documentation is necessary for clinical treatment as well as legal evidence.
Assess for symptoms of forced vaginal/anal penetrations.	Rape is a common form of partner abuse.
Assess for sexually transmitted diseases.	Even though the victim may be feeling very vulnerable at this time, a complete assessment is critical.
Implement treatment plan for each identified injury.	
Provide information on contraception.	Pregnancy does not stop—and sometimes exaggerates—battering.

Nursing Interventions	Rationales
Document: 1. location and extent of all injuries: • inform patient of existence of this information in medical record • advise patient of availability of this information for use in court or with law enforcement agencies	
2. treatment and the existence of any permanent or long-term damage caused by the injuries.	Again, this information is required for appropriate medical management and successful legal process.
3. consent for any photographs taken.	
4. surgeries and treatments performed/required for treatment of abuse.	
5. description of abuse event in victim's own words.	This will be useful in the event that the medical record is subpoenaed for court.
6. referrals/information/resources provided to the patient.	To document that the health care provider has complied with legal imperatives requiring that the patient be informed of resources.
7. interactions with partner/perpetrator.	Care provider needs to be aware that couple may have reconciled. A threatening situation may not be apparent to an observer, yet may still be present.

DISCHARGE PLANNING/CONTINUITY OF CARE

- Provide information about shelters and alternatives available by calling the Domestic Violence Hotline at 1–800–333–SAFE.
- Provide pamphlets that include resource lists, hotlines and legal rights.
- Refer for psychological counseling.
- Refer for ongoing medical treatment as indicated.
- Refer to support group.

REFERENCES

Bergman, B. & Brismar, B. (1991). A 5-year follow-up study of 117 battered women. *American Journal of Public Health, 81*(11), 1486–1489.

Bohn, D. K. (1990). Domestic violence and pregnancy: implications for practice. *Journal of Nurse-Midwifery, 35*(2), 86–98.

Council on Scientific Affairs. (1992). Violence against women. *Journal of the American Medical Association, 267*(23), 3184–3189.

Furniss, K. K. (1993). Screening for abuse in the clinical setting. *AWHONN's Clinical Issues in Perinatal and Women's Health Nursing, 4*(3), 402–406.

Hadley, S. (1992). Working with battered women in the emergency department. *Journal of Emergency Nursing, 18*(1), 18–23.

King, M. C. (1993). Changing women's lives: The primary prevention of violence against women. *AWHONN's Clinical Issues in Perinatal and Women's Health Nursing, 4*(3), 449–457.

King, M., Torres, S., Campbell, D., Ryan, J., Sheridan, D., Ulrich, Y., & McKenna, L. (1993). Violence and abuse of women: A perinatal health care issue. *AWHONN's Clinical Issues in Perinatal and Women's Health Nursing, 4*(2), 163–172.

Parker, B. & McFarlane, J. (1991). Identifying and helping battered pregnant women. *American Journal of Maternal-Child Nursing, 16*(3), 161–164.

Sampselle, C. M. (1991). The role of nursing in preventing violence against women. *Journal of Obstetric, Gynecologic, and Neonatal Nursing, 20*(6), 481–487.

▼

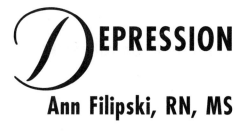

$\mathscr{D}$EPRESSION

Ann Filipski, RN, MS

Depression is an affective disturbance characterized by feelings of sadness, discouragement, and negativity. Such emotions may be experienced in relation to oneself, a given situation, or the future in general. Distinguished from the "normal" depressed reaction to a loss or disappointment, "clinical depression" is more serious and prolonged but may go unreported and therefore untreated. A significant incidence of morbidity and mortality is associated with depression, making its recognition and appropriate intervention extremely important. A disproportionate number of women suffer from depressive disorders, including major depression, dysthymia, and adjustment disorder with depressed mood.

ETIOLOGIES

- Personal or familial history of affective disorders
- Recent or cumulative losses or changes in life circumstances
- Physical illness and/or metabolic and hormonal imbalance
- Limited coping skills
- Inadequate social support system
- Repeated frustration in ability to attain goals or experience success
- Exposure to noxious or threatening situations the individual is unable to escape

CLINICAL MANIFESTATIONS

- Loss of interest in usually pleasurable activities
- Disturbance in sleep, appetite, energy, activity, elimination, and other biological rhythms (not attributable to other factors, such as endocrine disturbance, medication, or environmental circumstances)
- Verbal or behavioral helplessness/hopelessness
- Neglect of physical self (health, appearance, safety)
- Preoccupation with negativity
- Apathy, withdrawal, or difficulty in concentrating

11

▼

NURSING DIAGNOSIS: ALTERED HEALTH MAINTENANCE

Related To
- Impaired judgment
- Low self-esteem
- Inability to comply with treatment regime
- Limited coping skills
- New or coexisting physical illness
- Lack of knowledge

Defining Characteristics
Change in frequency of health-seeking behavior
Decline in health status
Multiple somatic complaints
Noncompliance
Low energy level
Suicidal ideation/intent
Risk-taking behaviors
Substance use/abuse
Overeating/undereating
Inadequate rest/sleep

Patient Outcomes
Patient will
- identify one problematic health behavior for modification.
- verbalize impact of emotional factors upon overall health state.

Nursing Interventions	Rationales
Review and document patient's past and present health behaviors with particular attention to: 1. general health history 2. frequency and types of injuries and illnesses 3. risk-taking behavior 4. adherence to health regimens and or treatment plans 5. frequency/nature of contacts with health resources/ professionals 6. health knowledge 7. other factors influencing health beliefs/practices (cultural, social, developmental, religious).	Eliciting factual and behavioral information is useful because when someone is depressed, his/her perceptions are often distorted. Recognition of one's actual health practices can aid the identification of needed changes.

Nursing Interventions	Rationales
Assess for signs/symptoms of depressive illness (see Clinical Manifestations).	
Note absence or presence of other identified health problems and somatic symptoms.	Many physical illnesses are accompanied by some depressive features or emotional sequelae. Further, some patients may not describe themselves as "depressed" but seek evaluation/ treatment for associated somatic complaints (insomnia, fatigue, weight change, anxiety, etc.).
Review with patient changes in health maintenance pattern. Explore patient's perception as to etiology and willingness/ability to address these issues at present.	Depressive symptoms generally represent a change from previous functioning, which may develop gradually or suddenly.
Educate the patient regarding the influence of physiological and emotional factors on health.	An understanding of the interrelationships between the body, mind, and emotions promotes insight into health needs and practices.
Emphasize the importance of good health practices in the address of depressive signs and symptoms: 1. structured daily routine 2. adequate sleep/rest 3. regular exercise 4. adequate nutrition 5. avoidance of use/abuse of tobacco, alcohol, or other drugs 6. opportunity for meaningful work and/or interaction with others.	Engaging in healthy behaviors promotes improved mood, self-esteem, and sense of mastery.
Assist patient in identifying and prioritizing health needs, and in developing a structured plan to address identified health needs.	Since depressed individuals tend to feel overwhelmed, it helps to divide tasks into small component parts. This also helps overcome distractions to concentration.

Nursing Interventions	Rationales
Offer support and positive reinforcement for patient's use of health promotion strategies and follow-through.	Depressed patients tend to disqualify or minimize their actual accomplishments.
Make appropriate referrals for evaluation of identified problems as needed.	Sometimes specific professional assistance may be warranted in problem areas.

▼

NURSING DIAGNOSIS: SELF-ESTEEM DISTURBANCE

Related To
- Illness, injury, or disability
- Significant loss(es)
- Repeated, cumulative stress
- Decreased level of independence
- Past/current relationship difficulties
- Excessively high standards/expectations
- Ineffective or limited coping skills
- Inadequate support system
- Cognitive/perceptual distortions

Defining Characteristics
Negative verbalizations about self
Neglect of appearance, hygiene, or personal needs
Anxious or guilty rumination
Excessive focus upon perceived flaws/failings
Fear of failure or rejection
Excessive reliance on opinions of others
Poor eye contact
Difficulty accepting compliments or positive feedback
Self-destructive behavior
Minimal verbalization

Patient Outcomes
Patient will
- increase frequency of participation in potentially pleasurable activities.
- Utilize positive self-statements to interrupt negative automatic thinking.

Nursing Interventions	Rationales
Review and document past and current level of functioning (i.e., physical, emotional, social intellectual, etc.).	This gives a perspective of how depression has impacted on the patient's life and the degree to which the patient is able to mobilize internal resources to function despite the depression.
Note relevant observations and monitor patient's verbalizations about self (see Defining Characteristics).	Once a patient learns to recognize the common cognitive distortions associated with impaired self-esteem (i.e.; overgeneralization, catastrophizing, all-or-nothing thinking, etc.) he/she can begin to challenge distorted self-critical thoughts.
Assist patient in verbalizing concerns/difficulties. Communicate willingness to listen without judging or minimizing the experience.	While this is a routine aspect of therapeutic nurse/patient communication, the depressed patient may have great difficulty in viewing his/her situation as "deserving" of the nurse's attention.
Assist patient in a gentle but realistic appraisal of strengths/assets. Acknowledge factors that may exist beyond the patient's control. Convey acceptance of human limitations to help decrease tendency to catastrophize and assume blame.	Paradoxically, the depressed person often assumes total responsibility for poor outcomes while refusing to take credit for success. This person feels powerless in the face of new challenges.
Aid patient in developing a list of positive self-statements as a concrete tool to use in overcoming negative thinking.	Depressive thinking is often characterized by the tendency to focus immediately and solely upon the negative and minimize or ignore strengths.
Encourage patient involvement in a variety of activities that offer opportunities to experience success and pleasure.	Depressed individuals often think motivation must precede action, and tend to wait until they "feel like it" to do something. However, changing behavior first is actually an effective way to challenge impaired self-esteem.

▼

NURSING DIAGNOSIS: HOPELESSNESS

Related To
- Severe/prolonged stress
- Repeated frustrations
- Ineffective coping skills
- Limited experience with success
- Cognitive/perceptual distortions
- Low self-esteem
- Coexisting physical illness/symptoms
- Decline in functional abilities

Defining Characteristics

Verbalized sense of failure, pessimism
Decreased affect or overly controlled affective expression
Sadness, resignation
Apathy, passivity
Poor eye contact
Decreased verbalization
Decreased energy and initiative
Difficulty with decision-making
Minimally responsive to stimuli
Decreased involvement in care
Views self as ineffectual, powerless
Describes self, future as hopeless

Patient Outcomes

Patient will
- verbalize "feeling statements" regarding current situation.
- identify one goal and desired outcome for the immediate future.

Nursing Interventions	Rationales
Explore with patient past sources of support, gratification, and hope.	When patients are feeling hopeless, they are so caught up in their present pain that they may completely forget that they ever felt better in the past and don't expect to ever feel better again.
Observe for presence or absence of subjective/objective indications of hopelessness (see Defining Characteristics).	An all-pervasive sense of hopelessness is often present in individuals who attempt suicide.

Nursing Interventions	**Rationales**
Assess and document degree of despair with particular attention to patient's ideas about outcome of current situation, plans for the future, and potential for self-directed harm/violence. Include: 1. presence of suicidal ideation or intent (active or passive) 2. any plan 3. potential lethality of plan/method 4. availability of means to carry out plan 5. any prior history of attempts	When depressed individuals have suicidal thoughts, it is important to assess their risk and get professional intervention if risk is high. As many as 5% of depressed patients do actually commit suicide.
Encourage recognition and verbalization of feelings.	The despairing patient often avoids this, since they believe there is no hope of change and fear burdening or depressing others. However, patients tend to feel relief if allowed to talk about their feelings.
Assist the patient with reality testing. Note distortions in thinking and gently restate or reframe these to help encourage flexibility in thinking.	Depressed people tend to confuse their feelings with facts, such that if they "feel" hopeless, they assume their situation actually "is" hopeless.
Assist the patient in realistic goal setting. Keep in mind past values, meanings, and purposes the patient has espoused and focus on how these may still play a role in the present and future. Provide anticipatory guidance in reviewing possible outcomes.	This aids patient in preparing for a range of options and may prevent the common "giving up" syndrome seen in the despairing.

Nursing Interventions

Make appropriate referrals and assist in mobilizing both patient and outside resources.

Rationales

Patients at-risk for self-directed harm or violence *must* be provided with immediate assistance. Assure the patient you are taking action on their behalf because you take their situation and feelings seriously, are concerned about their well-being, and believe that they can be helped (i.e., are *not* hopeless).

▼

NURSING DIAGNOSIS: INEFFECTIVE INDIVIDUAL COPING

Related To
- Change in personal circumstance
- Loss of close ties/relationships
- Limited/inadequate support system
- Overwhelming environmental stressors
- Poor self-esteem
- Emotional conflicts

Defining Characteristics

Subjective complaints of being "overwhelmed"
Decreased functional abilities
Inappropriate behavior
Self-destructive behavior
Difficulty with decision-making/problem-solving
Increasing self-absorption
Anxiety
Psychological immobilization.

Patient Outcomes

Patient will
- demonstrate enhanced coping skills as in solving problems.
- see alternatives and options.

Nursing Interventions	**Rationales**
Explore with patient his/her perceptions of current situation. Note: 1. number and type of stressors 2. events preceding onset of symptoms 3. subjective/objective indicators of stress 4. tendency to distort 5. impact upon patient's self-esteem	Depressed individuals may fail to recognize the "normalness" of having difficulty coping with a stressful situation. They may put unrealistic and unreasonable expectations on themselves without being aware of doing so.
Assist patient in mobilization of internal and external coping resources. 1. Review and document past and current strategies utilized by patient (qualitatively and quantitatively). 2. Note situations in which positive outcomes were achieved. 3. Emphasize the effectiveness of these strategies and their possible utility in the present.	Patients who are coping ineffectively may fail to recognize and give themselves credit for past successes in coping.
Discuss the problem-solving process. 1. Aid the patient in developing a problem list, concreting goals and setting priorities. 2. Help patient to break down large problems/tasks into a series of small, more manageable steps. 3. Consider strategies for resolution and the positive and negative aspects of each.	Facilitating a patient's move through the problem-solving process by identifying concrete steps can increase sense of personal mastery.
Facilitate patient's efforts to carry out selected strategies. Avoid reinforcing unrealistic expectations.	Depressed individuals may tend to be overly dependent or pseudoindependent because of their desire to please others and sense of low self-esteem.

Nursing Interventions	Rationales
Reinforce positive coping behaviors. Review plans with patient in ongoing fashion to help ensure success and build self-esteem.	Patients may not see the many ways throughout the day that they do successfully resolve conflicts and manage to be productive despite the debilitating effects of their depression.

▼

DISCHARGE PLANNING/CONTINUITY OF CARE

- Make appropriate referrals for evaluation of identified problems as needed:
  - primary nurse/nurse practitioner/clinical specialist
  - primary care physician
  - registered dietitian
  - mental health provider
  - health educator
  - support groups
- Make appropriate referrals and assist in mobilizing both patient and outside resources. Consider:
  - patient's family and friends
  - support groups
  - clergy or other spiritual resources
  - local mental health center
  - crisis units
  - inpatient psychiatric setting

REFERENCES

Calarco, M. M. & Krone, K. P. (1991). An integrated nursing model of depressive behavior in adults. *Nursing Clinics of North America, 26*(3), 573–584.

Hauenstein, E. J. (1991). Young women and depression: Origin, outcome, and nursing care. *Nursing Clinics of North America, 26*(3), 601–612.

Paykel, E. S. (1991). Depression in women. *British Journal of Psychiatry, 158*(10) (Suppl.), 22–29.

▼

$\mathcal{E}$ATING DISORDERS: ANOREXIA NERVOSA AND BULIMIA NERVOSA

Ursula Brozek, RN, MS

Anorexia nervosa and bulimia nervosa are classified as eating disorders. The population at greatest risk for these disorders is the young adult female, with onset at 12 to 23 years of age, and is increasing frequency in the older age groups. These disorders are seen in individuals at all socioeconomic levels.

ETIOLOGIES

- Need for control
- Distorted body image
- Inability to cope with physical and sexual maturation
- Minimal control over most aspects of personal life
- Food used to control a personal environment that may be experienced as chaotic

CLINICAL MANIFESTATIONS

Anorexia nervosa
- Strict self-control of food and fluid intake
  to lose weight
- Fear of gaining weight
- Preoccupation with weighing oneself
- Distorted perception of one's own body weight
  – believing one is "fat" even when one is emaciated
  – denial of thinness or emaciated appearance.
- Self-loathing
- Electrolyte imbalances due to decreased food/fluid intake

- Preoccupation with food
- Fasting and starvation
- Weight loss between 20% and 25% of original body weight
- Gastrointestinal disturbances resulting from decreased food/fluid intake
  - constipation
  - nausea

Bulimia nervosa

- Weight loss remains under 20% of original body weight
- Extremely impulsive behavior
  - binging and purging
  - excessive use of laxatives and diuretics
- Preoccupation with food
  - eating becomes a private rather than a social activity
- Social withdrawal
  - purging is done alone and social meals are avoided to decrease risk of "being found out"
- Gastrointestinal disturbances resulting from the binging/purging
  - bloating
  - abdominal distention
  - esophageal abrasions
  - dental cavities and buccal erosion

▼

NURSING DIAGNOSIS: ALTERED NUTRITION—LESS THAN BODY REQUIREMENTS

Related To

- Intensive fear of becoming obese (unrelated to actual body weight
- Preoccupation with food, body weight, and shape
- Disturbed body image
- Excessive exercising and dieting
- Recurrent binge eating and self-induced vomiting/purging

Defining Characteristics

Loss of weight

Inadequate food intake

Aversion to eating

Severe electrolyte imbalances

Missing a menstrual cycle for at least 3–4 months

Gastrointestinal disturbances: bloating, abdominal distention, esophageal abrasions, dental cavities, and buccal erosion due to self-induced vomiting

Patient Outcomes

Patient will

- participate in psychotherapy to gain some understanding of her abnormal eating habits.

- participate in nutrition counseling.
- cease losing weight.
- gain weight.

Nursing Interventions	Rationales
Assess patient's eating patterns and what foods means to her. Ask questions in a direct and nonaccusing manner.	This information will help differentiate between the disorders. Anorexics starve, whereas bulimics gorge, then purge.
Assess patient's weight loss in past 1–2 months.	This will help differentiate between anorexia and bulimia. Weight loss is progressive in anorexia, and fluctuates in bulimia. Knowledge of the severity of recent weight loss helps determine the need for inpatient treatment and stabilization.
Assess electrolyte status.	This information determines the severity of malnutrition and likewise the need for hospitalization.
Determine the caloric intake and type of nutrients needed to meet nutritional requirements. (This is done in conjunction with a nutritional consultation). Determine the need for nasogastric tube feeding.	The patient's interest in participation in this decision-making process plays a significant role in determining whether or not feeding will occur independently or through tube and intravenous feedings
Discuss the meaning of food to the patient and the important role it is playing in her life.	Food—or lack of food—becomes an obsession to patients as a means for escaping/controlling the stresses of life.
Monitor the patient's intake of calories and nutritional foods. Instruct patient to keep a food diary, and document relationship of binging and purging to feelings/activities.	Self-monitoring assists patient to see a relationship between feelings and binging and purging activity.

Nursing Interventions	Rationales
Weigh patient at scheduled visits in a matter-of-fact manner.	This reduces the emphasis on being weighed too often, yet provides information on patient's progress. Ensure that weight is accurate and that the patient has not secreted objects on her body or fluid-loaded prior to scheduled weighing to mimic weight gain.
Assess current use of any prescription and/or over-the-counter medication.	Information about the use of laxatives and diuretics helps differentiate bulimia from anorexia.
Stress importance of psychological counseling to help patient work out strategy for mealtimes.	
Encourage patient not to eat alone.	Mealtime and the period immediately following a meal are anxiety-provoking. A patient with an eating disorder has minimal ability to set interval limits and requires external limits placed on her.

▼

NURSING DIAGNOSIS: BODY IMAGE DISTURBANCE

Related To inability to cope with the physical and sexual maturation process

Defining Characteristics

Distorted perception of one's body weight, preoccupation with one's weight and shape

Intense fear of gaining weight and becoming obese unrelated to actual weight

Denial of thin or emaciated appearance

Negative feelings about body

Self-loathing

Patient Outcomes

Patient will
- describe a positive aspect about her body.
- identify a positive means to cope with her stresses.

Nursing Interventions	Rationales
Assess patient's image of self and the role her weight plays in her body image.	This aids in determining the degree of mind-body distortion.
Monitor patient's comments that identify relationship between body image and body shape and weight.	It is not unusual for the patient's distorted sense of self to pervade all aspects of her self-concept.
Assist patient in identifying the parts of her body about which she feels positive.	Verbalization of positive attributes of her body helps the patient strive to maintain a balanced self-image. It also helps the patient develop more realistic expectations of her body image and decreases self-loathing.
Instruct patient regarding harmful side effects/complications associated with excessive behavior: 1. Dieting can result in starvation, malnutrition, even death. 2. Excessive exercising is sometimes utilized as a means of controlling weight. 3. Purging can result in severe/life-threatening electrolyte imbalances. 4. Laxative abuse can result in laxative dependence.	Complications of malnutrition and electrolyte imbalances can occur. Patient needs to understand the *physical* consequences of her behavior. This does not always result in a reduction of binging and purging behaviors, but it provides a framework from which further information and feedback can be provided.
Refer patient for psychotherapy.	Eating disorders are a complex psychiatric condition that require specialized counseling.
Encourage attendance at support groups available to patient and family.	Recovery from binge eating and purging is difficult. Groups that come together for mutual support and guidance can be helpful.

▼

NURSING DIAGNOSIS: SOCIAL ISOLATION

Related To
- Extreme anxiety and conflict surrounding food
- Self-loathing

Defining Characteristics

Avoidance of social interactions and engagements involving food; inability
  to see meals and eating as a social activity
Social withdrawal from family and friends; need to "hide" the binging and
  purging from others for the bulimic
Seeks to be alone
Impaired ability to maintain interpersonal relationships

Patient Outcomes

Patient will
- begin to verbally communicate with family/significant others.
- identify interests/social activity to engage in that is not related to food.

Nursing Interventions	Rationales
Assess patient's level of energy and activity, as well as the kinds of activities in which the patient routinely engages.	This helps evaluate the degree of social interaction, as well as the patient's ability to focus on interests other than food.
Assess the patient's ability to interact with those around her, and the degree of spontaneity in these interactions.	This provides information on the patient's comfort level with those around her. Patients with these disorders are generally withdrawn and minimally spontaneous.
Interact verbally with the patient. Structure interaction so that it requires a verbal response.	Asking open-ended questions will encourage increased verbalization. Verbal engagement provides patient with the opportunity to socially interact without the pressure of initiating contact.
Encourage patient to focus on interests and engage in activities not related to food. Assist in setting goals that are non-food-related.	Focusing on non-food-related interests and activities will help redirect and reintegrate the patient into a larger social context.
Provide positive feedback when the patient initiates social contact and reaches out to others.	Initiating social contacts with others is anxiety-provoking.
Provide feedback about patient's strengths and limitations in communicating with others.	Feedback will increase the patient's self-awareness and insight.

Nursing Interventions	**Rationales**
Use role-playing as a therapeutic activity to teach communication skills. Function as role model to demonstrate effective communication.	

▼

DISCHARGE PLANNING/CONTINUITY OF CARE

- Ongoing scheduled visits with internist and nutritionist for evaluation of nutritional status
- Ongoing family therapy to deal with issues of control within the family
- Ongoing individual therapy to continue to examine issues related to body image and sexuality

REFERENCES

Merlin, R. (1992). Understanding bulemia and its implications in pregnancy. *Journal of Obstetrical, Gynecologic, & Neonatal Nursing, 21*(3), 199–205.

Nottingham, J. P. & Emerson, R. J. (1991). Anorexia nervosa in the older adult: A case study. *Clinical Nurse Specialist, 5*(2), 79–85.

Nusbaum, J. G. & Drever, E. (1990). Inpatient survey of nursing care measures for treatment of patients with anorexia nervosa. *Issues of Mental Health Nursing, 11*(2), 175–184.

Palmer, T. A. (1990). Anorexia nervosa, bulemia nervosa: Causal theories and treatment. *Nurse Practitioner, 15*(4), 12–18, 21.

Plehn, K. W. (1990). Anorexia nervosa and bulemia: Incidence and diagnosis. *Nurse Practitioner, 15*(4), 22, 25, 28.

Stuart, G. & Sundeen, S. (1991). *Principles and practice of psychiatric nursing* (4th ed). St. Louis, MO: C. V. Mosby.

White, J. (1993). Women and eating disorders. *AWHONN's Clinical Issues in Perinatal and Women's Health Nursing, 4*(2), 227–235.

▼

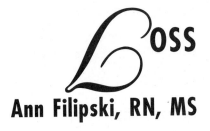

Loss

Ann Filipski, RN, MS

Loss is a subjectively defined phenomenon during which an individual encounters an actual or perceived disruption in the ability to accomplish a goal, achieve a hoped-for outcome in life, or maintain a healthy self-concept. Normally, loss is followed by a predictable grieving process.

ETIOLOGIES

- Death of a spouse or child
- Change in health status
- Change in personal or familial role
- End of a close relationship
- Unattained lifelong goal
- Loss of a highly prized personal attribute
- Loss of several friends or relatives
- Multiple physical injuries
- Traumatic or life-threatening diagnoses
- Recent versus past loss

CLINICAL MANIFESTATIONS

Patients may exhibit a number of behavioral signs and symptoms:
- Shock, disbelief, denial
- Emotional numbing or extremes, including anger, sorrow, tearfulness
- Rigid adherence to structured plans or the inability to function without guidance
- Preoccupation with loss in thought, focus of conversation, and activity
- Self-doubt and loss of confidence
- Immobilization (brief or prolonged)
- Need for support

▼

NURSING DIAGNOSIS: ANXIETY

Related To
- Change in function/role(s)
- New or unfamiliar situation
- Lack of clear goals/expectations
- Changes in level of independence
- Limited or ineffective coping skills
- Alteration in living circumstances.

Defining Characteristics
Change in autonomic indicators
Increased blood pressure, respiratory rate, heart rate
Palpitations, dry mouth, increased perspiration
Diarrhea and/or gastrointestinal distress
Behavioral/emotional manifestations
Irritability
Restlessness
Distractibility
Decreased concentration
Hypervigilance
Subjective reports of distress, such as "nervousness" or sense of foreboding
Diffuse somatic complaints

Patient Outcomes
Patient will
- recognize and describe signs and symptoms of anxiety.
- experience reduced anxiety as evidenced by calmer appearance and subjective reports of decreased distress.

Nursing Interventions	Rationales
Anticipate possible responses to changes in health status or life situation.	
Observe for manifestations of anxiety (physical, emotional, and cognitive/behavioral) and/or reports of changes in functional abilities.	Patients may not be aware of the relationship between their circumstances or emotional concerns and anxiety. Symptoms may provide information for the patient.
Explore and document circumstances preceding or following onset of signs and symptoms.	Recognition and exploration of such factors facilitate the development of alternative responses.

Nursing Interventions	Rationales
Assist patient to verbalize concerns/complaints and to gain awareness of symptoms of anxiety.	Patients frequently are focused upon the symptoms or ongoing manifestations of anxiety and may not recognize these as part of the larger phenomenon.
Normalize patient's experience without minimizing subjective distress or uniqueness of their perceptions.	Though a common experience, anxiety is highly subjective in its manifestations. Acknowledgment of the patient's experience is validating and communicates acceptance, thus reinforcing a sense of security for the patient.
Educate patient regarding means of managing anxiety at mild/moderate level: 1. exercise and/or involvement in focused activity 2. relaxation techniques 3. reduction in extraneous stressors 4. need to verbalize 5. creative visualization	This enhances sense of being able to cope effectively.
Educate patient to avoid reliance on somatic/chemical means of decreasing manifestations of anxiety, such as alcohol, over-the-counter sleep aids, prescription drugs, or other chemicals.	While properly used medications may be a useful adjunct for patients with disabling anxiety, anxiety management skills (see preceding intervention) promote a sense of personal mastery.
Refer to appropriate psychosocial resources.	Patients dealing with anxiety may benefit from resources (counseling, support, educational) that offer additional services to improve personal coping skills, problem-solving skills, and life-transition coping skills.

▼

NURSING DIAGNOSIS: HIGH RISK FOR SELF-ESTEEM DISTURBANCE

Risk Factors
- Uncertain outcome
- Threats to sense of personal competence
- Changes in level of independence

Patient Outcome
Patient will verbalize positive statements regarding self-worth.

Nursing Interventions	Rationales
Gather baseline data as to previous level of functioning and perceptions of self.	Having a baseline makes it easier to assess or interpret the significance of changes in the patient.

Assess for signs of self-esteem disturbance:
1. changes in reported/observed affect (blunted, sad, angry, etc.)
2. changes in usual levels of confidence, motivation, or verbalizations regarding self
3. deterioration in appearance/self-care skills
4. decline in cognitive functioning
  • difficulty in making decisions
  • poor concentration, lack of good judgment
5. behavioral changes
  • noncompliance
  • inability to follow through on establishing plan
  • denial
  • decline in functioning	

Explore patient's perceptions of current situation and sense of personal competence. Provide opportunity for verbalization of feelings and communicate recognition of impact of loss on patient's usual coping style.	Exploration and acknowledgment of the patient's perceptions and feelings validates the patient as worthwhile and important, thus promoting self-esteem.

Nursing Interventions	Rationales
Provide anticipatory guidance by sharing common responses to experience of loss.	Normalizing experience helps patient to reality-test and decreases sense of isolation and powerlessness.
Discuss normalcy of need for support and assistance.	Patient may not be aware of the normalcy of having reactions to loss that require assistance.
Encourage involvement in activities that promote sense of worth and competence.	Such behavioral changes are often the first step toward achieving a more positive sense of self-esteem.
Assure patient of availability of resources to deal with disruption in life circumstances. Make referral to appropriate support/self-help groups as needed.	Utilizing supportive resources counters isolation, and provides models of others who are coping.

▼

NURSING DIAGNOSIS: HIGH RISK FOR SOCIAL ISOLATION

Risk Factors
- Disruption in social support system
- Social withdrawal
- Decreased self-esteem
- Experience of loss

Patient Outcome
Patient will participate in social interactions as appropriate.

Nursing Interventions	Rationales
Explore patient's past and current pattern of social interactions. Identify impact of loss upon perception of self in relation to others.	To effectively deal with loss, a patient needs to take a realistic look at the actual and perceived social changes associated with the loss.

Nursing Interventions	Rationales
Assess for signs of social isolation: 1. decreased attendance at social functions 2. decreased frequency of patient-initiated social contacts 3. reluctance to see or talk with others 4. verbalized sense of isolation 5. references to having "little in common" with others 6. decreased energy level 7. exclusive focus on loss in conversation 8. perceived lack of acceptance/rejection by others.	
Support patient in verbalizing feelings related to experience of loss.	This promotes the appropriate grieving process.
Discuss role of social contacts in maintaining unique sense of self and connectedness to others. Assist patient in formulating concrete plan for meaningful interaction with others.	This may enhance patient's motivation and provide opportunity to challenge cognitive distortions (overgeneralization, all-or-none thinking, etc.) if present.
Assist patient in identifying and planning means of addressing actual/potential impediments to social contacts (i.e., transportation difficulties, changes in living circumstances, etc.).	Providing concrete problem-solving assistance and helping patient "rehearse" through planning, anticipating, visualizing success, and problem-solving obstacles will increase patient's confidence and mastery.
Review plan with patient to realistically ascertain progress. Revise plan as needed to capitalize upon positive experiences.	Patient may tend to be more keenly aware of how social contacts are "different" following a loss and, thereby, reinforce their sense of isolation. Feelings about the contacts should be shared and may facilitate the ability to grieve the loss.

▼

NURSING DIAGNOSIS: HIGH RISK FOR DYSFUNCTIONAL GRIEVING

Risk Factors
Inability to adequately mourn loss

Patient Outcomes
Patient will
- verbalize knowledge of grieving process.
- display appropriate signs of grieving as evidenced by ability to talk about loss.

Nursing Interventions	Rationales
Explore and document history of patient's response to identified loss.	This aids a patient in developing a sense of self-understanding. It can help a patient understand his/her response to a loss as an ongoing process rather than a static event.

Assess for signs of dysfunctional grief:
1. avoidance of emotional content in discussion of loss
2. distortion of affective expression
  • sad
  • blunted
  • emotional numbing
  • tearfulness
3. inability to acknowledge loss
4. avoidance of topics related to lost individual, role, or state
5. preoccupation with thoughts of lost person, object, or ability	

Offer support but avoid false reassurance and minimization of impact of loss.	False reassurances and minimizations give patients the message that the nurse is unwilling or unable to tolerate the reality of the patient's loss. This inhibits a patient's ability to feel understood and free to talk about the loss as needed.

Nursing Interventions	**Rationales**
Explore barriers to effectively grieving loss: 1. lack of adequate support system 2. distortion of familial/social roles 3. ambivalence toward loss 4. cumulative unresolved losses 5. other intervening stressors 6. lack of knowledge about grieving.	This will help patient become aware of the many factors that might add up or interact in a way to make it difficult to accomplish an effective resolution of grief.
Educate patient regarding "normal" process of grief and human desire to "avoid" pain: 1. a process must be experienced and involve "working through" painful feelings • anger • sorrow • shock • disbelief • numbness 2. not time-limited; may take weeks to years 3. believed to occur in predictable phases but order of occurrence not static: • denial • anger • ambivalence • acceptance 4. patient overwhelmed at times or absorbed and preoccupied 5. stress produced by *any* loss or change—not just those seen as "undesirable"	Although most persons recognize grief as a reality, many harbor unrealistic expectations of how it should occur and/or resolve.

Nursing Interventions	**Rationales**

Educate patient regarding signs/ symptoms of pathologic grieving:
1. prolonged or marked
  • isolation
  • neglect of personal needs
  • difficulty with judgment
2. acting-out behavior
  • destruction of property
  • self-injury
  • episodes of rage
3. immobilization and inability to function
4. altered thought processes
  • delusions
  • frank hallucinations
	Awareness of the differences between appropriate and dysfunctional grieving can help a patient identify when to seek out or accept professional assistance.

▼

DISCHARGE PLANNING/CONTINUITY OF CARE

- Refer to appropriate psychosocial resources as needed:
  - Psychiatric nursing consultant
  - Outpatient mental health agency
  - Social service department
  - Psychiatric inpatient unit
- Refer to appropriate support/self-help groups as needed:
  - Compassionate Friends
  - Resolve
  - Parents Without Partners
  - Emotions Anonymous

REFERENCES

Assimacopoulos, L. (1987). Realizing empathy in loss. *Journal of Psychosocial Nursing and Mental Health Services, 25*(11), 26–29, 35.

Bateman, A., Broderick, D., Gleason, L., Kardon R., Flaherty, C., & Anderson, S. (1992). Dysfunctional grieving. *Journal of Psychosocial Nursing and Mental Health Services, 30*(12), 5–9.

Haylor, M. J. (1987). Human response to loss. *Nurse Practitioner, 12*(5), 63–66.

Jacob, S. R. (1991). Facing it alone: Preholiday grief. *Journal of Psychosocial Nursing and Mental Health Services, 29*(11), 20–24, 36–37.

Kizilay, P. E. (1992). Women's health: Predictors of depression in women. *Nursing Clinics of North America, 27*(4): 983–993.

Remondet, J. H. & Hansson, R. O. (1987). Assessing a widow's grief: A short index. *Journal of Gerontological Nursing, 13*(4), 30–34.

Wingerson, N. (1992). Psychic loss in adult survivors of father-daughter incest. *Archives of Psychiatric Nursing, 6*(4), 239–244.

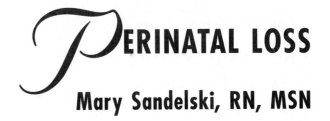

ERINATAL LOSS

Mary Sandelski, RN, MSN

Perinatal loss is an involuntary termination of pregnancy accompanied by grief, mental distress and sorrow.

ETIOLOGY

Death of fetus/neonate

CLINICAL MANIFESTATIONS

- Shock, disbelief, emotional numbing or extremes, including anger, sorrow, tearfulness
- Preoccupation with loss
- Self-doubt
- Need for support

▼

NURSING DIAGNOSIS: HIGH RISK FOR DYSFUNCTIONAL GRIEVING

Risk Factors
- Absence of anticipatory grieving
- Actual loss of fetus/neonate
- Thwarted grieving response to the loss

Patient Outcomes
Patient will
- verbalize knowledge of grieving process
- display appropriate signs of grieving, as evidenced by ability to talk about loss.
- identify support person/resource to aid in recovery process.

Nursing Interventions	Rationales
Assess impact of the loss on the patient and her significant other.	
Assess patient and significant other's stage in the grieving process.	
Code room and chart with a sign reflecting that family is in grief.	This will prevent auxiliary personnel from making inappropriate comments to the patient concerning the pregnancy.
Offer patient a room on a nonmaternity unit if available.	Some patients will feel uncomfortable on an obstetric unit with other women with healthy infants. However, if transferred, patient should be prepared for a staff less prepared to care for obstetrical patients.
Encourage free verbalization of feelings by patient/family.	This will help the patient and her family start to work through their grief and get their important questions answered and misconceptions corrected.
Acknowledge loss and verify reality of situation.	This will help the patient accept the reality of her loss. Patients appreciate staff that doesn't avoid them or the discussion of their loss.
Allow patient/family to hold/view fetus/neonate if of appropriate gestational age.	The viewing of the fetus makes the fetus itself and the subsequent loss of that fetus more of a reality for the patient/family. This will aid them in the grief process. Also, what the patient/family imagines the fetus to look like is often worse than reality.
Provide patient with footprint sheet, lock of infant's hair, picture of infant, infant hat and blanket if infant is of appropriate gestational age and patient desires the mementos; otherwise file for future.	In later stages of grief, these mementos validate the pregnancy and loss for the patient. To patients the pregnancy was part of the family and the mementos are treasured along with other family memorabilia.

Nursing Interventions	Rationales
Provide information on alternatives for the disposition of the infant/fetus body if appropriate.	Burials and memorial services are available for young fetuses. Since some patients regard a fetus as a person and a member of the family, these customs are important to them, and provide closure.
Refer to Social Services, Compassionate Friends as needed.	These services provide important support to patients in need.
Discuss autopsy if appropriate.	Autopsy is indicated if the patient has a history of loss, the fetus appears malformed, or the patients desire more definitive answers for the loss.
Contact the patient's or hospital clergy as needed for spiritual support.	
Increase contact time with patient/family.	These patients are acutely aware of and resent being avoided. These patients and their families have many questions and feelings that need additional contact time to adequately deal with the loss
Discuss usual physical/emotional grief responses.	This provides preparation for and validation of the patient's responses/feelings.
Facilitate functional coping responses of patient and family.	This provides support to and encourages continuation of positive behaviors displayed by patient and family.
Educate the patient regarding signs of pathological grief responses: 1. prolonged isolation, neglect of personal needs 2. acting-out behavior 3. immobilization, inability to function	Awareness of the differences between appropriate and dysfunctional grieving can help the patient identify when to seek out or accept professional assistance.
Administer medications for sleep and physical pain as ordered.	Inability to sleep is a possible grief reaction. Fatigue will lessen the patient's ability to cope with the grief.

Nursing Interventions	Rationales
Discuss the impact the loss has on patient/family (roles, siblings).	This will help prepare the patient for possible issues evolving from the loss and give her ideas on coping.
Assess patient's ability to function.	
Assess other factors that may affect patient's grieving process (e.g, religion, culture, other losses, etc).	Individual's coping methods are affected by many factors.

▼

NURSING DIAGNOSIS: HIGH RISK FOR SPIRITUAL DISTRESS

Risk Factors
- Loss of anticipated pregnancy
- Anger toward God or other spiritual entity

Patient Outcome
Patient will verbalize acceptance of the loss.

Nursing Interventions	Rationales
Assess patient's response to loss.	
If elective termination, assess how this decision fits into the patient's belief system.	Patients have a right to their beliefs, even if they conflict with the nurse's beliefs.
Encourage and accept any feelings of anger. Arrange for baptism or other appropriate religious ritual for fetus/neonate if requested.	A patient will draw strength and consolation from religion and its customs.
Allow for verbalization of feelings, remaining nonjudgmental.	A patient needs to express feelings of doubt and anger to begin to work through and get past these feelings.
Work with funeral director to meet patient's burial needs.	A funeral is a custom of closure and often has significant religious meaning. The staff should facilitate this procedure if the patient desires it.

▼

NURSING DIAGNOSIS: POWERLESSNESS

Related To poor pregnancy outcome

Defining Characteristics

Verbalization of loss of control
Dependency
Withdrawal
Expression of doubt regarding role performance
Antagonistic attitude
Uncooperative manner

Patient Outcomes

Patient will
- exercise ability to make choices when given the opportunity.
- verbalize an understanding of the uncontrollable circumstances.

Nursing Interventions	Rationales
Assess patient's level of independence and usual level of control over her life.	
Assess patient's perception of her role in the loss.	Patient may experience different feelings if abortion was spontaneous vs. elective.
Explain normalcy of patient's feelings.	Patient cannot control all the feelings she experiences. Explaining that this is normal will decrease her sense of powerlessness.
Encourage independence to increase the sense of control.	
Give patient options as often as possible in choice of treatments, time procedures carried out, etc.	This will create a sense of power over her care.
Explain the uncontrollable circumstances of the loss if the abortion was spontaneous.	The patient must realize she never had control of the situation, therefore she didn't have control to lose. There are no interventions available to prevent first trimester loss.

Nursing Interventions	Rationales
Encourage patient's family to allow her to decide what will be done with any infant/nursery items already obtained.	The power of this decision is often taken away from the patient by well-meaning family and friends and can add to her feeling of loss of control.

▼

NURSING DIAGNOSIS: HIGH RISK FOR SITUATIONAL LOW SELF-ESTEEM

Risk Factors
- Pregnancy loss
- Change in role as "mother"
- Feelings of inadequacy

Patient Outcomes
Patient will
- verbalize positive feelings of adequacy.
- recognize need to integrate loss into daily life.

Nursing Interventions	Rationales
Assess patient's/family's response to loss.	
Observe for expressions of shame, guilt, failure, or inadequacy.	
Allow patient to verbalize emotions.	Working through feelings will hasten the psychological healing process and then allow the performance of expected/desired roles.
Help patient differentiate her own responses from those of other people.	The patient needs to define herself and build her self-esteem regardless of others' responses. Positive outside responses can add to the patient's self-esteem, though.
Aid patient/family in identifying needs and concerns.	With needs identified and met, the patient can work on her self-esteem. Sometimes her needs will be related to her self-esteem.

Nursing Interventions	Rationales
Discuss normalcy of need for support and assistance.	Patient may not be aware of the normalcy of having reactions to loss that require assistance.
Allow/aid patient to discuss expected changes after the loss.	The patient is experiencing the loss of an anticipated role and the loss may affect her other role performances. Preparation will help her alter what she needs to continue in her roles. Ability to perform desired roles will positively affect her self-concept.
Reinforce positive feelings/statements about self/situation/others made by patient/family.	This will bring this support into the patient's conscious awareness.
Reinforce positive coping skills in patient/family.	This identifies positive practices to patient/family.
Help patient with activities that will give impetus to her progress on to independence and ultimately, the assumption of her routine role.	
Aid patient in prioritizing activities and help plan for their accomplishment.	This will help the patient assume the responsibilities of her roles, which will aid her self-concept.

NURSING DIAGNOSIS: HIGH RISK FOR ALTERED SEXUALITY PATTERNS

Risk Factors
- Fear of future pregnancies
- Expressed desire to immediately replace lost fetus/neonate
- Anger toward partner
- Altered self-concept
- Traumatic experience of pregnancy loss

Patient Outcomes
Patient will
- verbalize an understanding of the impact of loss on her reproductive function/sexuality.
- describe satisfaction with current expressions of sexuality.

Nursing Interventions	**Rationales**
Assess patient's interests in/concern about sexuality and future sexual practices.	Patient's feelings may range from avoidance of sex in the future to interest in getting pregnant right away.
Dispel myths or misinformation.	These could negatively affect the patient's practices and decision concerning resumption of sex and attempts with future pregnancies.
Educate patient/family on incidence and common causes of early and late losses.	Normal sexual expression may be diminished by grief. This may affect a decision for future pregnancies.
Explain grief reaction in relation to sexuality.	The patient/couple needs to anticipate a change to lessen the stress.
Provide an open discussion concerning resumption of ovulation/ fertility.	Unprotected sex may result in pregnancy.
Refer to physician for education on resumption of sex and fertility control.	With a vaginal delivery or D&C, intercourse may be delayed for several weeks. It may be suggested that future pregnancy be postponed for a certain time frame.
Educate patient on alternative sexual gratification.	Sex is an important part of a relationship; if intercourse is contraindicated, other means of gratification can be employed. These means may need to be introduced to the couple.

DISCHARGE PLANNING/CONTINUITY OF CARE

- Refer for psychological counseling as needed.
- Refer to "support" group/Compassionate Friends.
- Assist with contacting funeral director as needed.
- Refer for birth control education.

REFERENCES

Page-Lieberman, J. & Hughes, C. B. (1990). How fathers perceive perinatal death. *Maternal-Child Nursing, 15*(5), 320–323.

Parkman, S. E. (1992). Helping families say good-bye. *MCN American Journal of Maternal-Child Nursing, 17*(1), 14–17.

Ryan, P. F., Cote-Arsenault, D., & Sugarman, L. L. (1991). Facilitating care after perinatal loss: A comprehensive checklist. *Journal of Obstetrical, Gynecologic, & Neonatal Nursing, 20*(5), 385–389.

Szgalsky, J. B. (1989). Perinatal death, the family, and the role of the health professional. *Neonatal Network, 8*(2), 15–19.

▼

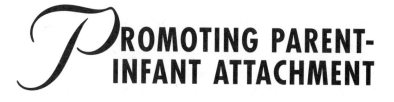

PROMOTING PARENT-INFANT ATTACHMENT

Catherine Folker-Maglaya, RN, MSN, IBCLC, Kathy Stewart, RN, and Mary Therese Rinzel, RN, MS

Attachment is a gradual process, which develops through the reciprocal interaction between the parent(s) and infant. This affectional tie endures for a lifetime. "Promoting" refers to interactions that assist the parent(s) in the attachment process.

ETIOLOGY

N/A

CLINICAL MANIFESTATIONS

N/A

▼

NURSING DIAGNOSIS: ALTERED PARENTING

Related To new experience with the childbearing process, infant care and nurturing, or parenting role

Defining Characteristics
Prenatal
Parent shows acceptance of pregnancy
Parent converses about gender and appearance
Parent fantasizes about baby's future
Parent considers/selects name
Parent rubs abdomen and talks to fetus
Parent calls fetus by pet name
Parent purchases clothing and rearranges home in preparation for baby

Parent reads about child development/attends prenatal classes
Parent expresses concern/anxiety for baby's well-being

Postdelivery
Parent holds baby closely to body
Parent establishes eye contact with baby
Parent calls baby by name and talks in soothing voice
Parent shows pleasure during nurturing activities (sings, smiles, rocks)
Parent readily receives baby
Parent asks questions about baby's behavior/care
Baby is content/soothed in parent's arms

Patient Outcome
Patient will achieve a positive parent-infant interaction as manifested by the presence of the following defining characteristics.

Nursing Interventions	Rationales
Prenatal Assess for maternal behaviors that imply attachment.	
Assess father for behaviors that imply attachment. Assist in activities that promote attachment whenever present.	
Encourage father's attendance at prenatal visits.	Recognize that the mother begins to attach to the infant early in pregnancy as she experiences physical changes and feels the baby move. The father's attachment progresses more slowly.
Assess for factors that may interfere with the mother (father) in preparing for the baby: 1. role conflict 2. past experiences with own parents 3. lack of knowledge about nurturing an infant 4. unplanned pregnancy 5. inadequate support systems 6. financial constraints	Depending on the cause, a variety of treatment strategies may be indicated.

Nursing Interventions	Rationales
Refer to the fetus as "the baby," or, if sex has been determined, "he/she" when conversing with mother (parents). Discuss the developmental stage of the fetus at each office visit. Use Doppler ultrasonography for obtaining fetal heart tones, enabling the mother (father) to hear the baby's heart rate.	This allows the parent to identify baby as "real" and personifies the fetus.
Provide opportunities for the mother (father) to talk about and make preparations for the baby.	
Discuss feeding choice with mother (father), early in pregnancy, sharing benefits of breast vs bottle feeding.	Breast feeding promotes a unique closeness between mother and infant.
Discuss birthing options and possibilities for continuous/daytime rooming-in as pregnancy progresses.	Rooming-in allows the parent time to learn to care for and get acquainted with the baby.
Provide information regarding community parenting groups.	Expectant parents can observe first-hand (prior to the baby's birth) other parents caring for their children.
Encourage attendance of childbirth preparation/infant care classes. Provide listing of community classes offered.	
Intrapartum Place mirror and position mother to enable optimal view of the baby's birth.	
Involve father in birthing process, if he is present. Assist him to comfort mother and support her with breathing exercises. Allow him to cut the umbilical cord if desired.	These activities provide the father with an active role in the delivery.

Nursing Interventions	Rationales
Allow mother (father) to hold and inspect the baby immediately post-delivery. Allow for skin-to-skin contact.	This activity facilitates attachment and allows the parent(s) to get acquainted with the baby through touch. The baby can hold the parent's fingers and be comforted by the parent's touch. This contact may alleviate anxieties/concerns regarding infant's well-being.
Assess the level of anxiety in mother (father) when holding/carrying the baby. Assist parent to obtain a comfortable position and to establish eye contact with baby.	
Assist mother as needed if she is breast-feeding.	Immediately after birth, the baby is in a quiet, alert state and apt to suckle with minimal assistance, which promotes confidence in the mother's ability to nurture her infant. In addition, the release of the lactation hormones (prolactin and oxytocin) enhances motherly feelings.
Allow the baby to remain with mother (parents) throughout the recovery period.	
Postpartum Provide mother extended contact with the baby. Encourage father to visit as much as possible.	This fosters a sense of connectedness.
Provide opportunities for/and assist mother (parents) with infant care (diaper changing, bathing, etc). Praise her efforts.	These activities promote confidence in the mother's ability to care for the baby.
Encourage attendance at baby care classes.	
Observe/assist with mother-infant interactions; explore the infant's entire body using the fingertips.	
Provide positive reinforcement, acknowledging positive maternal behaviors. Compliment mother.	Compliments enhance feelings of self-esteem.

Nursing Interventions	**Rationales**
Assess the father's participation in the baby's care. Assist with caretaking activities.	It is important to assess both parental anxiety levels regarding infant care. Lack of confidence and anxiety may be misinterpreted as disinterested or unaffectionate behavior.
Instruct the mother (parents) regarding normal infant behaviors, which are in response to inner drives and not a rejection of her caretaking capabilities: 1. regurgitates feedings frequently 2. grimaces and gurgles 3. maintains periods of sleeplessness 4. cries during changing, dressing, or bathing	Preparatory information reduces uncertainty.
Provide examples of positive infant feedback, and instruct mother to recognize these.	
Assess infant in mother's (parents') presence to help acquaint her with infant's response to stimuli. Provide mother (parents) with information on methods to provide infant stimulation.	This provides positive role modeling.
Provide additional interventions in the birth of a premature or sick infant or a baby with congenital malformation: 1. Show acceptance of the baby and emphasize the positive features. 2. Allow the parents to see and touch the baby as soon as possible.	If there is a long interval between the time the parent(s) are informed of the complication and the moment they actually see the baby, fantasies worse than the actual situation may develop. There is then the burden of eliminating the fantasies before they can begin relating to the reality of the baby.
Invite the parents to perform caretaking activities.	
Allow the parent(s) to hold and caress the stillborn baby.	

Nursing Interventions	Rationales
Involve adoptive parents in the baby's care as soon as possible. However, the relinquishing parent should have the opportunity to hold, inspect, and even breast-feed the baby if she desires.	

▼

DISCHARGE PLANNING/CONTINUITY OF CARE

- Telephone 1 week postdischarge to assess for familial adaptation to newborn and lifestyle change.
- At routine postpartum and serial pediatric visits, assess family adjustment.
- If problems or difficulties regarding familial adjustment, ability to care for infant, or coping are identified, or if there are signs of emotional or physical abuse/neglect, provide appropriate referrals (e.g., the social service agency, for counseling and/or supplemental nutrition program).
- Provide information on community parenting groups.

REFERENCES

Anderson, A. & Anderson, B. (1990). Toward a substantive theory of mother-twin attachment. *American Journal of Maternal-Child Nursing, 15*(6), 373–377.

Martell, L. K. (1990). Postpartum depression as a family problem. *American Journal of Maternal-Child Nursing, 15*(2), 90–93.

Norr, K. F. & Roberts, J. E. (1991). Early maternal attachment behaviors of adolescent and adult mothers. *Journal of Nurse-Midwifery, 36*(6), 334–342.

Symanski, M. E. (1992). Maternal-Infant bonding: Practice issues for the 1990s. *Journal of Nurse-Midwifery, 372*(Suppl), 675–735.

▼

RAPE–TRAUMA SYNDROME

Ursula Brozek, RN, MS

Rape is forced, assaultive sexual contact, which includes sexual penetration. The survivor may sustain significant physical trauma.

Rape-trauma syndrome involves a set of behaviors that develop in response to an attempted or actual rape. The acute response includes multiple physical and emotional symptoms. The long-term phase involves reorganization of the survivor's life and recovery from the trauma.

ETIOLOGY

Physical and emotional response to rape

CLINICAL MANIFESTATIONS

May include physical injury, emotional trauma, and lifestyle changes:
- acute phase
  - pain
  - sleep disturbances
  - muscle tension
  - genitourinary discomfort
  - fear
  - anger
  - embarassment
  - self-blame
- long-term phase
  - changes in lifestyle and relationships
  - recurrent nightmares and phobias
  - guilt
  - anxiety
  - sexual dysfunction

▼

ACUTE PHASE

NURSING DIAGNOSIS: PAIN

Related To injury sustained during the rape and/or attempted rape as a result of physical struggle/trauma

Defining Characteristics

Physical signs of bodily trauma as evidenced by bruises, swelling, lacerations, bleeding
Verbal reports of generalized soreness throughout body
Verbal reports of pain in areas of body targeted during the assault
Self-protective, guarded behavior
Alteration in muscle tone (may span from listless to rigid)
Autonomic responses; changes in blood pressure, pulse rate, respiratory rate

Patient Outcomes

Patient will
• appear more comfortable and relaxed.
• verbalize relief or ability to tolerate discomfort/pain.

Nursing Interventions	Rationales
Assess degree of injury sustained during the assault.	Both genital and extragenital injuries may occur. Some survivors require hospitalization.
Ask survivor to point to areas of body that sustained trauma, or that hurt, if survivor is unable to articulate clearly.	
Prepare woman for need for physical and pelvic examination. Attempt to reduce the invasive feeling of physical examination by reassuring survivor that physical examination is necessary to ensure her safety and health.	Laboratory tests are especially important to verify presence of semen and rule out venereal disease or pregnancy.

Nursing Interventions	Rationales
Describe clearly all components of physical examination and manner in which examination will proceed. Allow survivor to control the pace of the examination as much as possible. Ensure privacy.	Since the pelvic exam can trigger a flashback of the rape, the nurse needs to comfort/support patient throughout. Continuous dialogue in a gentle, nonintrusive manner will help survivor participate in complete examination.
Provide medical care/analgesics as ordered.	

▼

NURSING DIAGNOSIS: IMPAIRED VERBAL COMMUNICATION
Related To psychological barriers

Defining Characteristics
Impaired articulation
Inability to speak in complete sentences, or find words
Incessant verbalization
Dyspnea
Stuttering, slurring, inability to modulate speech
Disorientation

Patient Outcome
Patient will be able to communicate pertinent data and feelings.

Nursing Interventions	Rationales
Assess survivor's ability to identify and describe the event and assailant.	Often, a description of the assailant and nature of the assault helps determine the kind of experience the survivor had. Also, the manner in which the survivor is approached and worked with in the first 24 hours of the assault can have a tremendous impact on the survivor's resolution and recovery from the assault.

Nursing Interventions	Rationales
Assess contributing factors to difficulty/hesitancy in discussing rape: 1. fear of being killed (attacker's threat) 2. shame/humiliation/ embarrassment.	The survivor will often feel dirty, guilty, and shameful, and blame herself for bringing on the assault, or for behavior related to survival. Frequently, she will feel guilty for engaging in behaviors required for survival during the assault: "I had no choice. He said he would kill me."
Encourage verbalization of feelings by questioning the survivor in a gentle, non-intrusive manner.	The survivor will experience a profound loss of control over herself and her body. As a result of the assault, using the word, "survivor," communicates that she did everything necessary to survive the assault, and that this is the most important point.
Validate meaning of any non-verbal communication.	
Be nonjudgmental when interacting with patient.	

▼

NURSING DIAGNOSIS: POSTTRAUMA RESPONSE

Related To
• Shock and stress sustained during sexual assault
• A sustained, painful response to traumatic event

Defining Characteristics
Reports of appetite and sleep disturbances
Reports of feeling anxious, fearful, shameful, embarrassed, humiliated and out of control
Reexperience of traumatic event (flashbacks, nightmares/repetitive dreams, intrusive thoughts)
Verbalization of survival guilt and/or guilt about behavior required for survival.
Confusion, amnesia, constricted affect, dissociation, impaired ability for reality-testing.
Changes in lifestyle; development of phobias, impaired interpersonal relationships, poor impulse control; irritability.

Patient Outcomes

Patient will

- verbalize positive statements, such as "I was not responsible for the rape"; "I did not cause the rape."
- verbalize that rape is a crime of violence, not a sexual act.

Nursing Interventions	Rationales
Assess impact of survivor's religious and cultural beliefs on her experience of the assault.	The survivor's religious and cultural orientation will have a tremendous impact on her degree of self-blame, shame, and guilt. In addition, the nurse's religious and cultural orientation will likewise have an impact on her ability to relate to, and understand, the patient.
Emphasize to the survivor, that sexual assault is a crime, and that she is not responsible for this crime of violence.	The survivor's race and economic and marital status often influence the nurse's perception of the "reasons" for the assault; i.e., a single, unemployed, minority woman assaulted by someone she met at a bar is less likely to receive the unquestionable empathy, than the employed, married white female.
Emphasize to survivor that she *survived* the assault, and did everything possible to maintain control during the assault. Emphasize that she "did every thing right." Use the word, "survivor," rather than "victim:" Emphasize that the survivor did not "cause" the assault.	

▼

LONG-TERM PHASE

NURSING DIAGNOSIS: BODY IMAGE DISTURBANCE

Related To feelings of shame, guilt, self-loathing resulting from the trauma of a sexually violent act

Defining Characteristics

Reports of changes in lifestyle and relationships (relocation, sudden or gradual withdrawal from friends/family, social isolation)
Inability to look at or touch body parts
Hiding body parts
Negative feelings about body
Depersonalization of body parts through use of impersonal pronouns

Patient Outcome

Patient will begin to reorganize her life, as evidenced by return to work and engaging in some social activities.

Nursing Interventions	Rationales
Assess the survivor's ability to reorganize various aspects of her life: 1. social activity 2. sexual activity 3. return to work	A survivor often continues to experience guilt, depression, and a loss of control during the phase following the acute trauma. She often experiences a generalized loss of self-esteem. In addition, she frequently experiences stress in her interpersonal relationships and sexual relations.
Remind survivor that there is no outwardly visible sign that she was raped.	
Work with survivor to dispel myths about sexual assault.	Rape is an act of violence, not a sexual encounter.
Continue to evaluate survivor's degree of social isolation and her affect. Evaluate for potential depression and/or suicidal ideation.	
Assess family/significant other's response to rape.	How they respond will have a strong impact on the survivor's coping ability. The survivor's significant other may also exhibit emotional problems secondary to the rape and may require counseling.

▼

NURSING DIAGNOSIS: HIGH RISK FOR SEXUAL DYSFUNCTION

Risk Factors
- Altered body image
- Guilt
- Vulnerability resulting from the trauma of the rape or attempted rape

Patient Outcomes
Patient will
- verbalize some satisfaction with ability to express self sexually.
- exhibit sexually appropriate behavior.
- utilize support/counseling services as indicated.

Nursing Interventions	Rationales
Use survivor's pretrauma sexual history as baseline to assess any degree of dysfunction.	
Encourage discussion of current sexual interactions: 1. compatibility with partner 2. frequency of activity 3. comfort level	The survivor may experience physical pain during sexual activity, or may have difficulty relaxing and enjoying it.
Empathize with and respect survivor's anxiety about sexual relationships and activity.	The survivor may find sexual contact physically repulsive, be frightened by it, or be indifferent. The survivor's experience of a sexual encounter will be different because sex was used in a violent and aggressive manner to humiliate and control the survivor.
Encourage survivor to describe feelings, rather than label them.	

▼

DISCHARGE PLANNING/CONTINUITY OF CARE

- Refer to Rape Crisis Center and support group.
- Refer for individual/family counseling.
- Refer for sexual counseling.

- Make medical referrals as needed for venereal disease/injury follow-up.
- Refer for legal consultation.
- Suggest future self-defense classes to help rebuild confidence.

REFERENCES

Candell, S. (1988). *Crisis Intervention and Sexual Assault: An Advocate's Guide.* Chicago: Rape Victim Advocates.

DeLorey, C. & Wolf, K. A. (1993). Sexual violence and older women. *AWHONN's Clinical Issues in Perinatal and Women's Health Nursing, 4*(2), 173–179.

Ledray, L. E. (1992). The sexual assault examination. *Journal of Emergency Nursing, 18*(3), 223–232.

Ledray, L. E. (1992). The sexual assault nurse clinician: A 15-year experience in Minneapolis. *Journal of Emergency Nursing, 18*(3), 217–222.

Ledray, L. E. (1990). Counseling rape victims: The nursing challenge. *Perspectives on Psychiatric Care, 26*(2), 21–27.

Muram, D. (1992). Child sexual abuse. *Obstetrics and Gynecology Clinics of North America, 19*(1), 193–207.

Ruckman, L. M. (1992). Rape: How to begin the healing. *American Journal of Nursing, 92*(9), 48–51.

▼

$\mathcal{S}$UBSTANCE ABUSE

Joan Klein, RN, MS

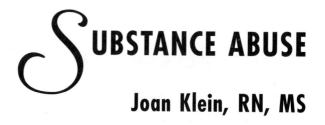

$\mathbf{A}$buse refers to a deviation from the norm and varies according to each society. Substance abuse includes continued use of any mood-altering substance despite negative, personal, familial, or social consequences. Commonly abused substances may include alcohol, prescribed or over-the-counter medications (e.g., narcotic analgesics, minor tranquilizers, or sleep aids) as well as illegal (street) drugs or any combination thereof.

ETIOLOGIES

- Excessive and/or compulsive use
- Powerful immediate reinforcement
- Low self-esteem
- Dysfunctional family
- Family history of abuse
- Illness related to abuse pattern
- Inadequate coping skills
- Genetic predisposition

CLINICAL MANIFESTATIONS

- Continued use despite knowledge of a persistent problem that is caused or aggravated by use of psychoactive substances
- Recurrent use in situations when such use is physically hazardous

DIAGNOSTIC FINDINGS

Positive blood/urine screening

▼

NURSING DIAGNOSIS: DEFENSIVE COPING

Related To
- Addiction process
- Inadequate coping skills
- Sense of shame/guilt
- Threatened self-esteem

Defining Characteristics
Denial
Defensiveness
Lack of follow-through in therapy
Projection of blame

Patient Outcomes
Patient will
- begin to identify/acknowledge existence of drug problem.
- seek treatment in appropriate program.

Nursing Interventions	Rationales
Assess for signs of substance abuse.	The person who is abusing a substance may present to an ambulatory setting offering a variety of complaints.
Attempt to assess how long patient has been using/abusing substance.	Denial is the most prominent defense mechanism used, and only skillful questioning by the nurse about the use of drugs will lead to confirmation.
Initiate a drug screen.	Screening verifies type and amount of drug ingested.

Nursing Interventions	Rationales
Administer alcohol screening tools, or refer, as appropriate.	Several methods/tools are available, such as the MAST (Michigan Alcohol Screening Test), the AUDIT (Alcohol Use Disorders Identification Test, put out by the World Health Organization) and the CAGE. CAGE is a mnemonic for the following questions: 1. Have you felt the need to *cut* down on your drinking? 2. Have you ever felt *annoyed* by criticism of your drinking? 3. Have you ever had *guilty* feelings about drinking? 4. Have you ever taken a morning *eye*-opener? Positive findings may provide objective evidence of a problem and assist the patient in accepting the reality of the situation.
Provide an opportunity for verbalization of feelings of anxiety, shame, or guilt. Avoid use of guilt-producing criticism.	The use of nonjudgmental approach by health care provider enhances patient's willingness to respond.
Provide information on the nature of substance abuse and the medical consequences associated with it.	Most drugs abused produce some form of physical dependence and/or medical complications.
Assist client in identifying the effect substance abuse is having on his family, social life, and occupation.	Focusing on the impact and consequences of substance use in patient's unique situation helps minimize defensiveness and discourages stereotyping (i.e., "alcoholic," "skid row bum," "crack head," etc).
Identify environmental and situational factors that may contribute to the problem.	
Assist patient in improving self-esteem.	
Encourage participation in appropriate support group/treatment programs.	Self-help and treatment groups offer patients alternative means of coping, support, and peer role models.

▼

NURSING DIAGNOSIS: ALTERED HEALTH MAINTENANCE

Related To
- Lack of ability to make thoughtful judgments
- Ineffective coping
- Lack of support systems

Defining Characteristics
Demonstrated lack of knowledge regarding health practices

Patient Outcomes
Patient will
- seek treatment for physical complaints.
- enter treatment program/participate in support group.
- identify early signs of relapse.

Nursing Interventions	Rationales
Obtain a thorough health history, including questions specifically related to substance abuse.	Patients do not seek treatment for substance abuse per se, but rather for complaints that may be related to it (i.e., nonspecific gastrointestinal problems, sleep disorders, anxiety, restlessness, dysrhythmia, stress-related illnesses [e.g., migraine headaches], sinusitis, reproductive dysfunction).
Assess for factors that contribute to altered health maintenance: 1. support systems 2. financial constraints 3. binging habits	
Perform comprehensive physical examination.	The physical examination identifies/verifies related pathophysiology.
Provide information about effects of substance abuse on health status.	
Provide patient with rationales for importance of health-maintaining behavior.	Understanding facilitates compliance.

Nursing Interventions	Rationales
Stress importance of ongoing participation in treatment program and consequences of continuing present lifestyle.	Emphasizing the personal consequences of substance use helps decrease reliance on denial and power struggles associated with abuse pattern relationships.
Teach early warning signs of relapse.	The powerful nature of substance abuse as a short-term source of gratification and means of coping makes it a difficult pattern to interrupt. Despite a strong resolve to "quit," patients often find themselves in situations that may encourage relapse. Being prepared to recognize these signs and offering other options or sources of assistance enhance the patient's ability to cope and minimize relapse episodes.
Emphasize the importance of participating in support groups.	
Refer to appropriate medical practitioner for specific medical problem.	
Consider detoxification for the patient currently under influence of a substance.	Considerable morbidity and mortality may accompany unsupervised substance withdrawal.
Engage family/significant other in treatment program.	

▼

NURSING DIAGNOSIS: HIGH RISK FOR INJURY/TRAUMA

Risk Factors
- Impaired cognition
- Involvement in abusive relationships
- Psychological dysfunction

Patient Outcome
Patient will begin to verbalize understanding of possibility of physical trauma to self or others related to substance abuse practices.

Nursing Interventions	Rationales
Assess for signs of trauma: 1. bruises on arms and legs 2. burns on hands or chest related to cigarette use	
Obtain history from patient to ascertain any hospitalizations related to trauma: 1. domestic violence 2. automobile accidents 3. fire	Influence of substances upon level of consciousness, judgment, coordination, place such patients at high risk for accidental trauma and injury. Secondary medical problems related to substance abuse may also lead to delayed healing and bleeding disorders.
Interview patient about current risks for trauma/injury related to: 1. domestic situation 2. driving while intoxicated 3. careless use of smoking materials	
Assess for any suicidal ideation.	Substance abusers are at increased risk for both depression and suicide.
Determine if patient is pregnant. If so, make appropriate referral for prenatal care.	Pregnant women should be classified as high-risk, since substance abuse may complicate outcome of pregnancy (increased risk of fetal anomalies, small for gestational age births, premature labor).
Explain the importance of seeking medical care/substance abuse treatment.	This is necessary to prevent further/future medical/physical consequences.
Inform patient of legal options available for an abusive situation. 1. restraining order 2. filing of charges	Patients usually need counseling to explore options available for removing themselves from abusive relationships.

▼

NURSING DIAGNOSIS: SELF ESTEEM DISTURBANCE

Related To
- Pattern of substance abuse
- Negative interpersonal relationships
- Previous failures with treatment program

Defining Characteristics

Self-negating verbalization
Expressions of guilt and shame
Declining level of functioning (social, familial, occupational)
Dependent on opinions of others
Nonassertive/passive
Excessively seeks reassurance

Patient Outcomes

Patient will begin to verbalize positive feelings about self.

Nursing Interventions	Rationales
Assess for signs of disturbed self-concept.	Most substance abusers suffer from low self esteem and a distorted sense of their own abilities and competence.
Support patient in verbalizing feelings.	Most patients have difficulty acknowledging and/or verbalizing feelings.
Assess for suicidal thoughts or plans. If present, refer to inpatient treatment program.	Substance abusers are at increased risk for both depression and suicide.
Avoid use of guilt-producing criticism.	The use of nonjudgmental approach by health care provider enhances patient's willingness to respond.
Explore availability of support groups or programs. Provide positive reinforcement in initiating/following through with treatment plans.	Assisting patient to abandon a powerful source of gratification and/or means of tension reduction (whatever the drug) requires considerable external support and reinforcement.

▼

NURSING DIAGNOSIS: HIGH RISK OF ALTERED NUTRITION—LESS THAN BODY REQUIREMENTS

Risk Factors

- Desire for food replaced by substance use
- Poor nutritional choices
- Altered gastrointestinal absorption
- Social isolation

Patient Outcomes

Patient will
- identify good nutritional food choices.
- gain weight.

Nursing Interventions	Rationales
Obtain nutritional history.	
Assess for signs of nutritional deficit: 1. 10–20% below intended body weight 2. documented inadequate intake 3. skin changes: • flushed appearance • jaundice • poor skin turgor • thinning of hair	Substance abusers often experience primary or secondary appetite suppression and changes in eating habits. This, coupled with possible changes in digestion and metabolism, may lead to varying degrees of weight loss and malnutrition.
Request patient to keep a record of regular weight checks.	
Assist patient with meal planning.	Educating patient regarding role of nutrition in health maintenance can facilitate self-care skills and enhance sense of well-being.
Discourage use of "junk foods."	
Refer to nutritionist.	
Assist patient in identifying the effects of substance abuse.	

▼

DISCHARGE PLANNING/CONTINUITY OF CARE

- Refer patient/family to appropriate self-help groups (Alcoholics Anonymous, Narcotics Anonymous, AL-Anon, Al-A-Teen).
- Refer to inpatient substance abuse program.
- Refer to outpatient substance abuse program.
- Refer to nutritionist.

REFERENCES

Hughes, T. & Fox, M. (1993). Patterns of alcohol and drug use among women: Focus on special populations. *AWHONN's Clinical Issues in Perinatal and Women's Health Nursing, 4*(2), 203–212.

Kinney, J. (1991). *Clinical Manual of Substance Abuse.* St. Louis, MO: Mosby-Year Book.

Leibenluft, E., Fiero, P., Bartko, J., Moul, D., & Rosenthal, N. (1993). Depressive symptoms and the self-reported use of alcohol, caffeine, and carbohydrates in normal volunteers and four groups of psychiatric outpatients. *American Journal of Psychiatry, 150*(2), 294–301.

Miller, W. R., Leckman, A. L., Delaney, H. D., & Tinkcom, M. (1992). Long-term follow-up of behavioral self-control training. *Journal of Studies on Alcohol, 53*3), 249–261.

Rodin, J. & Ickovics, J. R. (1990). Women's health: Review and research agenda as we approach the 21st century. *American Psychologist, 45,* 1081–1034.

Schultz, J. & Dark, S. (1990). *Manual of Psychiatric Nursing Care Plans,* 3rd. Ed. Glenview, IL: Scott, Foresman/Little, Brown.

Steele, C. M. & Josephs, R. A. (1990). Alcohol myopia: Its prized and dangerous effects. *American Psychologist, 45,* 921–933.

Thomas, E. J. (1991). Reaching the uncooperative alcohol abuser through a cooperative spouse: The unilateral approach. Paper presented at the NIDA National Conference on Drug Abuse Research and Practice, Washington, D.C.

Tweed, S. H. & Ryff, C. D. (1991). Adult children of alcoholics: Profiles of wellness amidst distress. *Journal of the Study of Alcohol, 52*(2), 133–141.

Tweed, S. H. (1989). Identifying the alcoholic client. *The Nursing Clinics of North America, 24*(1), 13–32.

▼

Gynecological Medical Concerns

▼

$\mathcal{P}$ROSTAGLANDIN-INDUCED ABORTION (SECOND TRIMESTER)

Janet Williams, RN, BSN

Midtrimester abortions are performed from 12 to 20 weeks gestation. They may be done electively or for therapeutic indications. Regardless of the reasons for abortion, the mother faces labor (which is often protracted), the birth of her child, and the grief associated with the loss of the fetus. Other descriptive terms for second trimester abortion are therapeutic abortion, elective abortion, prostaglandin induction. Prostaglandins may be used alone or together with other agents including: laminaria/dileteria, or oxytocin.

INDICATIONS

- Mother chooses not to maintain pregnancy
- Fetus has anomalies incompatible with life
- Extreme medical, psychiatric, or pregnancy-related complications that compromise maternal life

▼

NURSING DIAGNOSIS: HIGH RISK FOR INJURY TO MOTHER

Risk Factors
- Violent labor leading to ruptured uterus
- Hemorrhage, hypovolemic shock, sepsis

Patient Outcome
Risk of injury is reduced by early assessment and treatment.

Nursing Interventions	Rationales
Monitor vital signs.	Elevated temperature may indicate sepsis. Prostaglandin normally causes a small increase in temperature. Blood pressure, pulse, and respiration changes may indicate shock/hemorrhage.
Assess and document status of membranes. Notify physician when bag of water ruptures or of presence of foul-smelling amniotic fluid.	Risk of infection increases the longer the membranes are ruptured.
Assess and document strength, length, and intensity of contractions as well as relaxation between contractions. Determine whether contractions return to baseline.	Hypertonicity may precipitate abruption. Sudden tearing pain and then absence of pain may indicate uterine rupture.
Assess and document amount of vaginal bleeding.	Excessive vaginal bleeding may indicate rupture/perforation of uterus/cervix.
Assess for signs and symptoms of shock: 1. decreased blood pressure 2. increased heart rate 3. changes in level of consciousness 4. diaphoresis	
If shock occurs: 1. Notify physician. 2. Elevate right hip to avoid supine hypotensive syndrome. 3. Increase intravenous drip rate. 4. Insert airway for oxygen administration. 5. Monitor vital signs.	
Assess and document fluid return from intra-amniotic injection as physician injects the prostaglandin.	Clear fluid indicates proper placement of needle in amniotic sac; blood return may indicate needle placement in blood vessel.
Notify physician of shortness of breath, wheezing, chest pain, or tightness.	These symptoms may indicate severe reaction to prostaglandin.

Nursing Interventions	Rationales
Assess integrity of cervix after removal of laminaria to rule out lacerations.	

▼

NURSING DIAGNOSIS: HIGH RISK FOR FLUID VOLUME DEFICIT

Risk Factors
- Side effects of prostaglandin administration
  - nausea
  - vomiting
  - diaphoresis

Patient Outcome
Optimal fluid volume will be maintained, as evidenced by normal specific gravity and urine output of at least 50 mL/hr.

Nursing Interventions	Rationales
Assess for excessive diaphoresis.	Fluid loss through diaphoresis may be substantial.
Monitor severity of nausea and amount of vomiting.	This measure will determine how much fluid needs to be replaced intravenously.
Give antiemetic as ordered.	An antiemetic may be needed to decrease the amount of nausea and vomiting.
Administer fluids intravenously as ordered. Evaluate need for electrolyte replacement.	Severe vomiting and diarrhea will result in significant deficiencies even in the healthy patient.
Monitor intake and output.	
Assess urine amount, color, and concentration. Dipstick urine for specific gravity.	High specific gravity indicates dehydration.
Note number and consistency of bowel movements. Give antidiarrheal agents as ordered.	Medication may be indicated to reduce diarrhea associated with prostaglandin.

▼

NURSING DIAGNOSIS: PAIN

Related To uterine concentrations

Defining Characteristics
Grimaces
Hyperventilation
Moaning/crying
Muscle tension
Thrashing about in bed
Verbalizes pain

Patient Outcome
Patient verbalizes ability to cope with pain.

Nursing Interventions	Rationales
Elicit patient's perception of discomfort related to uterine contractions.	The patient undegoing an abortion should be adequately medicated for pain. Patient-controlled analgesia (PCA) pumps have been effectively used with this population. The effect of the pain medication on the infant is not a consideration here.
Evaluate the mechanisms patient uses to manage discomfort (e.g., talking/silence, rocking).	Supporting the patient's efforts to use familiar measures to manage pain is the first step.
Explain the cyclic nature of uterine contractions and the role of these contractions in terminating pregnancy. Keep patient informed of labor progress.	This information may help patient understand and cope with labor process.
Use nonpharmacologic comfort measures when appropriate: 1. position changes 2. relaxation techniques 3. breathing techniques 4. distraction 5. presence of support person 6. emotional support as needed	

Nursing Interventions	Rationales
Reduce/eliminate other factors that may contribute to discomfort, e.g., encourage frequent voiding.	Bladder distention can add to discomfort.
Provide emotional support and personal contact.	Abortions, elective or therapeutic, are stressful. Giving emotional support helps lessen stress, promotes atmosphere of comfort.

▼

NURSING DIAGNOSIS: ANTICIPATORY GRIEVING

Related To
- Loss of pregnancy by abortion
- Loss of fetus to whom attachments may have formed
- Loss of perfect image of baby if fetus is malformed
- Concern about ability to become pregnant/parent again
- Feelings of guilt

Defining Characteristics
Crying
Shock/disbelief
Defensiveness
Anger
Denial

Patient Outcome
Patient will display beginning signs of coping with grief as evidenced by ability to cry and express feelings/sadness.

Nursing Interventions	Rationales
Assist patient in identifying and verbalizing feelings about abortion.	Abortion, elective or therapeutic, is experienced as a loss of a potential future. Allowing patient to verbalize/act out grief (safely) will enhance the patient's ability to process the abortion event so that reconciliation can be reached. Other family members may also feel the loss; aiding them to express their grief might help them to be more emotionally available to the patient. Their support in helping patient cope with grief is critical. Note defense mechanisms patient may use.
Assess the mother's level of maturity and her attachment to the pregnancy.	These factors will affect how she experiences and manages her grief.
Assess the influence of cultural/religious beliefs on grieving process.	Guilt/remorse may interfere with the patient's ability to grieve.
Assess patient's stage in grieving process.	This will determine the type of support the patient will require. Grief work may begin long before the actual termination, or long after it.
Assess patient's support system.	Family and friends may be available to assist the patient in her grief work. Encourage client to think of someone with whom she can share her concerns and feelings.
If the abortion is for therapeutic indications: 1. Assess patient's knowledge of clinical conditions that resulted in decision to have therapeutic abortion. 2. Assess how bearing an imperfect child influences how she feels about herself.	

Nursing Interventions	Rationales
Avoid minimizing the event.	For some people who elect to abort, the decision is very difficult and may be painful.
Accept behaviors that are not self-destructive/injurious to others.	Sadness and stress may produce behavior deviating from normal, which may be part of the patient's way of coping with situation.
Encourage the presence of father/significant other throughout procedure.	The presence and support may provide comfort and help patient cope with experience. Father's participation may diminish possible recriminations at a later time.
Give patient/significant others opportunity to view fetus. When helping a family view their dead, defected fetus, focus on the traits which are not aberrant, e.g., the perfectly shaped hands or tiny ears or soft skin.	Viewing fetus helps with separation of fetus from self; also helps decrease possibility of later forming false mental images of fetus. This is important, particularly when abortion is being done for fetal anomalies. The real fetal anomalies are rarely as bad as what the patient imagines.
Accept patient's decision not to view fetus.	A patient's aversion to this should be respected. Reassure the woman that until disposition of the infant's body takes place, seeing the infant remains an option should she change her mind. Photograph the infant and make these pictures available to the family if they desire. If they are not interested at this time, remind them that the pictures will be kept on file.
Facilitate baptismal rites/last rites if patient desires.	
Proceed with postmortem care with respect.	It is especially important to respect family wishes about religious ceremonies. Even when termination is elective, grief is natural; all measures to facilitate the grieving process are critical.

▼

NURSING DIAGNOSIS: KNOWLEDGE DEFICIT ABOUT CONTRACEPTION

Related To
- Lack of information
- Lack of motivation
- Cultural/religious barriers

Defining Characteristics

Lack of questions
Multiple abortions
Multiple questions
Requested information about contraception

Patient Outcome

Patient will verbalize understanding of types of contraceptives available, their actions, and effectiveness ratings.

Nursing Interventions	Rationales
Assess patient's maturation level and influence, if any, of cultural/religious beliefs about birth control.	The nurse may need to discuss abstinence or maternal-family planning with someone who is morally opposed to other types of contraception.
Describe different medications/devices for contraception and how they are used: 1. intrauterine devices (IUDs) 2. diaphragm 3. pills 4. condoms and foam 5. suppositories 6. sponges 7. implants	This knowledge will relieve fears and dispel myths associated with birth control, and will allow patient to choose suitable birth control freely.
Stress importance of carefully following instructions for birth control method used.	
Explain effectiveness of each method.	

Nursing Interventions	Rationales
Formulate with patient a plan for contraception: 1. listings of family planning clinics 2. information about payment/ funding for family planning services	

▼

DISCHARGE PLANNING/CONTINUITY OF CARE

- Schedule postabortion checkup in 2 to 4 weeks.
- Instruct patient to place nothing in the vagina (no tampons, douching, or intercourse), until after postabortion checkup.
- Instruct patient to call physician if
  - bleeding becomes excessive
  - temperature becomes elevated
  - foul-smelling discharge from vagina is noted
  - tissue or clots are expelled from vagina
- Refer patient to support group for families who sustain a fetal/ neonatal loss (SHARE).
- Encourage family to utilize friends, clergy, and family during grief period.

REFERENCES

Faulkner, A. (1990). Antinatal care: Forgotten mothers. Women who choose a termination because of fetal abnormality. *Community Outlook, 8*, 11–12.

Frye, B. (1993). Abortion. *AWHONN's Clinical Issues in Perinatal and Women's Health Nursing, 4*(2), 265–271.

Mueller, L. (1991). Second-trimester termination of pregnancy: Nursing care. *Journal of Obstetrical, Gynecologic, and Neonatal Nursing, 20*(4), 284–289.

▼

$\mathcal{S}$PONTANEOUS ABORTION (FIRST TRIMESTER)

Mary Sandelski, RN, MSN

$\mathbf{S}$pontaneous abortion is an interruption of a pregnancy during the first 12 weeks. For psychosocial aspects of nursing care, see Perinatal Loss.

ETIOLOGIES

Spontaneous abortion is not well understood, and most often is attributed to:
- anomalies incompatible with life in the developing embryo
- placenta and implantation anomalies

CLINICAL MANIFESTATIONS

Patient may complain of mild to severe abdominal cramping with or without vaginal bleeding. Part or all of the products of conception may be expelled:
- threatened abortion
  - vaginal bleeding with or without cramping in the presence of a live fetus
- inevitable abortion
  - vaginal bleeding accompanied by cervical dilation and/or rupture of membranes
- complete abortion
  - complete expulsion of the products of conception before the tenth week
- incomplete abortion
  - occurs after 10 weeks gestation, usually marked by incomplete expulsion of the products of conception, and necessitating a dilatation and curettage (D&C)
- missed abortion
  - retention of the products of conception after the pregnancy has ceased developing and the embryo/fetus has died

- septic abortion
  - legal or illegal pregnancy termination resulting in massive systemic infection

CLINICAL/DIAGNOSTIC FINDINGS

- Ultrasound evaluation may reveal an empty gestational sac or a pregnancy that ceases development
- Human chorionic gonadotropin levels may fall

▼

NURSING DIAGNOSIS: PAIN

Related To uterine cramping, contractions

Defining Characteristics

Crying
Moaning
Restlessness
Verbal reports of discomfort
Requests for pain relief medication
Grimacing

Patient Outcomes

Patient will
- verbalize decreasing levels of discomfort.
- appear relaxed and comfortable.

Nursing Interventions	Rationales
Monitor occurrence and characteristics of cramping.	Knowing the frequency and severity of pain enables nurse to meet patient's pain management needs.
Use therapeutic communication strategies to acknowledge the pain experienced and to convey understanding of the patient's response to pain.	
Assess past experiences with pain, and prior successful coping strategies.	

Nursing Interventions	Rationales
Encourage use of nonpharmaceutical coping mechanisms such as relaxation breathing, imaging, position changes, massage, heating pad, clean linen, cool cloth.	Pharmaceutical pain management may be contraindicated or not completely effective.
Encourage presence of significant other(s) and support these persons in their role.	Patients often receive much consolation/support from significant others in their lives. Caregivers need to recognize this and validate visitors' presence.
Minimize/eliminate distracting stimuli such as bright lights, noise, frequent interruptions.	Unpleasant environmental factors can compound physical discomfort.
Administer analgesics as ordered.	
Assess effectiveness of interventions.	

▼

NURSING DIAGNOSIS: HIGH RISK FOR FLUID VOLUME DEFICIT

Risk Factors
- Vaginal bleeding
- Nausea, vomiting, diarrhea

Patient Outcome
Patient will display signs of normovolemia: heart rate and blood pressure within normal limits, urine output > 30 mL/hr.

Nursing Interventions	Rationales
Assess vaginal bleeding for amount, color, presence of clots/tissue.	
Save all tissue passed.	It allows for better estimation of amount of products of conception passed.
Implement a perineal pad count.	This allows for a more quantitative, objective estimation of bleeding.

Nursing Interventions	Rationales
Monitor heart rate, blood pressure, and urinary output.	These measurements provide information as to the degree of fluid volume deficit. Severe hypovolemia may precede kidney shutdown. Pitocin has antidiuretic effect.
Assess for nausea, vomiting, or diarrhea. Treat with antiemetics and antidiarrheals as needed.	Nausea, vomiting, and diarrhea are a common reaction to prostin use, which is given to induce labor.
Initiate IV lines as needed.	These can be used to transfuse blood products, maintain hydration, and as access for medications.
Maintain NPO status if ordered.	If abortion necessitates a D&C, general anesthesia may be used and an NPO status is required to help avoid aspiration of gastric contents.
Record uterine height and tone.	A boggy, displaced uterus is common with increased vaginal bleeding and measures need to be taken to increase uterine tone.
Postexpulsion, administer oxytocin as ordered.	Oxytocin causes uterine contraction and decreases vaginal bleeding.
Order/obtain laboratory work as ordered.	Laboratory findings, such as a decreased hemoglobin (Hb) or hematocrit (Hct), are indicative of bleeding. An electrolyte imbalance may indicate dehydration from the nausea and vomiting.
Administer blood as ordered.	Severe vaginal bleeding will reduce blood volume.

Nursing Interventions	Rationales
Document blood type and Rh factor of patient (and male partner if possible).	An Rh-negative mother and an Rh-positive father may produce an Rh-positive fetus. If Rh-negative fetal red blood cells enter maternal circulation, the mother might develop a sensitivity to Rh-positive blood. These antibodies could be transmitted to a future Rh-positive fetus and result in Rh isoimmunization.
Document blood type and Rh factor of fetus if possible.	If fetus is Rh-negative, RhoGAM is not needed.
Administer RhoGAM intramuscularly as appropriate within 72 hours.	If fetus is Rh-positive or Rh factor is undetermined, RhoGAM will be needed. A delay in administration increases the likelihood of antibody formation and threatens subsequent pregnancies.
Provide patient with identification card supplied with RhoGAM and stress the importance of RhoGAM with future pregnancies/losses.	
Prepare patient for a D&C if ordered.	If all the products of conception are not expelled with a spontaneous abortion, a D&C is performed to empty the uterus, thereby avoiding hemorrhage and sepsis.

▼

NURSING DIAGNOSIS: HIGH RISK FOR INFECTION

Risk Factors
- Retention of products of conception
- Operative procedures (D&C)

Patient Outcome
Patient will not display signs and symptoms of infection.

Nursing Interventions	Rationales
Monitor patient for elevated temperature and increased heart rate.	These are early signs of infectious process.
Assess for foul-smelling vaginal discharge or bleeding.	
Assess for abdominal tenderness.	This may indicate developing intrauterine infection.
Monitor laboratory work: C-reactive protein, white blood count, blood cultures.	These allow for the diagnosis of infection and will dictate the antibiotic used as determined by sensitivity through cultures.
Administer antibiotics as ordered.	
Administer antipyretics as ordered.	
Prepare patient for D&C if products of conception are retained.	Retained products may cause sepsis if not removed.

▼

NURSING DIAGNOSIS: KNOWLEDGE DEFICIT

Related To new experience

Defining Characteristics
Expressed confusion concerning current event(s)
Multiple questions
Antagonism
Dependency
Uncooperativeness
Withdrawal

Patient Outcomes
Patient will.
• verbalize an understanding of events.
• verbalize knowledge of treatment plan.

Nursing Interventions	Rationales
Assess perception of events surrounding pregnancy loss.	Patient's experience of events leading up to miscarriage may be colored by/distorted by grief, fear, and guilt.

Nursing Interventions	Rationales
Dispel any "myths" patient/family may have as to the cause of the loss.	Lay persons have many misconceptions. Perpetuation of these may delay effective grief work.
Repeat/reinforce teaching.	Information may not all be assimilated at one time. Repetition will help ensure information is imparted to the patient in a manageable form. The complexity of information may be too great to impart at once.
Include family in teaching.	The family will have questions and the patient may not be up to or may prefer that health care providers provide crucial information. A patient is part of a family and should not be isolated from that system but cared for within it.
Provide patient/family with loss information pack.	This can be taken home and referred to later.

▼

DISCHARGE PLANNING/CONTINUITY OF CARE

- Instruct patient not to place anything in vagina until the physician has seen patient for four-week checkup.
- Instruct patient to report temperature, severe abdominal pain, foul-smelling vaginal secretions.
- Remind patient that unprotected sex may result in pregnancy.
- Monitor hemoglobin and hematocrit if blood loss was significant.

REFERENCES

Armstrong, B., McDonald, A., & Sloan, M. (1992). Cigarette, alcohol and coffee consumption and spontaneous abortion. *American Journal of Public Health, 82*(1), 85–87.

Bansen, S. & Stevens, H. (1992). Women's experience of miscarriage in early pregnancy. *Journal of Nurse Midwifery, 37*(2), 84–90.

Niebyl, J. R. (1990). Detecting signs and symptoms of incompetent cervix. *Contemporary Obstetrics and Gynecology*, October:37–46.

Reed, K. S. (1992). The effects of gestational age and pregnancy planning status on obstetrical nurses' perceptions of giving emotional care to women experiencing miscarriage. *Image: Journal of Nursing Scholarship, 24*(2), 107–110.

Stewart, A., Harker, L., & Ford, J. (1992). An unfinished story: Helping people to come to terms with miscarriage. *Professional Nurse, 7*(10), 656–660.

▼

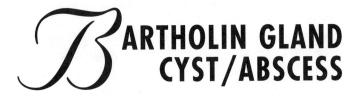

BARTHOLIN GLAND CYST/ABSCESS

Denise Wheeler, RN, MS, CNM

Bartholinitis is an infection of the Bartholin gland(s). Cysts or abscesses of the Bartholin gland(s) may represent an acute or chronic infection.

ETIOLOGIES

- *Escherichia coli*
- *Neisseria gonorrhoeae*
- *Chlamydia*
- *Proteus mirabilia*
- Mixed bacteria

CLINICAL MANIFESTATIONS

- Vulvar or vaginal pain and/or swelling
- Drainage from the Bartholin gland(s)
- Dyspareunia
- Fever and chills

CLINICAL/DIAGNOSTIC FINDINGS

N/A

▼

NURSING DIAGNOSIS: PAIN
Related To Bartholin gland cyst/abscess

Patient Outcomes

Patient will

- verbalize knowledge of comfort measures.
- express some relief of pain.

Defining Characteristics

Vulvar or vaginal pain
Pain with intercourse
Nonverbal expressions of pain, e.g., facial contortions, crying
Slow walking or other movements
Pain with urination or defecation
Tender, often palpable, inguinal lymph nodes

Nursing Interventions	Rationales
Obtain history of pain. Assess patient's level of discomfort; determine effects of pain on usual activities.	
Assess degree of edema and swelling of the vulva and vaginal area, and for presence of any visible discharge from the vagina.	Diagnosis is made by examination of external genitalia and by culture.
Determine which, if any, comfort measures have been tried, and with what degree of success.	
Anticipate need for and provide analgesia as appropriate prior to pelvic examination.	Examination of the infected area will cause the patient additional discomfort. Proper pain control is important for patient cooperation during the examination and any procedures that may be required.
Assist the physician in obtaining any specimens, including gonorrhea, chlamydia, anaerobic and aerobic genital cultures.	Cultures may be done to identify the infecting organism and initiate appropriate antibiotic treatment. Treatment of partners may be indicated.
Prepare for possible incision and drainage in the office or hospital setting.	Some physicians prefer to place Ward catheters in the ambulatory surgical setting rather than office. Frequently, Bartholin gland cysts can only be resolved by surgical incision followed by antibiotic therapy. In chronic infections, removal of the Bartholin glands may be recommended.

Nursing Interventions	Rationales
Teach about comfort measures. Provide information about sitz baths at home, warm packs, and ice packs.	
Instruct patient in proper use of antibiotics or pain medication at home if ordered. Encourage patient to complete entire antibiotic course.	Many people stop taking antibiotics when they begin to feel better. Incomplete treatment of the infecting organism increases the likelihood of recurrence.

▼

NURSING DIAGNOSIS: KNOWLEDGE DEFICIT

Related To
- New experience
- Embarrassment about infection

Defining Characteristics

Many questions regarding origins of infection, transmission route, diagnosis and treatment
Concern about possible sexually transmitted nature
Concern about spread of infection, impact on fertility
Nonverbal communication: failure to make eye contact, tension, no questions, anger

Patient Outcomes

Patient will verbalize understanding of the infectious process as it relates to Bartholin cyst infection.

Nursing Interventions	Rationales
Assess present level of understanding about anatomy of the vagina and vulva, Bartholin gland infections, diagnosis, and treatment, and source of information.	

Nursing Interventions	Rationales
Accept patient's diagnosis in a nonjudgmental and supportive manner.	Infections of the reproductive organs may be embarrassing for the patient (and nurse). It is critical to remember that not all Bartholin cyst infections are caused by organisms that are sexually transmitted. It should never be implied that the condition was caused by the patient's behavior or her sexual partner's. Such implication defeats the nurse's attempts at patient education.
Obtain a history of the current problem, if not already done; include sexual history.	Changes in sexual behavior or partners may contribute to bartholinitis. Recent resumption of intercourse following a period of abstinence may cause inflammation. The sexual history will also help the nurse to assess the possibility that the patient's sexual behavior resulted in infection.
Teach patient about anatomy of the vulva and vagina, using pictures and diagrams when indicated.	The patient must understand the location of the Bartholin glands and their relationship to the other reproductive organs to understand the infection and comply with treatment.
Explain infection of the Bartholin glands, including possible causes of infection. Organisms may include: *Escherichia coli*, *Neisseria gonorrhoeae*, *Chlamydia*, *Proteus mirabilia*, and mixed bacteria. Include partner in discussion if appropriate.	Both partners need to be aware that bartholinitis is not always a sexually transmitted event. Public health concerns require that this topic be addressed.
Reassure and explain procedures for examination.	
Instruct patient in care of Ward catheter if placed in office. The catheter is left to drain and is removed in 2–3 weeks. It will frequently fall out prior to that.	The patient should be aware that if the catheter falls out, it will not need to be replaced if the cyst continues to drain and does not recur.

Nursing Interventions	Rationales
Provide instruction in personal hygiene. Include information about 1. cleansing and wiping techniques 2. normal vaginal secretions 3. signs and symptoms of infection 4. vulvar self-examination.	

▼

NURSING DIAGNOSIS: SEXUAL DYSFUNCTION

Related To
- Physical discomfort
- Confusion
- Fear about venereal disease
- Anger

Defining Characteristics
Concern about ability to resume sexual relationship with partner
Concern about social or sexual habits
Concern about required period of abstinence as cyst drains and heals

Patient Outcomes
- Patient and her partner will discuss the effects the infection has had on their relationship, emotionally and sexually.
- Patient will verbalize methods of prevention of sexually transmitted diseases

Nursing Interventions	Rationales
Question patient about her relationship with her sexual partner and the effects of her condition on their relationship.	
Allow patient to verbalize her concerns, anger, doubts, and other emotions about this diagnosis.	Infections of the reproductive organs may cause the patient to question her own self-esteem and self-respect and perhaps that of her partner. Maintaining a supportive, nonjudgmental manner will communicate to the patient that she is a victim of this organism, and her value as a person in unchanged.

Nursing Interventions	Rationales
Assure confidentiality.	Discussing her sexuality may be uncomfortable for the patient. The nurse's obvious comfort with the discussion will encourage the patient to verbalize her concerns and thoughts more readily.
Remind patient that abstinence is not required; she may resume sexual activity as comfort allows (even with Ward's catheter in place). Suggest that condoms may be appropriate.	
Inform patient that infertility should not be a concern with simple bartholinitis; however, if chlamydia occurs, or gonorrhea is involved, there could be a problem.	

▼

DISCHARGE PLANNING/CONTINUITY OF CARE

Follow-up
- Gynecologist: 2 weeks
- If STD, test of cure will be necessary
- Sexually transmitted disease clinic: if partner needs treatment (chlamydia, gonorrhea)

REFERENCES

Byyny, R. & Speroff, L. (1990). *A Clinical Guide for the Care of Older Women*. Baltimore, MD: Williams & Wilkins.
Lichtman, R. & Papera, S. (1990). *Gynecology: Well Woman Care*. E. Norwalk, CT: Appleton & Lange.

▼

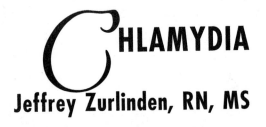

CHLAMYDIA

Jeffrey Zurlinden, RN, MS

Chlamydia is a sexually transmitted disease (STD). It may cause a localized infection of the urethra, endocervical canal, rectum, or pharynx. The patient may have one site of infection or many sites. The infection is spread by sexual contact with the infected site. Untreated infections may lead to pelvic inflammatory disease (PID) and reproductive difficulties due to scarring.

ETIOLOGY

Infection with the bacteria *Chlamydia trachomatis*

CLINICAL MANIFESTATIONS

- Often asymptomatic
- Endocervical infections
  - yellowish discharge
  - dysuria
  - spotting between menstrual periods
- Rectal infections
  - itching
  - changes in bowel habits
  - blood or mucus in stool

CLINICAL/DIAGNOSTIC FINDINGS

- Cultures or ELISA (enzyme-linked immunosorbent assay) tests are positive.
- If a discharge is present, smears can rule out gonorrhea.

▼

NURSING DIAGNOSIS: INFECTION

Related To presence of infectious organisms

Defining Characteristics

Positive tissue culture from urethra, endocervical canal, throat, or rectum
Gram stain with polymorphonuclear leukocytes and no gram-negative intracellular diplococci on smear
Positive chlamydia ELISA results from endocervical, urethral, or throat specimens
History of sexual contact with an infected person
Persistent symptoms despite treatment for gonorrhea and negative gonorrhea cultures

Patient Outcome

Patient will exhibit no signs of infection, as evidenced by resolution of discharge.

Nursing Interventions	Rationales
Determine date of last sexual contact, number of sexual partners, and description of recent sexual activities.	This provides information regarding behavior that increases risk of sexually transmitted diseases.
Obtain cultures from all sites of possible infection.	Patients may present with multiple sites of infection.
Obtain smears from discharges.	
Obtain history of previous STDs.	Though chlamydial infections are easily cured with antibiotics, they do tend to recur.
Assess: 1. urethral or cervical discharge 2. urinary frequency 3. pain or burning when urinating 4. spotting between menstrual periods or after intercourse 5. rectal discharge 6. mucus or blood in stools 7. rectal spasms 8. change in bowel movements	About 80% of women are asymptomatic. If symptomatic, mucoid yellowish discharge, less profuse than with gonorrhea, occurs within 21 days after infection.

Nursing Interventions	Rationales
Screen for other STDs, hepatitis B, and human immunodeficiency virus (HIV).	Patients with one STD are at higher risk for a concomitant STD.
Obtain menstrual history, including date of last period.	It can be difficult to obtain culture during menstruation; results are less accurate, especially with tampon use, and there will be increased number of false negatives.
Determine method and compliance with birth control.	Acquiring STDs suggests no use/improper use of condoms. Women may be at higher risk for pregnancy. Nurse should use this opportunity for health screening/education.
Perform pregnancy test.	This is necessary for early detection of pregnancy. Some drugs have teratogenic effect. Tetracycline is contraindicated for use with pregnant women.
Administer antibiotics as ordered.	Treatment for chlamydia frequently changes in response to new antibiotics, usually doxycycline, tetracycline, azithromycin, or ofloxacin. Follow the current guidelines from the Center for Disease Control (CDC) or your local Health Department.
Observe for possible anaphylactic reaction if antibiotics are given intramuscularly during clinic visit.	
Dispense condoms.	The use of latex condoms is the most effective means of preventing the spread of disease during sexual contact.
Instruct patient to inform all sexual partners within the last three weeks of possible exposure to chlamydia and need for treatment.	Untreated asymptomatic sexual partners are a common source of reinfection.

▼

NURSING DIAGNOSIS: KNOWLEDGE DEFICIT

Related To new diagnosis

Defining Characteristics

Many questions
Few questions
History of repeated infections
Unable to state the causes, treatment, and prevention of chlamydia

Patient Outcomes

Patient will state
- medication schedule
- medication side effects
- date of return visit for test of cure
- how to use condoms to prevent future infections

Nursing Interventions	Rationales
Assess patient's present level of understanding.	Misconceptions can increase anxiety/fear and foster spread of sexually transmitted disease.
Instruct patient about medication schedule and side effects of antibiotics used to treat chlamydia.	Treatment for chlamydia frequently changes in response to new antibiotics. Follow the current guidelines from the CDC or your local Health Department. (If a tetracycline, take on an empty stomach, avoid dairy products, and screen from the sun.)
Instruct patient to refrain from vaginal, rectal, and pharyngeal sexual intercourse until partners are treated and results are reported from test of cure.	
Instruct patient on mode of transmission: local inoculation of bacteria from partner's penis to patient's throat, vagina, or rectum.	
Instruct patient to use latex condoms or use other nonintercourse sexual methods to prevent future infection.	Latex condoms are an effective barrier against chlamydia.

Nursing Interventions	Rationales
Inform patient of the possible consequences of untreated chlamydia.	Pelvic inflammatory disease or difficulty conceiving due to scarred fallopian tubes are common complications

▼

NURSING DIAGNOSIS: INEFFECTIVE MANAGEMENT OF THERAPEUTIC REGIMEN

Related To
- Complexity of treatment
- Unwillingness to comply with treatment, prevention, or informing sexual partners

Defining Characteristics
Persistent infection not caused by antibiotic-resistant strains
Missed return visit for test of cure
Incorrect pill count at return visit
Inadequate blood level of antibiotic

Patient Outcomes
Patient will
- complete course of treatment.
- notify sexual partners.
- use condoms to prevent infection.

Nursing Interventions	Rationales
Compare actual effect and expected therapeutic effect.	
Plot patient's pattern of returning for follow-up visits.	
Determine social support system and presence of significant others.	Interpersonal influences can impact on compliance with treatment regimen.
Assess patient's and significant other's beliefs about current illness and treatment plan.	How one perceives susceptibility, severity, and threat of disease impacts on health behavior.
Assess quality of relationship between patient and health care workers and health care facility.	

Nursing Interventions	Rationales
Role-play to practice informing sexual partners of possible exposure to gonorrhea.	Role-playing gives the patient opportunity to rehearse the situation and allows nurse to provide feedback.
Suggest short-term therapy if patient has a history of not taking oral medication.	Less complex therapies facilitate compliance. Azithromycin is a single dose.
Role-play to practice new behaviors in situations leading to reinfection (such as saying "no" or using condoms.)	
Develop a positive relationship with the patient that encourages participation with treatment decisions. (The nurse-patient relationship is based on recognition of patient's right to self-determination and capacity for self-management with focus on decision-making and goal attainment.)	
Determine with the patient the plan of treatment she is most likely to complete.	Involving the patient in planning the regimen improves compliance.

▼

NURSING DIAGNOSIS: ALTERED SEXUALITY PATTERNS

Related To
- Imposed restrictions
- Fear
- Risk of spread of infection

Defining Characteristics
Patient or significant other expresses concern about the effect chlamydia and treatment has on their expressions of physical intimacy.

Patient Outcomes
Patient will state ways of expressing physical intimacy during treatment.

Nursing Interventions	Rationales
Determine patient's or significant other's concerns.	Diagnosis of STDs may provoke feelings of guilt, shame, the need for punishment, or other anxiety-provoking thoughts unique to patient.
Determine if concerns are also related to fears about acquired immunodeficiency syndrome (AIDS).	STD diagnosis may provoke fear of AIDS that alters sexual behavior.
Assess perception of meaning of chlamydia infection.	Provides opportunity to correct misconceptions.
Elicit patient's feeling about limits on sexual behavior.	
Interview patient in a quiet, private, distraction-free environment.	Most women are hesitant to discuss personal sexual matters. The proper setting may facilitate discussion.
Explore ways to express physical intimacy during treatment excluding vaginal, rectal, and pharyngeal intercourse.	Restrictions on sexual activity should not deprive the couple of other activities that convey the message that they are loved and desired.
Explore ways to express physical intimacy that do not lead to reinfection.	Barrier contraception with latex condoms are effective.

▼

DISCHARGE PLANNING/CONTINUITY OF CARE

- Instruct patient to return for routine screening if high-risk sexual behavior continues.
- Instruct patient to report persistence or recurrence of symptoms.
- Refer for human immunodeficiency virus (HIV) counseling and testing.
- Refer to family planning clinic.

REFERENCES

Graham, J. M. & Blanco, J. D. (1990). Chlamydial infections. *Primary Care, 17*(1), 85–93.

Handsfield, H. H. (1991). Recent developments in STDs: I. Bacterial diseases. *Hospital Practice, 26*(7), 47–56.

Handsfield, H. H. (1991). Recent developments in STDs: II. Viral and other syndromes. *Hospital Practice, 27,* 175–200.

Handsfield, H. H. & Hammerschlag, M. (1992). Chlamydia: A diagnostic challenge. *Patient Care, 26,* 69–84.

Noble, R. C. (1990). Sequelae of sexually transmitted diseases. *Primary Care, 17*(1), 173–181.

▼

Chapter adapted with permission from Gulanick M., et al. (Eds) (1990). *Nursing Care Plans: Nursing Diagnosis and Intervention.* (2nd ed). St. Louis, MO: C.V. Mosby Company.

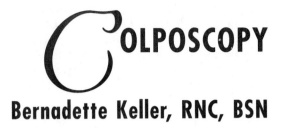

COLPOSCOPY

Bernadette Keller, RNC, BSN

Colposcopy is a procedure in which the visible part of the cervix is observed under lighted, low-power magnification. Areas for biopsy are isolated after evaluating visualized changes in the vulva, vagina, and cervix, especially in women with abnormal Pap smears and following radiation therapy.

INDICATION

- Abnormal Pap smear

▼

NURSING DIAGNOSIS: KNOWLEDGE DEFICIT REGARDING INDICATIONS FOR PROCEDURES

Related To
- New experience/procedure
- Lack of information resources

Defining Characteristics
Multiple questions or lack of questions
Overly anxious
Inability to discuss procedure
Apparent confusion
Expressed need for more information

Patient Outcome
The patient will express understanding of condition requiring a colposcopy and steps involved in the procedure.

Nursing Interventions	Rationales
Assess knowledge regarding colposcopy procedure.	
Explain information obtained from colposcopy: 1. visualization of lesion 2. extent of lesion 3. biopsy for histological examination	

Instruct patient regarding specific procedures:
 	
1. usually performed in physician's office
2. douching prohibited for 24 hours prior to procedure
 	
3. only light meal 2–3 hours prior to procedure
4. analgesics, if necessary, 30–60 minutes prior to procedure to reduce discomfort
5. patient usually placed in lithotomy position
6. some discomfort possible during procedure:
  • perineal pressure from speculum placed in the vagina
  • pulling sensation and brief sharp pinching from the cervix as biopsy is being taken (tissue sampling lasts only 1–2 minutes)
7. patient discharged home after a brief observation period
	Information about the unknown procedure provides a sense of adequacy in confronting fear.
	
	Douching may wash away vaginal secretions, and it may distort findings.
	This diminishes risk of nausea and vomiting.

▼

NURSING DIAGNOSIS: PAIN

Related To uncomfortable procedure

Defining Characteristics
Verbalized pain
Facial expressions of discomfort

Guarding behavior
Crying/moaning

Patient Outcomes

Patient will experience reduced discomfort, as evidenced by
• relaxed facial and body expressions
• statements of comfort

Nursing Interventions	Rationales
Determine factors contributing to patient's discomfort and attempt to eliminate or reduce them.	
1. Have patient void prior to procedure.	This serves to minimize discomfort from bladder distention.
2. Assist patient into lithotomy positioning; ensure legs and head are supported.	Proper positioning reduces muscle tension.
3. Make certain patient has private, secure surroundings and is properly draped to provide privacy and permit minimal exposure.	
4. Encourage use of relaxation methods and diversional techniques to help patient not to concentrate on pain. • Teach slow-rhythmic deep chest breathing. • Teach use of guided imagery, use of focal points. • Engage patient in conversation.	Patient will experience brief episode of pain as tissue sample is taken and may feel several minutes of cramping afterward. Distraction may reduce perception of discomfort.
5. Instruct patient to take analgesics as prescribed if there is any cramping or tenderness subsequent to the examination.	

▼

NURSING DIAGNOSIS: HIGH RISK FOR FLUID VOLUME DEFICIT

Risk Factors
Excessive or prolonged vaginal bleeding

Patient Outcomes
The patient will verbalize knowledge of signs of excessive bleeding, and when to notify health care provider.

Nursing Interventions	Rationales
Note any abnormalities in bleeding during or immediately following the procedure.	Early assessment will guide treatment. An applicator or sponge is applied directly to the biopsy site to tamponade the bleeding that might follow.
Instruct patient to: 1. anticipate vaginal bleeding/spotting, which should diminish over 1–2 days. 2. avoid lifting heavy objects for 1–2 days. 3. report an increase over and above the vaginal bleeding described here.	Knowledge facilitates compliance.

▼

NURSING DIAGNOSIS: HIGH RISK FOR INFECTION

Risk Factors
Surgical alteration of an intact system

Patient Outcomes
The patient will verbalize recognition of early signs and symptoms, and when to notify health care provider.

Nursing Interventions	Rationales
Instruct patient to avoid intercourse or inserting anything in the vagina for 7–14 days following procedure.	It is important to avoid introducing pathogens during healing of the cervix.
Encourage and instruct patient on taking prophylactic antibiotics if prescribed.	
Instruct patient to: 1. check for persistent elevated temperature, which may indicate presence of infection. 2. report presence of malodorous vaginal discharge, and/or yellow-green discharge, which may indicate infection at the biopsy site. 3. report onset, location, duration, intensity of abdominal pain, which may be indicative of pelvic infection. 4. report all signs and symptoms of infection.	Infection is a rare complication of this procedure, but it has been reported.

▼

DISCHARGE PLANNING/CONTINUITY OF CARE

- Secure an appointment for patient to return to office to discuss results of colposcopy.

REFERENCES

Barsevick, A. M. & Johnson, J. E. (1990). Preference for information and involvement, information seeking and emotional responses of women undergoing colposcopy. *Research in Nursing and Health, 13*(1), 1–7.

Barsevick, A. M. & Lauver, D. (1990). Women's informational needs about colposcopy. *Image: Journal of Nursing Scholarship, 22*(1), 23–26.

Deitch, K. V. & Smith, J. E. (1990). Symptoms of chronic vaginal infection and microscopic condyloma in women. *Journal of Obstetrical, Gynecologic, & Neonatal Nursing, 19*(2), 133–138.

Marteau, T. M., Walker, P., Giles J., & Smail, M. (1990). Anxieties in women undergoing colposcopy. *British Journal of Obstetrics & Gynaecology, 99*(9), 859–861.

Nugent, L. & Tamlyn-Leaman, K. (1992). The colposcopy experience: What do women know? *Journal of Advanced Nursing, 17*(4), 514–520.

▼

CONDYLOMA ACUMINATA (GENITAL WARTS)

Mary McGoldrick–Charleza, RN, MPH

Condyloma acuminata (genital warts) is the most common sexually transmitted disease. It is estimated that as many as 20% of women have been exposed to condyloma acuminata. Once infected, there may be an incubation period of 1 to 6 months before warts develop. Lesions are contagious even before they are evident. There are incidences of infection that remain subclinical, exhibiting no symptoms. Options for treatment include keratolytic agents, cryotherapy, laser therapy, and interferon therapy. Condyloma acuminata disease can be resistant to treatment or can recur.

ETIOLOGY

Human papillomavirus (HPV)

CLINICAL MANIFESTATIONS

- Cauliflowerlike lesions: (warts)
  - usually soft, pink-gray
  - alone or in multiple groupings
- Lesions occur on:
  - external genitalia
  - vagina
  - cervix
  - rectum
- Pain
- Itching
- Discharge
- Odor

DIAGNOSTIC FINDINGS

- Pap smear showing HPV virus identified by cytology testing
- Biopsy showing HPV
- DNA testing identifies presence and type of virus

▼

NURSING DIAGNOSIS: IMPAIRED SKIN INTEGRITY

Related To
- Contact with HPV virus
- Condyloma lesions

Defining Characteristics

Single or multiple raised lesions: located on the perineum, around the rectum, in the vagina or on the cervix. See also clinical manifestations

Patient Outcome

Patient will verbalize the rationale for the treatment process and her role in it.

Nursing Interventions	Rationales
Assess patient's perception of lesions: 1. discomfort 2. odor 3. discharge	Genital warts are usually painless.
Visually inspect lesions.	Lesions may be isolated warts or coalesce to form a large mass.
Assist with diagnostic procedures as needed: 1. Pap smear 2. biopsy 3. colposcopy	Many sexually transmitted diseases (STDs) have similar lesions. Diagnosis is confirmed by these procedures.
Explain the rationale for selected treatment, common side effects, need for follow-up as indicated.	It is difficult to treat HPV. Several approaches may be indicated, often necessitating frequent treatment/follow-up visits.

Nursing Interventions

Assist with treatments as needed.
1. keratolytic agents:
   - *podophyllin:* Apply to lesions and allow to dry. Instruct patient to wash off 4 to 6 hours after application. May require weekly application. Instruct patient to watch for systemic hypersensitive reaction to this agent: nausea, diarrhea, malaise, coma.
   - trichloroacetic acid: Causes tissue to slough over a few days. Application may be repeated in a few weeks.
   - *5–fluorouracil:* Not FDA-approved. Apply to lesion(s) according to prescribed schedule. Instruct patient to wash off as instructed (in tub or sitz bath). May cause pain and erythema at site. Instruct patient not to have intercourse for 24 hours after use of cream. Requires colposcopy 6 to 8 weeks after therapy is finished.
2. cryotherapy with liquid nitrogen: may require several (3 to 6) treatments
3. electrocautery
4. surgical removal or laser surgery (usually done in hospital)
5. immunotherapies (e.g., Interferon):
   - administered intramuscularly or subcutaneously
   - three times per week for approximately 6 weeks
   - most common side effect: fever with the first dose
   - occasionally headache or fatigue
   - may be used in conjunction with other therapies

Rationales

Knowing what to expect during and after treatments can decrease anxiety and increase sense of control and ability to monitor for adverse reactions.

Nursing Interventions	Rationales
Instruct patient that several treatment options require more than one session.	STDs are very difficult to treat.
Instruct patient regarding the following self-care measures:	
1. use of condoms	The condom is the only contraceptive device that offers prophylaxis to STDs.
2. treatment of partner(s) to prevent reinfection	
3. obtaining treatment when lesions recur	
4. avoidance of multiple sex partners	This is associated with increased risk for both STDs and cervical cancer.
5. perineal hygiene after intercourse.	Postcoital voiding, cleansing, and douching may be beneficial.
6. relationship between human papillomavirus and cervical cancer • need for Pap smear or colposcopic screening every 6 to 12 months	There is a strong association between specific types of warts (Types 16, 18, and 31) and cervical cancer. It is possible for malignant changes to occur as early as 12 to 24 months after infection.

▼

NURSING DIAGNOSIS: INEFFECTIVE INDIVIDUAL COPING

Related To diagnosis of a lifelong viral condition that is sexually transmitted, often recurrent, and possibly resistant to treatments.

Defining Characteristics
Depression
Anger, resistance, frustration
Missed follow-up appointments
Inappropriate affect
Non-compliance with treatment

Patient Outcomes
The patient will
• describe her feelings and what lifestyle adjustments she is making.

- be "proactive" in initiating follow-up care as needed with recurrences, pregnancy, etc.

Nursing Interventions	Rationales
Assess level of frustration, anger, or presence of paralyzing concern.	Dealing with STDs that are difficult to treat can make the patient feel angry and powerless.
Assess readiness to accept diagnosis.	Denial may result in inadequate treatment and reinfection.
Assess factors that may interfere with adjustment.	Inadequate support systems, low self-esteem, immaturity, and grieving over changed health status are examples of factors that can impede coping.
Assess coping mechanisms for dealing with a lifelong, possibly recurrent infection with no absolute cure presently available.	
Assess perception of significant other's response/support.	
Assess self-care practices in use (condoms, Pap smears, and follow-through with treatment). Reaffirm their use.	Reinforcing areas in which patient can take control may help decrease frustration and helplessness.
Provide information regarding: 1. cause/transmission of infection 2. signs/symptoms of infection 3. possible sites of infection	
Encourage expression of concerns, questions, frustrations.	

▼

NURSING DIAGNOSIS: HIGH RISK FOR INJURY TO FETUS

Risk Factors
Increase or recurrence of condyloma often noted during pregnancy.

Patient Outcome
Patient will verbalize appropriate self-care measures to reduce risk of fetal injury during pregnancy.

Nursing Interventions	Rationales
Assess for presence/change in lesions at regular intervals throughout pregnancy.	Genital warts spread more rapidly during pregnancy.
Provide information regarding changes in pregnancy and possible effects on fetus/baby: 1. The lesions may recur during pregnancy. 2. The lesions may require different treatments if prior therapy (podophyllin or 5–fluorouracil) is contraindicated in pregnancy. 3. Large vascular condyloma may create a barrier to vaginal delivery or cause excessive bleeding. 4. Some mother-to-infant transmission of human papillomavirus has been noted.	Electrocautery, laser therapy, cryosurgery, or trichloroacetic acid are used during pregnancy instead to decrease risk of teratogenesis. Mother needs to be advised of possibility of cesarean section.

▼

DISCHARGE PLANNING/CONTINUITY OF CARE

- Make sure the woman has a follow-up appointment and phone numbers to contact her health care provider for questions and concerns.
- Refer to STD clinics.
- Refer to support group.
- Provide written material/pamphlets to patient and partner.

REFERENCES

American College of Obstetricians and Gynecologists. (1990). *Precis IV: An Update in Obstetrics & Gynecology*. Washington, DC: ACOG.

Handsfield, H. H. (1992). Recent developments in STDs: II. Viral and other syndromes. *Hospital Practice*, 27(1), 175–182, 187, 191–192.

Kelley, K. F., Galbraith, M. A., & Vermund, S. H. (1992). Genital human papillomavirus infections in women. *Journal of Obstetrical, Gynecologic, & Neonatal Nursing*, 21(6), 503–515.

Tinkle, M. J. (1990). Genital human papillomavirus infection. A growing health risk. *Journal of Obstetrical, Gynecologic, & Neonatal Nursing*, 19(6), 501–507.

Toole, K. A. & Vigilante, P. (1990). Cervical dysplasia and condyloma as risks for carcinoma. *American Journal of Maternal-Child Nursing*, 15(3), 170–175.

▼

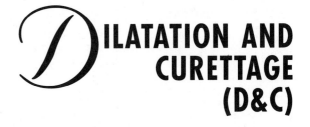

DILATATION AND CURETTAGE (D&C)

Mary McGoldrick-Charleza, RN, MPH

Dilatation and curettage (D&C) is a surgical procedure, often performed on an outpatient basis, that involves dilation of the cervical os and curettage (or scraping) of the uterine lining.

INDICATIONS

It can be performed for diagnostic or therapeutic reasons.

Diagnostic D&C:
- To rule out endometrial cancer
- To secure a biopsy
- To treat menstrual irregularities
- To investigate congenital malformations

Therapeutic D&C:
- To remove retained products of conception
- To terminate a pregnancy
- To aid the diagnosis of endometrial cancer, dysmenorrhea, or menstrual derangements.

▼

NURSING DIAGNOSIS: HIGH RISK FOR INFECTION

Risk Factors
- Intrauterine procedure
- An open cervical os

Patient Outcomes
Patient will
- describe signs of infection and report them if manifested.
- reduce risk of infection by following instructions for hygiene and absence of sexual activity.

Nursing Interventions	Rationales
Assess vital signs, including temperature.	
Assess color, odor, and amount of vaginal drainage.	
Assess for severe uterine tenderness.	Uterine infections can be seeded as instruments are passed from the nonsterile vagina into the normally sterile uterine environment.
Instruct patient in proper perineal care (wiping from front to back) after voidings/elimination.	
Instruct patient to avoid tampons, douching, and intercourse until healed.	These activities may increase the risk of infection while the cervical os may still be open.

▼

NURSING DIAGNOSIS: PAIN

Related To uterine cramping before or after procedure

Defining Characteristics
Verbal expression of abdominal pain or discomfort
Restlessness
Facial expression/body language suggesting presence of pain

Patient Outcome
Patient will verbalize minimal or no pain/discomfort.

Nursing Interventions	Rationales
Assess patient's perception of discomfort, ability to cope with discomfort, and need for relief.	Each individual perceives pain differently.
Evaluate for anxiety or responses to the procedure that may affect coping with pain/discomfort.	
Provide comfort with bed rest, change of position, or relaxation techniques while awaiting effects of analgesia.	Muscle tension and activity may precipitate/enhance pain.

Nursing Interventions	Rationales
Medicate with analgesics as ordered.	The need for pain medication is usually fairly short term. Once cramping ceases (usually does not exceed 24 hours), medications will not be required.

▼

NURSING DIAGNOSIS: KNOWLEDGE DEFICIT

Related To
Unfamiliar procedure
Need for follow-up with self-care and assessment at home

Defining Characteristics
Questions/lack of questions regarding:
- procedure
- care
- what to expect after leaving health care site

Patient Outcomes
Patient will verbalize
- purpose of procedure
- self-care needs
- when to notify physician
- what follow-up is indicated

Nursing Interventions	Rationales
Assess patient's understanding of procedure and its purpose.	Determination of baseline knowledge guides development of teaching plan.
Assess patient's knowledge of her home care needs.	

Nursing Interventions	Rationales
Provide information as needed regarding self-care topics:	
1. Cramping sometimes occurs and may last 2–3 days after the procedure. It may be relieved with analgesics such as acetaminophen or ibuprofen. Severe pain should be reported to the physician immediately.	
2. Spotting or a small amount of vaginal bleeding may occur after a D&C. It may last 3–4 weeks or subside earlier. Peripads or pantyliners may be worn during this time.	Bleeding heavier than one's period is not usual and should be reported.
3. Activities may be resumed when the patient feels up to it (possibly 2–3 days).	
4. Intercourse, douching, and the use of tampons must be avoided until after the follow-up examination (usually 2 weeks).	Avoidance allows for healing and decreases the risk of infection.
5. A shower should be used for personal hygiene instead of a tub bath during the first few days.	
6. If ordered, medications should be taken as prescribed.	
7. A follow-up appointment must be made and kept to assess healing.	
8. The physician should be notified of: • moderate to large bleeding and/or clots • moderate to severe pain • oral temperature > 100.4° F • foul-smelling drainage	The patient must understand that she must not wait for her appointment if these symptoms occur, but should notify her physician immediately.

▼

DISCHARGE PLANNING/CONTINUITY OF CARE

- Refer to gynecologist, primary health care provider, in 2 weeks.
- Provide written information to read at home. Include medication instructions and follow-up appointment information.

REFERENCES

Pritchard, J. A. & MacDonald, P. C. (1989). *Williams Obstetrics*. E. Norwalk, CT: Appleton & Lange.

Stewart, F. H., Stewart, G. H., Guest, F., & Hatcher, R. (1987). *Understanding Your Body: Every Woman's Guide to a Lifetime of Health*. New York: Bantam Books.

▼

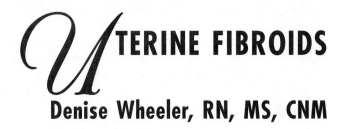

UTERINE FIBROIDS

Denise Wheeler, RN, MS, CNM

Myomas (fibroids, leiomyomas) are common tumors arising from smooth muscle and connective tissue of the uterus. The majority are benign, slow growing, and asymptomatic. Myomas are classified according to location:
1. Interstitial: within uterine wall
2. Submucosal: extends into uterine cavity
3. Subserosal: extends through uterine wall
4. Intraligamentous: within a ligament
5. Pedunculated: attached with a pedicule
6. Parasitic: extrudes from the uterus and develops own blood supply

ETIOLOGIES

Origins of fibroids are not well understood. They may develop from embryonic cell rests or in response to estrogen.

CLINICAL MANIFESTATIONS

- Pain
- Dyspareunia
- Menorrhagia
- Heavy menstrual bleeding
- Urinary incontinence
- Urinary frequency
- Back pain
- Infertility
- Recurrent pregnancy loss

DIAGNOSTIC FINDINGS

Abdominal sonogram reveals fibroids

▼

NURSING DIAGNOSIS: PAIN

Related To
- Manifestations of uterine fibroids
- May result from degeneration of a pedunculated fibroid, large tumors causing a sensation of heaviness or pressure, pressure of tumors on nerves, torsion of a pedunculated fibroid

Defining Characteristics
Cramplike pain occurring during menses (dysmenorrhea)
Pelvic pressure and discomfort
Dyspareunia
Sudden, severe pelvic pain

Patient Outcomes
Patient will
- verbalize the cause of pain and self-help measures available.
- verbalize relief or reduction of discomfort.

Nursing Interventions	Rationales
Assess level of patient's pain. Determine extent to which pain from fibroids affects patient's activities and lifestyle.	
Determine what self-help methods and/or medications the patient has previously used to cope with pain.	
Reassure patient that most fibroids are benign.	Women are frightened that fibroid tumors are dangerous or precancerous growths, and the pain accompanying menses appears to validate their fears.
Teach patient self-help comfort measures: 1. positioning 2. exercise 3. ice or heat packs 4. breathing and relaxation techniques 5. regular bowel function 6. frequent urination	These interventions may vary, depending on the number, size, and location of fibroids. Providing women with nonmedical comfort measures increases their sense of control over their pain. Relaxation and breathing techniques have been used successfully in many pain management programs.

Nursing Interventions	Rationales
Teach patients appropriate use of pain medications as ordered. Review any other medications being taken, allergies, potential drug interactions.	
Encourage the patient to discuss the effects that pelvic pain may have on her self-image and/or sexual functioning.	Disorders or perceived disorders of female reproductive organs frequently challenge a woman's concept of her femininity. In some cultures, and for some women, the ability to reproduce, therefore, healthy reproductive organs, is central to a woman's value.
Reassure patient that concerns about self-image and sexual function are common feelings that may be resolved with effective treatment of fibroids.	

▼

NURSING DIAGNOSIS: KNOWLEDGE DEFICIT

Related To unfamiliarity with diagnosis

Defining Characteristics
Expressed need for more information
Confusion, fear or anger
Repeated requests for reassurance regarding benign nature of the condition

Patient Outcomes
The patient and her partner will verbalize an understanding of the location, possible causes, treatment options (if indicated), and prognosis when diagnosed with uterine fibroids.

Nursing Interventions	Rationales
Determine what the patient already understands about myomas, and her expectations of treatment.	Gathering information assists in determining realistic approaches to current problem.
Teach patient about anatomy and physiology of the reproductive organs, using pictures and diagrams when possible.	A variety of teaching materials promotes interest.

Nursing Interventions	**Rationales**
Tell the patient that because estrogen stimulation of the uterus is thought to contribute to the growth of myomas, they do not disappear during the childbearing years but may shrink after menopause. In addition, nonhormonal methods of birth control may be recommended in women of childbearing age.	
Discuss fertility in women of childbearing age. 1. Myomas may be the cause of infertility, multiple miscarriages, preterm labor, and postpartum bleeding; most myomas, however, cause few problems during pregnancy. 2. Generally, pregnancies complicated by myomas only require consideration to the possibility of growth of the fibroid, teaching about preterm birth prevention, and careful postpartum attention.	Providing current accurate information will aid in diffusing unnecessary fears and misconceptions.
Reassure the patient that most fibroids are asymptomatic and require no treatment. They are a common finding in women over age 30. Myomas may be found in approximately 50% of women of color.	
Instruct the patient to contact her physician if her periods become heavy, are accompanied by severe pain or pressure, or if she develops accompanying symptoms (incontinence, back pain, dyspareunia, urinary frequency).	Many women have fibroids throughout their reproductive years which are asymptomatic. Some symptoms require treatment.

Nursing Interventions	**Rationales**
Discuss options for treatment of symptomatic uterine fibroids:	
1. suppression therapy; side effects may include: • hot flushes • headaches • joint pain • insomnia • vaginal dryness • acne • cessation of menses • irregular menses	Medications suppress production of estrogen by the ovaries, causing a temporary menopausal effect. Fibroids may shrink in the absence of estrogen. If surgical intervention is being considered, suppression therapy may first be used to shrink the fibroids, decreasing blood loss at the time of surgery.
2. surgical interventions: • myomectomy: surgical removal of the myoma(s) only. NOTE: This procedure may be done under general anesthesia with a scalpel or using laser surgery. Risks include the usual surgical precautions. A discussion of the long-term effects of uterine surgery should include: possible need for cesarean section delivery if pregnancy occurs, preterm labor, possible recurrence of fibroids.	Indications for surgery include: uterine size greater than 12–14 weeks gestational size (uterus is out of the pelvis); myoma extends into the cervix, broad ligament, or adnexa; pedunculated myomas; excessive pain, pressure, or bleeding.
• hysterectomy: surgical removal of the uterus (see Hysterectomy, p. 162.)	The patient and her partner should be aware of all possible treatment options to make an informed decision.
Prepare patient for diagnostic procedures as appropriate. Explain ultrasonography, and abdominal and vaginal approaches. Instruct patient to fill bladder (4–6 glasses of water one hour before examination).	If the patient has not previously had a pelvic ultrasound, she may be concerned about discomfort with the procedure. Filling the bladder will elevate the uterus and improve the visibility of the uterus.

NURSING DIAGNOSIS: HIGH RISK FOR FLUID VOLUME DEFICIT

Risk Factors

- Hyperplasia of the endometrium around a submucosal fibroid, which results in heavier blood loss
- Enlargement of the uterine cavity, which results in a larger surface area for blood loss
- Altered contractile mechanism caused by the presence of large fibroids
- Increased venous congestion

Patient Outcomes

Patient will describe why abnormal bleeding may occur in the presence of uterine myomas, and when to notify health professional.

Nursing Interventions	Rationales
Assess patient's present understanding of the role of fibroids and altered menstrual patterns.	Altered menstrual function is commonly caused by the presence of symptomatic myomas.
Obtain specimens as ordered to evaluate patient for anemia secondary to excessive menstrual blood loss. Provide iron supplementation as directed/indicated.	Excess blood loss during the menses may result in iron-deficient anemia.
Teach patient about expected blood loss during the menses. Women should be encouraged to contact their provider if blood loss exceeds saturation of two feminine hygiene pads per hour, bleeding lasts longer than 10 days, or bleeding occurs more frequently than every 23 days.	

▼

NURSING DIAGNOSIS: STRESS URINARY INCONTINENCE

Related To presence of uterine myomas and bladder pressure

Defining Characteristics

Involuntary loss of urine when sneezing, laughing, coughing, or other bearing-down activities
Frequency of urge to void

Patient Outcomes

Patient will
- describe why urinary incontinence and frequency may occur with myomas.
- verbalize satisfaction with nonsurgical treatments for stress urinary incontinence.

Nursing Interventions	Rationales
Inquire what affect stress urinary incontinence has had on the patient's lifestyle and what coping methods she has tried.	Gathering information assists in determining realistic approaches to current problem.
Determine patient's willingness to try new management techniques if surgical correction is not desired.	Patient cooperation is required for successful treatment.
Explain anatomy of the pelvis, including relationship of the uterus to the bladder. Use diagrams and pictures when appropriate.	
Teach patient Kegal exercises if she is not already aware of them.	While Kegal exercises do not alleviate the problem of the fibroid causing stress urinary incontinence, the improved vaginal and sphincter tone achieved may afford the patient some degree of control over her incontinence.
Encourage frequent bladder emptying.	Prevents overdistention of bladder.
Instruct to avoid bladder irritants (i.e., caffeine); teach signs and symptoms of urinary tract infection.	Irritants are frequently a cause of additional stress on bladder.

Nursing Interventions	Rationales
Instruct patient of the availability of protection for her clothing to reduce embarrassment.	Such information assists patient to maintain a positive self-image.

▼

DISCHARGE PLANNING/CONTINUITY OF CARE

- Gynecologist: 4–6 months unless symptoms increase
- Women's Support Group
- Incontinence Support Group
- American College of Obstetricians & Gynecologists (ACOG) pamphlets

REFERENCES

Byyny, R. & Speroff, L. (1990). *A Clinical Guide for the Care of Older Women*. Baltimore, MD: Williams & Wilkins.

Davis, J. L., Ray-Mazumber, S., Hobel, C. J., Baley, K., & Sassoon, D. (1990). Uterine leiomyomias in pregnancy: A prospective study. *Obstetrics and Gynecology, 75*(1), 41–44.

Lichtman, R., & Papera, S. (1990). *Gynecology: Well Woman Care*. E. Norwalk, CT: Appleton & Lange.

Podolsky, D. (1990). Saved from the knife. *US News and World Report, 109*(20), 76–77.

▼

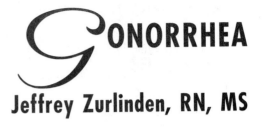

${\mathcal{G}}$ONORRHEA

Jeffrey Zurlinden, RN, MS

Gonorrhea is a sexually transmitted disease. It usually causes a localized infection of the urethra, endocervical canal, rectum, or pharynx. The patient may have one site of infection or many sites. The infection is spread by sexual contact with the infected site. Although symptoms abate without treatment, untreated gonorrhea may lead to septicemia, pelvic inflammatory disease, arthritis-dermatitis syndrome, and reproductive difficulties due to scarring.

ETIOLOGY

Infection with *Neisseria gonorrhoeae* bacteria

CLINICAL MANIFESTATIONS

- May be asymptomatic
- Thick white-yellow discharge 2 to 10 days after inoculation at site of infection
- Urinary frequency
- Pain or burning when urinating
- Sore throat
- Mucus or blood in stools
- Change in bowel movements

DIAGNOSTIC FINDINGS

- Smears from infected sites show gram-negative intracellular diplococci
- Cultures from infected sites grow *Neisseria gonorrhoeae.*

  NOTE: asymptomatic sexual partners of infected patients usually receive treatment regardless of culture results.

▼

NURSING DIAGNOSIS: INFECTION

Related To presence of infectious organisms

Defining Characteristics
Positive culture from urethra, cervix, throat, or rectum
Gram-negative intracellular diplococci on smear
History of sexual contact with an infected person

Patient Outcome
Patient will exhibit no signs of infection, as evidenced by resolution of discharge or negative test-of-cure culture.

Nursing Interventions	Rationales
Determine date of last sexual contact, number of sexual partners, and description of recent sexual activities.	This provides information regarding behaviors that increase risk of sexually transmitted disease.
Obtain cultures from all sites of possible infection.	Women frequently self-inoculate rectums with gonococci from urethral or endocervical discharges. Because cold culture medium is bactericidal, warm Thayer Martin culture plates to room temperature before inoculation. Store inoculated plates in CO_2-enriched environment to prevent death of *Neisseria gonorrhoeae* from room air O_2 concentrations.
Obtain smears from discharges.	
Obtain history of previous sexually transmitted diseases (STDs).	Though gonorrhea can be effectively treated with antibiotics, the cure will not prevent future recurrences of the disease.
Assess:	
1. urethral and/or cervical discharge	This condition is frequently asymptomatic. If symptomatic, thick yellow-white discharge occurs 2–10 days after infection.
2. urinary frequency	

Nursing Interventions	Rationales
3. pain or burning when urinating	
4. rectal discharge	
5. mucus or blood in stools 6. change in bowel movements	
7. sore throat	Pharyngeal gonorrhea is usually asymptomatic.
Screen for other STDs, including hepatitis B, and human immunodeficiency virus (HIV).	Patients with one STD are at higher risk for a concomitant STD; 30–40% of women with gonorrhea are also infected with chlamydia and may require treatment with additional antibiotics.
Obtain menstrual history, including date of last period.	It can be difficult to get cultures during menstruation; results are less accurate, especially with tampon use. There is an increase in false negatives.
Determine method and compliance with birth control.	The contraction of STDs suggests no use/improper use of condoms. Women may be at high risk for pregnancy. Nurse should use this opportunity for health screening/education.
Perform pregnancy test.	Necessary for early detection of pregnancy. Some drugs have teratogenic effect.
Administer antibiotics as ordered.	Treatment for gonorrhea frequently changes in response to new antibiotics and new resistant strains. Follow the current guidelines from the Centers for Disease Control (CDC) or your local Health Department.
Observe for possible anaphylactic reaction to antibiotics administered intramuscularly during clinic visit.	
Dispense condoms.	Latex condoms are the most effective means of preventing spread of disease during sexual contact.

Nursing Interventions	Rationales
Untreated asymptomatic sexual partners are a common source of reinfection.	Instruct patient to inform all recent sexual partners of possible exposure to gonorrhea and need for treatment.

NURSING DIAGNOSIS: KNOWLEDGE DEFICIT

Related To new diagnosis

Defining Characteristics
Many questions
Few questions
History of repeated infections
Unable to state the causes, treatment, and prevention of gonorrhea

Patient Outcomes
Patient will state
- medication schedule
- medication side effects
- date of return visit for test of cure
- how to use condoms to prevent future infections

Nursing Interventions	Rationales
Assess patient's present level of understanding.	Misconceptions can increase anxiety/fear and foster spread of sexually transmitted disease.
Instruct patient about medication schedule and side effects of antibiotics used to treat gonorrhea.	Treatment for gonorrhea frequently changes in response to new antibiotics and new resistant strains. Follow the current guidelines from the Centers for Disease Control or your local Health Department.
Instruct patient to refrain from vaginal, rectal, and pharyngeal sexual intercourse until partners are treated and results are reported from test-of-cure.	
Instruct patient on mode of transmission: local inoculation of bacteria from partner's penis to patient's throat, vagina, or rectum.	

Nursing Interventions	Rationales
Instruct patient to use latex condoms or use other nonintercourse sexual methods to prevent future infection.	Latex condoms are an effective barrier against gonorrhea.
Inform patient of the possible consequences of untreated gonorrhea.	Pelvic inflammatory disease (PID), ectopic pregnancy, or difficulty in conceiving due to scarred fallopian tubes are common complications.

▼

NURSING DIAGNOSIS: INEFFECTIVE MANAGEMENT OF THERAPEUTIC REGIMEN

Related To
- Unwillingness to comply with treatment, prevention, or informing sexual partners
- Complexity of treatment regimen

Defining Characteristics
Persistent infection not caused by antibiotic-resistant strains
Missed return visit for test of cure
Incorrect pill count at return visit
Inadequate blood level of antibiotic

Patient Outcomes
Patient will
- complete course of treatment.
- notify sexual partners.
- return for test-of-cure culture.
- use condoms to prevent infection.

Nursing Interventions	Rationales
Compare actual effect and expected therapeutic effect.	
Plot patient's pattern of returning for tests of cure or follow-up visits.	
Determine social support system and presence of significant others.	Interpersonal support and understanding can influence compliance with treatment regimen.

Nursing Interventions	Rationales
Assess patient's and significant other's beliefs about current illness and treatment plan.	How one perceives susceptibility, severity, and threat of disease affects health behavior.
Assess quality of relationship between patient and health care workers and health care facility.	
Role-play to practice informing sexual partners of possible exposure to gonorrhea	Gives patient opportunity to rehearse situation and allows nurse to provide feedback.
Suggest intramuscular medications or short-term therapy, if patient has a history of not taking oral medication.	Intramuscular medication eliminates the patient's need to participate in treatment.
Role-play to practice new behaviors in situations leading to reinfection (such as saying "no" or using condoms).	
Develop a positive relationship with the patient that encourages participation with treatment decisions.	The nurse-patient relationship is based on recognition of patient's right to self-determination and capacity for self-management with focus on decision-making and goal attainment.
Determine with the patient the plan of treatment she is most likely to complete.	Involving the patient in planning the regimen improves compliance.

▼

NURSING DIAGNOSIS: ALTERED SEXUALITY PATTERNS

Related To
- Imposed restrictions
- Fear
- Risk of contagion

Defining Characteristics
Patient or significant other expresses concern about the effects gonorrhea and treatment has on their expressions of physical intimacy.

Patient Outcomes
Patient will state ways of expressing physical intimacy during treatment.

Nursing Interventions	Rationales
Determine patient's or significant other's concerns.	STD diagnosis may provoke feelings of guilt, shame, the need for punishment, or other anxiety-provoking thoughts unique to the patient.
Determine if patient's or significant other's concerns are also related to fears about acquired immunodeficiency syndrome (AIDS).	An STD diagnosis may provoke fear of AIDS that alters sexual behavior.
Assess perception of meaning of gonorrhea infection.	This provides opportunity to correct misconceptions.
Elicit patient's feeling about limits on sexual behavior.	
Interview patient in a quiet, private, distraction-free environment.	Most women are hesitant to discuss personal sexual matters. The proper setting may facilitate discussion.
Explore ways to express physical intimacy during treatment excluding vaginal, rectal, and pharyngeal intercourse.	Restrictions on sexual activity should not deprive the couple of other activities that convey the message that they are loved and desired.
Explore ways to express physical intimacy that do not lead to reinfection.	Barrier contraception with latex condoms are effective.

▼

DISCHARGE PLANNING/CONTINUITY OF CARE

- Schedule patient to return to the clinic to obtain culture to demonstrate test-of-cure. (Antibiotic-resistant strains cause treatment failures that can only be detected by test of cure.)
- Instruct patient to return for routine screening if high-risk sexual behavior continues.
- Instruct patient to report persistence or recurrence of symptoms.
- Refer for HIV counseling and testing.
- Refer to family planning clinic.
- Refer to support group.

REFERENCES

Cates, W. & Tooney, K. E. (1990). Sexually transmitted diseases: Overview of the situation. *Primary Care, 17*(1), 1–27.

Custodio, D. E. & Henschen, R. R. (1991). Sexually transmitted diseases. *Topics in Emergency Medicine, 13*, 66–74.

Handsfield, H. H. (1991). Recent developments in STDs: I. Bacterial diseases. *Hospital Practice, 26*(7), 47–56.

Moy, J. B. & Clasen, M. E. (1990). The patient with gonococcal infection. *Primary Care, 17*(1), 59–83.

Noble, R. C. (1990). Sequelae of sexually transmitted diseases. *Primary Care, 17*(1), 173–182.

▼

Chapter adapted with permission from Gulanick, M., et al. (Eds.) (1990). *Nursing Care Plans: Nursing Diagnosis and Intervention,* (2nd ed). St. Louis, MO: C. V. Mosby Company.

$\mathcal{H}$ERPES

Jeffrey Zurlinden, RN, MS

Herpes is a sexually transmitted disease. It is a chronic viral infection that results in periodic outbreaks of blisters. The blisters shed virus that may cause new infections at the site of contact with traumatized skin or mucous membranes. Because herpes can cause serious, life-threatening infections in newborns, pregnant women require treatment for outbreaks, and may require cesarean birth.

ETIOLOGY

Herpes simplex virus (HSV) types I and II

CLINICAL MANIFESTATIONS

Characteristic lesions:
- clusters of itching, burning, painful vesicles that coalesce then erode

Patient may have prodromal symptoms of
- fatigue
- malaise
- headache
- enlarged or tender lymph nodes

DIAGNOSTIC FINDINGS

- Cultures can confirm diagnosis and differentiate type of herpes.
- Presence of infectious organisms.

▼

NURSING DIAGNOSIS: INFECTION

Related To presence of infectious organisms

Defining Characteristics
Painful vesicles
Culture positive for HSV

Patient Outcomes
- Patient's vesicles will heal.
- No additional sites of infection will develop.

Nursing Interventions	Rationales
Determine date of last sexual contact, number of sexual partners, and description of recent sexual activities.	Provide information regarding behaviors that increase risk of sexually transmitted disease (STD).
Obtain cultures (may be unnecessary).	Once diagnosis of HSV has been made via cultures, it may be unnecessary to culture subsequent outbreaks of vesicles.
Obtain history of previous STDs.	
Inspect the perineum, vagina, rectum, and mouth for vesicles.	

Ask about:
1. constitutional symptoms
  • fatigue
  • headache
  • malaise
  • muscle ache
2. localized symptoms
  • itching
  • burning
  • paresthesia
  • tender or swollen regional lymph nodes
	This will help to detect associated complications that may require treatment/intervention.

Screen for other STDs, hepatitis B, and human immunodeficiency virus (HIV).	Patients with one STD are at higher risk for a concomitant STD.
Obtain menstrual history, including date of last period.	It can be difficult to get cultures during menstruation; results are less accurate, especially with tampon use, and false negative cultures occur more frequently.

Nursing Interventions	Rationales
Determine method of and compliance with birth control.	Getting STDs suggests no use/improper use of condoms. Women may be at higher risk for pregnancy. Nurse should use this opportunity for health screening/education.
Perform pregnancy test.	Necessary for early detection of pregnancy. Some drugs have teratogenic effect. If the virus is active during a pregnancy, the baby can be at risk.
Administer acyclovir (Zovirax) as ordered.	The acyclovir dose is usually 200 mg five times daily for 10 days for initial outbreak. The patient with frequent outbreaks may receive chronic suppressive therapy with 200 mg three times daily.
For subsequent outbreaks, instruct patient to start medication at the time of the first sensation of tingling.	Medication is most effective if started early.
Dispense condoms.	Because virus continues to shed through healed lesions, condoms are necessary even after vesicles heal.
Instruct patient to wash hands upon waking and after using the bathroom.	Frequent handwashing during outbreaks prevents spreading of virus to new sites.
Instruct patient to wash genital lesions with mild soap and dry with a blow dryer.	

▼

NURSING DIAGNOSIS: KNOWLEDGE DEFICIT

Related To new diagnosis

Defining Characteristics
Many questions
Few questions
Unable to state the causes, treatment, and ways to prevent spreading HSV

Patient Outcomes

Patient will state
- medication schedule
- medication side effects
- how to use condoms to prevent new sites of infection
- how virus is transmitted and reactivated
- the effects of stress on outbreaks

Nursing Interventions	Rationales
Assess patient's present level of understanding.	Misconceptions can increase anxiety/fear and foster spread of sexually transmitted disease.
Instruct patient about medication schedule and side effects of acyclovir.	Oral medications may be prescribed for 5 days to 6 months, depending upon whether the infection is initial, recurrent, or chronic.
Instruct patient to refrain from sexual intercourse involving the infected part of the body during outbreaks, starting at the time of the first sensation of tingling.	
Instruct patient on mode of transmission: local inoculation of virus from the vesicles to the partner's traumatized skin or mucous membranes.	During outbreaks, the patient may also inoculate virus to new sites of her body, for example, by scratching vesicles then rubbing her eyes without first washing her hands.
Instruct patient to use latex condoms or use other nonintercourse sexual methods to prevent future infections.	Latex condoms reduce the risk of spreading the virus. Because the virus may be shed for many months through healed skin, condoms are necessary even after the vesicles heal.
Inform patient of the possible consequences of untreated HSV during pregnancy: infection of the newborn as it passes through the birth canal.	HSV may cause serious, life-threatening infections in newborns.
Inform patient that herpes is a chronic infection with periods of exacerbation and remission.	

Nursing Interventions	Rationales
Inform patient that stress may precipitate outbreaks.	Stress may be emotional or physical, such as other infections, menses, or prolonged exposure to the sun or heat.

▼

NURSING DIAGNOSIS: INEFFECTIVE MANAGEMENT OF THERAPEUTIC REGIMEN

Related To unwillingness to comply with, prevention, or informing sexual partners

Defining Characteristics
Frequent outbreaks
Transmission of infection to partners

Patient Outcomes
Patient will
• notify sexual partners.
• use condoms to prevent new sites of infection.

Nursing Interventions	Rationales
Compare actual effect and expected therapeutic effect.	
Determine social support system and presence of significant others.	Interpersonal support and understanding can influence compliance with treatment regimen.
Assess patient's and significant other's beliefs about current illness and treatment plan.	How one perceives susceptibility, severity, and threat of disease affects health behavior.
Assess quality of relationship between patient and health care workers and health care facility.	
Role-play to practice informing sexual partners of HSV infection.	Gives patient an opportunity to rehearse situation and allows nurse to provide feedback.

Nursing Interventions	Rationales
Role-play to practice new behaviors in situations leading to reinfection (such as saying "no" or using condoms).	
Develop a positive relationship with the patient that encourages participation with treatment decisions.	The nurse-patient relationship is based on recognition of patient's right to self-determination and capacity for self-management with focus on decision-making and goal attainment.
Determine with the patient the plan of treatment she is most likely to complete.	Involving the patient in planning the regimen improves compliance.

▼

NURSING DIAGNOSIS: ALTERED SEXUALITY PATTERNS

Related To
- Imposed restrictions
- Fear
- Risk of spread of infection

Defining Characteristics
Patient or significant other expresses concern about the effect of herpes on their expressions of physical intimacy.

Patient Outcome
Patient will state ways of expressing physical intimacy during a herpes outbreak.

Nursing Interventions	Rationales
Determine patient's or significant other's concerns.	STD diagnosis may provoke feelings of guilt, shame, the need for punishment, or other anxiety-provoking thoughts unique to patient.
Determine if concerns are also related to fears about AIDS.	An STD diagnosis may provoke fear of AIDS that alters sexual behavior.
Assess perception of meaning of herpes infection.	This provides an opportunity to correct misconceptions.

Nursing Interventions	Rationales
Explore ways to express physical intimacy during outbreaks, excluding vaginal, rectal, and pharyngeal intercourse.	Restrictions on sexual activity should not deprive the couple of other activities that convey the message that they are loved and desired.
Elicit patient's feeling about limits on sexual behavior.	

▼

DISCHARGE PLANNING/CONTINUITY OF CARE

- Instruct patient to report persistence or recurrence of symptoms.
- Refer for HIV counseling and testing.
- Refer to family planning clinic.
- Refer for stress management.
- Refer to support group.
- Instruct patient, if she becomes pregnant, to notify physician of history of herpes.

REFERENCES

Cates, W. & Toomey, K.E. (1990). Sexually transmitted diseases: Overview of the situation. *Primary Care, 17*(1), 1–27.

Dawkins, B. J. (1990). Genital herpes simplex infections. *Primary Care, 17*(1), 95–113.

Handsfield, H. H. (1991). Recent developments in STDs: II. Viral and other syndromes. *Hospital Practice, 27,* 175–200.

Keller, M. L., Jadack, R. A., & Mims, K. F. (1991). Perceived stressors and coping responses in persons with recurrent genital herpes. *Research in Nursing and Health, 14*(6), 421–430.

Nettina, S. L. & Kaufman, F. H. (1990). Diagnosis and management of sexually transmitted genital lesions. *Nurse Practitioner, 15*(1), 20–39.

▼

Chapter adapted with permission from Gulanick, M., et al. (Eds.) (1990). *Nursing Care Plans: Nursing Diagnosis and Intervention,* (2nd ed). St. Louis, MO: C. V. Mosby Company.

HUMAN IMMUNODEFICIENCY VIRUS DISEASE

Pat Moss, RN, MSN

Since human immunodeficiency virus (HIV) was first described in 1981, it has become one of the fastest growing viruses affecting women in the last several years. As HIV progresses and destroys the immune system, the person becomes at risk for developing an acquired immunodeficiency syndrome (AIDS). AIDS has become one of the ten leading causes of death for women of reproductive age in the United States as of 1987. Women represent 11% of all reported adult AIDS cases. However, one-third of all infected women have acquired HIV by heterosexual transmission. It disproportionately affects blacks and Hispanics; black and Hispanic women make up only 17% of all U.S. women, yet represent 73% of all reported AIDS cases among women. It is sometimes difficult to determine when a person is diagnosed with AIDS, but it is many times more difficult to diagnose HIV disease unless a person tests positive for the virus.

ETIOLOGY

Viral transmission

CLINICAL MANIFESTATIONS

These may differ depending on the stage of the disease or the presenting opportunistic infections indicating a diagnosis of AIDS. Common manifestations are:
- Fever
- Weight loss (>10% of body weight)
- Candidiasis, oral or vaginal
- Pelvic inflammatory disease
- Human papillomavirus (HPV)
- Genital ulcers

143

- Cervical dysplasia
- Genital warts
- Cough
- Pneumonias
- Herpes simplex virus
- Mental status changes

Some common opportunistic infections that indicate a diagnosis of AIDS are:

- Candidiasis (esophagus, trachea, bronchi, or lungs)
- Cryptosporidiosis, with diarrhea persisting >1 month
- Herpes simplex virus infection, causing a mucocutaneous ulcer in the vaginal or perineal area that persists >1 month
- Lymphoma of the brain, affecting women < 60 years of age
- *Mycobacterium aviumintracellulare* complex, disseminated
- *Pneumocystis carinii* pneumonia

CLINICAL/DIAGNOSTIC FINDINGS

- CD4 counts below 500 mm^3 (normal: 600–1400 mm^3)
- Decreased CD4/CD8 ratio
- Elevated erythrocyte sedimentation rate
- Elevated serum globulin (hypergammaglobulinemia)
- Elevated serum lactate dehydrogenase
- Low serum cholesterol
- Neutropenia
- Thrombocytopenia
- Anemia
- Positive serology for syphilis
- Anergy to antigens

An individual can test positive for HIV and still have a normal CD4 count. It has not been determined at which stage of the disease the CD4 count begins to drop. It is very difficult to determine when the individual became infected with HIV, because persons will be symptom-free and therefore never think of being tested for HIV.

▼

NURSING DIAGNOSIS: KNOWLEDGE DEFICIT

Related To unfamiliarity with disease, treatment, and complications

Defining Characteristics

Verbalizes many questions
Lack of questions
Verbalizes misinformation
Failure to comply with treatment

Patient Outcomes

Patient will

- verbalize accurate information about HIV and disease progression.
- describe ways to prevent the spread of HIV to others.
- be an active participant in the treatment regimen.

Nursing Interventions	Rationales
Assess for knowledge of HIV infection, disease process, and progression. Provide necessary explanation: 1. HIV invades the immune system and slowly destroys it. 2. As HIV destroys the immune system, the individual infected becomes at risk for many different opportunistic infections. 3. Presence of opportunistic infections leads to a diagnosis of AIDS.	The diagnosis of AIDS is made only when the individual presents with any of the AIDS-defining opportunistic infections such as pneumocystis pneumonia (PCP), *Mycobacterium avium intracellulare*, esophageal candidiasis, toxoplasmosis, or cytomegalovirus.
Provide information on infection control, safe sex techniques, risk of exposure to others and transmissibility: 1. HIV is transmitted sexually by the woman who is infected when she has unprotected (without a condom) vaginal or anal intercourse. 2. HIV is transmitted by sharing needles with someone who is HIV infected. 3. HIV cannot be transmitted by any casual contact like shaking hands, hugging, kissing on the lips, or living in the same house with an infected person. There has to be an exchange of body fluids (vaginal secretions, semen, blood, or breast milk) for the virus to be transmitted.	
Determine where patient obtained her information and whether it is accurate.	

Nursing Interventions	Rationales
Assess for any cultural beliefs or emotional fears that may hinder compliance with therapy.	There has been some negative information about azidothymidine (AZT) and its lack of effectiveness in African American persons. This has not been proven to have any validity. Some persons may feel that certain herbs can cure HIV/AIDS. It is not harmful for the patient to use herbal therapies; however, they should never be used in place of the recommended proven medical therapies.
Assess understanding about medication administration. Determine whether patient/family can participate in medication administration or in research drug protocols. Determine the family's previous experience with hospitals and health care professionals.	If the experience was positive, they are more likely to be supportive of the medical treatment. Research protocols usually require frequent visits and additional medications. The dosing schedules differ with each medication. Often patients do not want to participate in protocols for fear that more people will find out about their disease.
Instruct on need for Pap smears every 4–6 months to rule out cervical cancer.	It has been found that cervical cancer progresses more rapidly in HIV-positive women when compared to those who are not HIV infected.

▼

NURSING DIAGNOSIS: HIGH RISK FOR INFECTION

Risk Factors
Compromised immune system

Patient Outcomes
Patient will
- take all prescribed medications.
- return for all follow-up appointments.
- verbalize and practice safe sex with all sexual partners to avoid all types of infections.
- be aware of any changes in her body that could indicate a new occurrence of an infection and will immediately report for clinical follow-up.

Nursing Interventions	Rationales
Draw blood for rapid plasma reagin test (RPR).	
Do pelvic examination and send cultures for gonorrhea, chlamydia, herpes, or candidiasis. Send cervical smear for Pap test.	The presence of these infections indicates person has been sexually active without the use of a condom. Women will have symptoms with herpes and candidiasis, but may be asymptomatic with gonorrhea and chlamydia. The continual recurrence of sexually transmitted diseases (STDs) puts a woman more at risk for HIV mainly because the vaginal tissue and labia are infected and open to invasion of the virus.
Assess vagina and labia for any signs of genital ulcers, chancroids, vaginal pruritus, or discharge (clear or thick and white).	While yeast infections are common in women who are diabetic, pregnant, or using birth control pills, HIV should be ruled out in any woman with a consistent history of vaginal yeast infections.
If cultures are positive:	
1. Instruct patient on self-administration of acyclovir.	This is a common treatment for herpes simplex virus. This drug can be taken as an oral tablet or as a topical ointment.
2. Instruct patient on the importance of antibiotic therapies for treatment of syphilis, gonorrhea, and chlamydia.	The woman needs to take the full course of antibiotic treatment for complete resolution of the infection. It is also important that all sexual partners be treated concurrently for the STDs.
3. Instruct patient on use of anti-fungal medications to treat candidiasis: • miconanzole • nystatin • clotrimazole • ketoconazole • fluconazole	
4. Instruct patient in how to insert vaginal suppositories or creams.	

Nursing Interventions	Rationales
Obtain thorough history of patient's sexual behavior pattern and partner history.	If patient has been sexually active, all partners need to be tested and treated concurrently for STDs.
Instruct on use of condoms during sexual intercourse (vaginal, anal, or oral sex).	Whether the partner is HIV-positive or -negative the woman needs to protect herself from exposure to all types of bacteria.
Discourage use of intrauterine devices (IUDs) as a contraceptive device.	String from IUD serves as a wick for ascending infection.
Instruct women to 1. avoid tight-fitting pants. 2. wear cotton underpants. 3. wash hands after contact with genital ulcers to avoid infecting other areas of body (mouth, eyes, face).	Herpes virus is very contagious and can be easily spread to any part of the body.
Teach patient to assess for any signs of pelvic inflammatory disease (i.e., lower abdominal and/or pelvic pain).	Pelvic inflammatory disease has been indicative of HIV disease progression.

▼

NURSING DIAGNOSIS: HIGH RISK FOR ACQUIRING AN OPPORTUNISTIC INFECTION

Risk Factors
- Immunodeficiency
- Poor nutritional status

Patient Outcomes
Patient will
- participate in screening for opportunistic infections at scheduled times.
- take prophylactic/treatment medications as prescribed.

Nursing Interventions	Rationales
Assess for presence of immune response to antigens on patient's first outpatient visit.	

Nursing Interventions	Rationales
Do baseline laboratory screening for any evidence of cytomegalovirus, toxoplasmosis, hepatitis B, cryptococcus, *Mycobacterium aviumintracellulare* complex.	If patient is negative for hepatitis B antibodies, she should receive the hepatitis B vaccine series. Cytomegalovirus, toxoplasmosis, cryptococcus and *Mycobacterium aviumintracellulare* complex are opportunistic infections associated with AIDS. There is no vaccine for these infections; however, treatment is available.
Assess for any signs of respiratory compromise that would indicate *Pneumocystis carinii* pneumonia or tuberculosis: 1. cough 2. fever 3. night sweats 4. pulmonary infiltrates assessed by auscultation or chest x-ray	
Instruct patient on prophylactic therapies to prevent *Pneumocystis carinii* pneumonia (e.g., Bactrim and inhaled pentamidine).	Therapy is usually begun when CD4 count drops below 200 mm³.
Instruct patient on self-administration of antibiotics, antivirals, and immune modulators; side effects of drugs; and drug interactions.	Antivirals (zidovudine [AZT], ddI, or ddC), are begun when CD4 counts drop below 500 mm³.
Instruct on adherence to a nutritionally balanced diet and avoidance of raw foods (e.g., eggs, meat).	Raw foods could cause salmonella or other intestinal bacterial organisms.

▼

NURSING DIAGNOSIS: HIGH RISK FOR FLUID VOLUME DEFICIT

Risk Factors
- Human immunodeficiency virus
- A gastrointestinal infection, which can be caused by
  - *Giardia lamblia*
  - *Entamoeba histolytica*
  - *Salmonella*

- *Shigella*
- *Campylobacter*
- *Isospora belli*
- *Cryptosporidium*
- *Mycobacterium aviumintracellulare* complex
- Cytomegalovirus
- Herpes simplex
- Decreased fluid and nutritional intake
- Fluctuating body temperature
- Candidiasis of the throat or esophagus

Patient Outcomes
- Patient will maintain an adequate fluid intake.
- Electrolytes will be within normal range.
- Diarrhea will be decreased or controlled with medication.

Nursing Interventions	Rationales
Observe for changes in body weight. Monitor patient's weight daily.	Patients can keep their own record of daily weights and report any changes.
Monitor electrolytes, urine osmolarity.	
Monitor changes in vital signs.	
Observe for signs of dehydration: 1. output exceeds intake 2. increased weight loss (more than 10% of baseline body weight) 3. poor skin turgor 4. increase in serum sodium and urine specific gravity 5. dry mucous membranes	
Assess history of diarrhea.	
Assess for current drug therapy.	Some drugs, such as AZT, Bactrim, or pentamidine by intravenous injection, can cause nausea or loss of appetite.
Assess for food or fluid intolerance.	Difficulty swallowing food or fluids could be an indication of candidiasis of the throat or esophagus.
Encourage patient to increase oral fluid intake.	

Nursing Interventions	Rationales
If patients are dehydrated, administer intravenous fluids to compensate for fluid loss from diarrhea and decreased fluid intake.	
If diarrhea is the cause, administer medications and/or oral fluids.	

▼

NURSING DIAGNOSIS: HIGH RISK FOR MENTAL AND NEUROLOGICAL STATUS CHANGES

Risk Factors
- HIV infections
- Central nervous system infection
- Cerebral lesions

Patient Outcomes
Family/significant other will
- report changes in mental status.
- verbalize understanding of resources available to assist patient.

Nursing Interventions	Rationales
Assess for any mental status changes such as: 1. loss of short-term memory 2. changes in behavior pattern (depressed, withdrawn) 3. short attention span 4. inability to perform activities of daily living 5. decreased cognitive function 6. poor judgment	
Assess for any neurological status changes, such as: 1. impaired motor functioning 2. changes in speech pattern 3. visual changes or vision loss 4. poor coordination or loss of muscle tone or functioning 5. headaches	

Nursing Interventions	Rationales
Assess for presence of toxoplasmosis, malignancies of brain.	Blood cultures may sometimes be positive for toxoplasmosis; however, magnetic resonance imaging (MRI) or brain scan may be more definitive for either toxoplasmosis or malignancies.
Assess for electrolyte imbalance.	
Assess for CD4 count.	Mental status changes are more likely to occur when counts drop below 100 mm^3.
Assess for presence of any opportunistic infection.	
Determine the availability of support systems.	Patients will need help to cope with mental status changes.
Determine the presence of any previous psychiatric illnesses.	It is important to determine the patient's baseline metal status and behavior so that changes from the baseline can be evaluated.
If mental or neurological status changes are due to toxoplasmosis or malignancies, administer prescribed drugs to treat condition.	
If patient has problems with motor function, determine if caregiver is available to assist patient with activities of daily living (ADLs).	
Instruct patient's caregiver to be alert for any mental or neurological status changes 1. changes in speech pattern 2. poor coordination 3. weakness of any extremities 4. loss of memory	Changes should be reported to patient's health care provider as soon as possible.
Arrange for physical therapist and/or social worker to assess the patient's home environment for any possible hazards that could cause the patient potential injury.	

▼

NURSING DIAGNOSIS: ALTERED NUTRITION—LESS THAN BODY REQUIREMENTS

Related To
- Anorexia
- Difficulty in swallowing or chewing
- Decreased food intake due to side effects from medications
- Nausea and vomiting
- Oral or esophageal infections
- Systemic infections causing fever, hypermetabolism or catabolism
- Increased nutritional needs as a result of HIV infection

Defining Characteristics
Weight loss
Body weight 20% or more under ideal
Inadequate food intake

Patient Outcomes
Patient will
- maintain optimal nutritional state, as evidenced by loss of no more than 10% of body weight.
- verbalize understanding of necessary calorie intake.

Nursing Interventions	Rationales
Obtain history of nutritional intake, diarrhea, anorexia, difficulty swallowing, weight loss (i.e., amount lost over what period of time).	
Determine knowledge of nutritional needs.	
Evaluate for possible adverse reactions to drugs.	Intravenous pentamidine, trimethoprim-sulfamethoxazole (Bactrim), zidovudine (AZT) ampicillin, ciprofloxacin, clofazimine, ethambutol, ganciclovir, isoniazid, pyrazinamide, pyramethamine, and rifampin can cause anorexia, nausea, or weight loss.
Observe for any changes in weight.	
Assess for evidence of oral cavity infections.	These could affect patient's nutritional intake.

Nursing Interventions	Rationales
Encourage intake of high-caloric, vitamin-rich liquid supplements.	
Advise patient to arrange for in-home delivery of meals (Meals on Wheels) if unable to prepare meals.	
Instruct patient to take antiemetic before she begins meal preparation, or have someone else prepare meals, if nausea affects her nutritional intake.	
Instruct patient to restrict the amount of fluids taken before and during meals.	Excess amount of fluid taken before and during meals will cause a feeling of fullness, therefore decreasing the amount of calories taken in by solid food.
Instruct patient to eat frequent small meals. Eat high-calorie food when not nauseated.	
Instruct patient to avoid lying down immediately after eating.	This can cause indigestion or nausea.
Instruct patient to keep daily record of weight gain and loss.	

▼

NURSING DIAGNOSIS: HIGH RISK FOR INJURY (HIV COMPLICATIONS DURING PREGNANCY)

Risk Factors
Compromised immune system:
- decrease in CD4 cells
- CD4:CD8 ratio inverted
- interleukin-2 (IL-2) decreased
- natural killer (NK) cell number and activity decreased

Patient Outcomes
Patient will verbalize understanding of medical treatment necessary to avoid complications during the prenatal and postpartum period.

Nursing Interventions	Rationales
Prenatal	
Instruct HIV patient to seek prenatal care throughout pregnancy.	It is important to evaluate any change or complications that occur as they relate to HIV or pregnancy. There have not been large numbers of pregnant women with HIV available for study, therefore the medical information on the progression of HIV during pregnancy is limited.
Assess for occurrence of any sexually transmitted diseases during prenatal period (syphilis, gonorrhea, herpes, hepatitis B, chlamydia).	
Assess for signs of anemia.	It can occur normally during pregnancy, but is common in HIV-infected adults.
Initiate prenatal lab work: 1. CD4 lymphocyte count done every trimester, but monthly if CD4 count below 350 mm^3. 2. First visit: • blood drawn for antibodies to toxoplasma, cytomegalovirus (CMV), syphilis, VDRL (venereal disease research laboratory), or RPR (rapid plasma reagin) test.	Toxoplasma can be transmitted to the fetus and cause spontaneous abortion, stillbirth, or mental retardation. CMV can be acquired during pregnancy and passed on to the fetus. In the immunocompromised host, it can cause blindness, respiratory distress, or gastrointestinal disorders. If untreated, syphilis can be transmitted to the fetus.
• skin test for tuberculosis (TB).	TB not only causes respiratory problems for the mother, but is a health threat to everyone with whom the person comes into contact.

Nursing Interventions	Rationales
• cultures for gonorrhea and chlamydia. • blood drawn for presence of Hepatitis B surface antigens and cryptococcal antigens, beta-2 microglobulins, chemistry profile. • Pneumovax vaccine given.	
Evaluate CD4 count. If the CD4 count is above 500 mm^3, antiviral therapy (zidovudine [AZT]) is not needed. When CD4 count drops below 500 mm^3, antiviral therapy should be discussed with the patient.	It has not been determined in research studies if antiviral drugs have teratogenic effects on the fetus. The patient should be informed about the drug and allowed to make the decision to take antiviral drugs.
When the CD4 count drops below 200, pneumocystis pneumonia prophylaxis should be started.	
If treatment is indicated, draw a G6PD (glucose-6-phosphate dehydrogenase) level.	If the patient is G6PD-deficient, Bactrim is not the drug to be used because it can cause hemolysis, neutropenia, and liver disease. Dapsone is less toxic. G6PD deficiency is more common in patients of African American descent.
At Delivery Send urine to laboratory to be tested for presence of cytomegalovirus.	It is important to determine if the woman has had an exposure to CMV since initially tested.
Instruct the woman not to breast-feed her infant.	HIV is present in breast milk and HIV transmission through breast milk has been documented.
Postpartum Treat HIV disease in the postpartum patient as in any adult with HIV. When the patient is seen on the postpartum visit, evaluate the CD4 count, complete blood count, and chemistry profile.	Necessary to evaluate changes that may have occurred due to the pregnancy.

Nursing Interventions	Rationales
Anticipate antiviral therapy and pneumocytsis pneumonia prophy- laxis to be continued or started if the CD4 count is low enough.	
Instruct the mother that the infant should be followed by a pediatri- cian at least every 6 weeks for the first 18–24 months.	It takes approximately this long before HIV serostatus can be ac- curately determined. There is a 30% to 50% probability that an infant exposed during pregnancy will be infected with HIV.

▼

NURSING DIAGNOSIS: BODY IMAGE DISTURBANCE

Related To
- Changes in body image and function because of AIDS-related infections that can cause weight loss, motor dysfunction, and impaired cognitive functioning
- Stigma/public opinion regarding AIDS and how it is acquired

Defining Characteristics
Expressions of shame or guilt
Self-negating verbalization
Preoccupation with self

Patient Outcomes
Patient will
- express a more positive self-concept.
- identify situations that positively or negatively affect her self-concept.

Nursing Interventions	Rationales
Assist patient to identify sources of threats to self-concept (ie., changes in body image, alteration in roles, relationships).	
Identify signs of grieving and allow patient to verbalize the meaning of the change and/or losses related to her self-concept.	

Nursing Interventions	Rationales
Encourage her to think about all the positive things still able to be done, rather than only things she is unable to do.	
Assist in identifying activities that are suited to her ability and limitations.	This reinforces positive abilities.
Identify signs of depression and anxiety.	
Discuss safe sex practices so she may feel free to establish intimate relationship with partner.	

▼

NURSING DIAGNOSIS: ANTICIPATORY GRIEVING

Related To chronic and terminal illness

Defining Characteristics
Feelings of hopelessness
Suicidal thoughts
Spiritual emptiness
Feelings of being alone or abandoned
Anger
Sorrow

Patient Outcomes
Patient will
- discuss feelings regarding her disease and prognosis.
- utilize appropriate support services.

Nursing Interventions	Rationales
Assess knowledge of disease and medications.	Knowledge regarding medications that can help keep illness under control may offer some hope.
Determine support systems available for patient (family, friends, spouse, support groups).	Patients have a multitude of problems accompanying illness that are difficult to cope with.
Acknowledge any progress patient makes; offer hope.	

Nursing Interventions	Rationales
Allow patient to verbalize feelings of fear of dying.	
Emphasize that HIV disease is becoming a chronic disease and does not necessarily mean death will occur shortly after diagnosis.	

▼

NURSING DIAGNOSIS: HIGH RISK FOR IMPAIRED HOME MAINTENANCE MANAGEMENT

Risk Factors
- Chronic and/or terminal disease
- Insufficient finances
- Unfamiliarity with resources
- Inadequate support system
- Lack of role modeling
- Lack of knowledge

Patient Outcomes
- Patient/significant other will utilize appropriate support system/resources.
- Patient will receive necessary care services to maintain self-care needs.

Nursing Interventions	Rationales
Assess support systems available within the home or family/significant other who live nearby.	
Evaluate the patient's functional status, and whether there are any sensory or motor impairments that would interfere with preparing meals or performing activities of daily living (ADLs).	Some cities have a Meals on Wheels service. Patient may need a home health aide or homemaker to assist with ADLs.
Determine whether there are any safety concerns within the home (e.g., stairs to climb).	

Nursing Interventions	Rationales
Assess whether home health nurses will be needed to provide care within the home (e.g., administer intravenous medications, central line care, or dressing changes.	Most insurance companies and public aid will pay for some professional nursing care; however, the family or significant other may need education on medication administration.
Determine whether someone is available to care for any children within the home, if woman is too ill to maintain her role as mother.	
Evaluate need for any rehabilitation therapy (physical, occupational, or speech).	
Determine whether transportation is available or if it will need to be arranged for follow-up medical visits.	Many cities provide free (or very inexpensive) transportation for individuals who are unable to travel by public transportation.
Discuss whether the patient has insurance or public aid or is eligible to apply for disability.	Some insurance companies have limited benefits or any home care services.
Provide information on community services.	

DISCHARGE PLANNING/CONTINUITY OF CARE

- Refer to the many community organizations and services available in most major cities.
- Refer to HIV-positive female support group.
- Refer to social workers, psychologists, psychiatrists, and social support agencies.
- Refer to Meals on Wheels.
- Refer to Visiting Nurse Association (VNA), home health aide, homemaker.
- Refer to American Red Cross, the AIDS Foundation, and local health department for educational/community service information.
- Inform of AIDS Hotline (1-800-AID-AIDS).

REFERENCES

Allen, M. (1990). Primary care of women infected with the human immunodeficiency virus. *Obstetrics and Gynecology Clinics of North America, 17*(3), 557–569.

Coyne, B. & Landers, D. (1990). The immunology of HIV disease and pregnancy and possible interactions. *Obstetrics and Gynecology Clinics of North America, 17*(3), 595–606.

Ellerbrock, T. & Rogers, M. (1990). Epidemiology of human immunodeficiency virus infection in women in the United States. *Obstetrics and Gynecology Clinics of North America, 17*(3), 523–544.

Ellerbrock, T., Bush, T., Chamberland, M., & Oxtoby, M. (1991). Epidemiology of women with AIDS in the United States, 1981 through 1990. *Journal of the American Medical Association, 265*(22), 2971–2975.

Flaskerud, J. & Ungvarski, P. (1992). *HIV/AIDS: A Guide to Nursing Care.* Philadelphia, PA: Saunders.

Gee, G. & Moran, T. (1990). *AIDS: Concepts in Nursing Practice.* Baltimore: Williams & Wilkins.

Hoegsberg, B., Abulafia, O., Sedlis, A., Feldman, J., DesJalais, D., Landesman, S., & Minkoff, H. (1990). Sexually transmitted diseases and human immunodeficiency virus infection among women with pelvic inflammatory disease. *American Journal of Obstetrics and Gynecology, 163,* 1135–1139.

Jay, N. (1993). Gynecologic issues of women with human immunodeficiency virus with infection. *AWHONN's Clinical Issues in Perinatal Women's Health Nursing, 4*(2), 250–257.

Jones, D. (1991). HIV-seropositive childbearing women: Nursing management. *Journal of the Obstetrical Gynecologicand Neonatal Nursing, 20*(6), 446–452.

Minkof, H. & DeHovitz, J. (1991). Care of women infected with the human immunodeficiency virus. *Journal of the American Medical Association, 266*(16), 2253–2258.

Nanda, D. (1990). Human immunodeficiency virus infection in pregnancy. *Obstetrics and Gynecology Clinics of North America, 17*(3), 617–626.

Nanda, D. & Minkoff, H. (1992). Pregnancy and women at risk for HIV infection. *Primary Care, 19*(1), 157–169.

Notte, S., Sohn, M. A., & Koons, B. (1993). Prevention of HIV infection in women. *Journal of Obstetric Gynecologic and Neonatal Nursing, 22*(2), 128–134.

Stratton, P., Mofenson, L., & Willoughby, A. (1992). Human immunodeficiency virus infection in pregnant women under care at AIDS clinical trials centers in the United States. *Obstetrics and Gynecology, 79*(3), 364–368.

Tannenbaum, I. (1993). Women and HIV. *RN, 56*(5), 34–41.

▼

$\mathcal{H}$YSTERECTOMY

Denise Wheeler, RN, MS, CNM

Hysterectomy is the surgical removal of the uterus. Procedures that may accompany hysterectomy include oophorectomy (removal of the ovaries) and salpingectomy (removal of the fallopian tubes). These procedures may be done unilaterally or bilaterally. This care plan will be divided into two sections: Preoperative Care and Postoperative Care of the woman requiring hysterectomy (ambulatory setting).

INDICATIONS

- Presence of uterine fibroids
- Elective sterilization/abortion
- Reproductive malignancy
- Adherent placenta (placenta acreta)
- Uterine perforation/hemorrhage/rupture
- Endometriosis
- Persistent hydatidiform mole
- Infection
- Ectopic pregnancy

▼

PREOPERATIVE CARE

NURSING DIAGNOSIS: KNOWLEDGE DEFICIT

Related To
- Unfamiliarity with scheduled procedure
- Lack of resources

Defining Characteristics

Need for additional information
Few questions
Many questions
Fear or concern about having surgery

Patient Outcomes

The patient will
- verbalize what to expect regarding her preoperative and postoperative surgical phase.
- express an understanding of the need for surgery, techniques involved, expected changes in body function, potential need for hormone replacement therapy.

Nursing Interventions	Rationales
Inquire about the patient and her partner's understanding of the causes for hysterectomy, loss of reproduction potential, risks and benefits of the procedure.	
Determine if the physician has suggested an abdominal or vaginal approach to hysterectomy and if any additional procedures (oophorectomy/salpingectomy) are planned. If patient has reservations regarding abdominal or vaginal approach, refer to the physician.	The patient may desire either a vaginal or abdominal hysterectomy for her own reasons, but she may not have communicated that to her physician. The physician recommends the approach that will be the safest and most appropriate for each woman, depending on the nature of her problem. However, the physician may not have communicated this to the patient. Allowing her to discuss this with the surgeon will give her some sense of control over what is occurring.
Instruct the patient and her partner regarding routine preoperative instructions. Instruct patient how to administer medicated douche the evening before surgery (if ordered).	Douching is of particular importance to reduce risk of infection when vaginal approach is used.

Nursing Interventions	Rationales
Discuss what the patient can expect in terms of: 1. intravenous therapy 2. anesthesia evaluation 3. bladder catheterization 4. abdominal preparation 5. suprapubic catheterization, if indicated 6. hospital stay 7. food and fluid restrictions (if any) 8. pain relief 9. ambulation	
Teach patient the anatomy of the pelvis, using diagrams and pictures when necessary: 1. Describe the size and placement of the uterus and its adjacent structures. 2. Explain that when the uterus is removed, the other pelvic and abdominal organs will settle into the small space left. 3. Remind the patient that she may experience some vaginal bleeding for a few days after surgery.	Vaginal bleeding following hysterectomy comes from the vaginal cuff incision. Preparing the patient for vaginal bleeding in the absence of a uterus will make it less frightening when it happens.

Nursing Interventions

Discuss menopause and hormone replacement therapy (HRT) if appropriate:
1. advantages of HRT include protection against:
   - osteoporosis and heart disease
   - loss of breast tissue
   - loss of muscle tone (especially vaginal support of the bladder)
   - loss of skin integrity
   - facial hair growth
   - mood swings
   and prevention or relief of:
   - hot flushes
   - insomnia
   - vaginal dryness
2. side effects and disadvantages may include:
   - breast tenderness
   - bloating
   - mood swings
   - acne
   - potential for increased blood pressure and blood clotting disorders
3. The issue of breast cancer and HRT is unresolved. There is no evidence that HRT causes development of breast cancer, however, estrogen will stimulate growth of a breast cancer that is already present.

Rationales

Women need to make an informed choice about hormone replacement. Many women choose not to take hormones because it is not "natural." Unfortunately, women with surgically induced menopause may be a higher risk for osteoporosis than women who naturally reach menopause. Some of the side effects are uncommon, especially increased blood pressure and blood clotting, because the dosages for hormone replacement in menopause are significantly lower than those prescribed for birth control pills. Because women now spend about one-third of their lives after menopause, improvement in the quality of life is important.

Nursing Interventions	Rationales
Discuss possible changes in sexual response following hysterectomy.	The uterus contracts during orgasm. Movement of the cervix may also contribute to orgasm. Following removal of the uterus, the sensations of sexual pleasure may change. This does not imply a loss of sexual function, but a change. On the other hand, for women who have had pain with intercourse, heavy bleeding, or other problems that may interfere with sexual response, sexual function may be improved following hysterectomy.
Encourage the patient to discuss the effects that hysterectomy may have on her self-image and/or sexual functioning.	Disorders of the female reproductive organs frequently challenge a woman's concept of her femininity. This may be more of an issue when dealing with women in cross-cultural situations. In some cultures, the ability to reproduce—which requires healthy reproductive organs—is central to a woman's value.
Allow the patient and her partner to express their concerns regarding loss of the ability to reproduce, if appropriate.	For many women, the need for hysterectomy will occur after they have had children. However, for some women, the need for hysterectomy will deny them the possibility of ever conceiving and delivering their own children. It is important that the woman and her partner have the opportunity to discuss what this loss means to them, grieve that loss, and explore alternatives for having a family. Unresolved anger, confusion, and grief for infertility may disrupt the patient's relationships with her partner, friends, family, and other sources of support. Referral to a sensitive therapist may be appreciated.

Nursing Interventions	Rationales

Provide patient with information regarding self-help for pain relief during the postoperative period of abdominal surgery. Instruct her to
1. brace the surgical site when
  • moving
  • coughing
  • straining
2. ambulate
3. apply ice packs to the abdominal incision
4. use relaxation techniques
5. initiate over-the-counter and prescribed pain relief as needed
	Inadequate pain relief may delay the patient's recovery by prolonging her immobility.

Teach patient postsurgical self-care tips, including: 1. care of the suprapubic or urethral catheter, as appropriate 2. care of the incision, if abdominal 3. advice that loose clothing will be more comfortable than tight-fitting clothing initially	
Discuss preparation of the home for the early postoperative period: 1. Help with meal preparation, groceries, laundry, and housekeeping may be needed temporarily. 2. Patients who live in upstairs apartments or two-story homes should plan ahead to limit the number of times they must climb stairs. 3. Patients should be cautioned about heavy lifting (e.g., groceries, laundry baskets, children).	Postsurgical patients tire quickly and fatigue will prolong recovery.

POSTOPERATIVE CARE (AMBULATORY SETTING)

NURSING DIAGNOSIS: PAIN

Related To operative procedure

Defining Characteristics
Verbalizes discomfort
Grimaces
Walks slowly while guarding abdomen

Patient Outcomes
Patient will verbalize comfort and pain relief.

Nursing Interventions	Rationales
Question patient about her level of discomfort, and any improvement in her comfort levels since discharge from hospital.	Each person's perception of pain is unique. The patient's discomfort should be acknowledged, and her efforts to deal with her pain encouraged.
Review self-help pain control measures and reinforce those that she is already using.	
Allow the patient to move at her own pace. Assist her to be as comfortable as she can be during the postoperative examination.	
Assist her to see how her recovery has progressed since hospital discharge.	Patients need reassurance that their recovery is proceeding as expected, and that whatever pain they are experiencing will resolve.

▼

NURSING DIAGNOSIS: HIGH RISK FOR INFECTION

Risk Factors
- Abdominal or vaginal incision
- Bladder catheterization

Patient Outcomes
Patient will
- describe the potential for infection, and signs and symptoms for early detection.
- initiate self-care techniques that minimize the potential for infection.

Nursing Interventions	**Rationales**
Question patient about the appearance of any symptoms of infection: 1. fever 2. chills 3. malaise 4. reddened incision 5. increased drainage 6. difficulty voiding	Early detection facilitates early treatment.
Examine abdominal incision site, if appropriate, for redness, swelling, separation, drainage.	
Encourage patient to maintain adequate fluid intake, and to avoid bladder irritants (e.g., caffeine). Remind her to empty bladder frequently. Reinforce proper hygiene and wiping techniques.	Urinary tract infections are common postoperative problems following hysterectomy.
Obtain appropriate specimens or assist in obtaining specimens for culture and sensitivity: 1. urine 2. exudate or vaginal discharge 3. blood	
Discourage douching unless prescribed by physician.	There are no proven health benefits to douching. Following hysterectomy, there is a normal amount of vaginal bleeding (from the vaginal cuff incision), and vaginal discharge may be noted. Douching may further alter the acid balance in the vagina and promote the development of vaginitis. In addition, sutures are present in the vaginal cuff. Douching may damage the sutures, causing bleeding, and incision breakdown, which may require reparative surgery.
Instruct patient in: 1. inspection of the incision site 2. dressing changes 3. cleansing the incision with hydrogen peroxide, as appropriate	

Nursing Interventions	Rationales
Individualize the teaching for obese women.	Obese women may need assistance from family members for this. Additionally, obese women may require additional instruction in ways to keep the incision site dry (e.g., use of hair dryer)
Instruct patient in actions, proper dosage, frequency, and side effects of any antibiotics the physician may order. Review any other medications being taken, allergies, and potential drug interactions.	

▼

NURSING DIAGNOSIS: KNOWLEDGE DEFICIT REGARDING RESUMPTION OF USUAL ACTIVITIES

Related To
- New experience
- Lack of information/resources

Defining Characteristics
Need for more information
Lack of questions
Lack of compliance with prescribed activity plan
Resistance to follow-up treatment

Patient Outcomes
Patient will
- verbalize understanding of any activity restrictions.
- verbalize rationale for preventive health maintenance.

Nursing Interventions	Rationales
Question the patient about her level of activity and how quickly she tires.	Each patient will recover at a different rate.
Determine which activities patient feels ready to resume or would like to resume.	

Nursing Interventions	Rationales
Inform the patient that she may gradually increase her activity as tolerated. Remind her not to overdo stair climbing or lifting.	How much activity she can tolerate will be determined by how quickly she tires, any increase in pain with activity, and her previous physical state.
Stress importance of follow-up office visits.	Follow-up is necessary to assess the final outcome of the surgical intervention.
Instruct the patient in preventive health maintenance, including Pap smears.	Women mistakenly assume that Pap smears are no longer necessary following hysterectomy. Vaginal Pap smears are recommended every 2 to 3 years following hysterectomy. In addition, women need regular breast examinations, mammography, colon and rectal cancer screening, cholesterol checks. Annual bimanual pelvic examinations are critical if the ovaries have been left in place and useful to assess pelvic masses even if the ovaries have been removed.
Review patient response to hormone replacement therapy and reinforce preoperative teaching in this area.	

▼

DISCHARGE PLANNING/CONTINUITY OF CARE

- Instruct to see gynecologist in 2 and 6 weeks, then in one year unless problems occur.
- Refer to sex therapist if necessary.
- Distribute pamphlets available from the American College of Obstetricians and Gynecologists
- Suggest books on hysterectomy that can be found in libraries; videotaped discussions may also be available.
- Determine what assistance and support the patient will have at home following surgery

REFERENCES

Byyny, R. & Speroff, L. (1990). *A Clinical Guide for the Care of Older Women.* Baltimore, MD: Williams & Wilkins.

Lichtman, R. & Papera, S. (1990). *Gynecology: Well Woman Care.* E. Norwalk. CT: Appleton & Lange.

Williamson, M. L. (1992). Sexual adjustment after hysterectomy. *Journal of Obstetrical, Gynecologic, and Neonatal Nursing, 21*(1), 42–47.

▼

$\mathscr{I}$NFERTILITY

Janet L. Engstrom, RN, PhD, CNM

Infertility is defined as the inability to conceive after one year of regular, unprotected intercourse. Infertility can be classified as primary or secondary. Primary infertility applies to the couple who has never conceived; secondary infertility applies to the couple who has conceived in the past but who has been unable to conceive after 12 months of regular, unprotected intercourse, regardless of the number of previous pregnancies.

ETIOLOGIES

There are numerous factors that are associated with infertility. In the female, causes of infertility are:
- ovulatory disorders
- cervical factors
- uterine abnormalities
- tubal disorders
- peritoneal factors
- immunological disorders
- idiopathic

In the male, causes of infertility are:
- testicular disorders
- ejaculatory factors
- immunological disorders

DIAGNOSTIC FINDINGS

There are numerous diagnostic procedures that may be performed to evaluate a couple's infertility. The selection of diagnostic procedures will depend on the couple's reproductive and health histories, as well as findings on examination. Selected diagnostic procedures may include:

Female
- Basal body temperature
- Endometrial biopsy
- Evaluation of cervical mucous
- Post-coital test
- Cervical cultures
- Hysterosalpingogram
- Hysteroscopy
- Laparoscopy
- Endocrine assays:
  - FSH
  - LH
  - estradiol
  - progesterone
  - prolactin
  - TSH, T_3, T_4
  - androgen levels
- Immunological studies including tests for:
  - antisperm antibodies
  - autoimmune disorders

Male
- Semen analysis assessing sperm count
  - motility and morphology
  - semen volume and viscosity
- Sperm penetration assay
- Immunological studies, including tests for antisperm antibodies in blood and semen
- Endocrine assays, including:
  - FSH
  - LH
  - testosterone
  - prolactin
  - estrogens

▼

NURSING DIAGNOSIS: KNOWLEDGE DEFICIT

Related To unfamiliarity with the causes, diagnosis, and treatment of infertility

Defining Characteristics

Need for more information
Misconceptions and/or misunderstandings
Incorrect follow-through of instructions
Lack of compliance with treatment
Resistance to treatment

Patient Outcomes

Patient will
- verbalize correct information about the causes, diagnosis, and treatment of infertility.
- identify health care providers and community resources.
- verbalize realistic expectations of the success of infertility treatment and the demands of undergoing treatment.
- execute prescribed instructions/medications correctly.

Nursing Interventions	Rationales
Assess knowledge of normal reproductive anatomy and physiology.	
Assess knowledge of the causes, diagnosis, and treatment of infertility.	Gathering information facilitates development of appropriate teaching plan.
Assess the patient's changing need for information as she progresses through treatment.	

Provide information on:
1. Normal reproductive anatomy and physiology.
2. The pathophysiology related to the cause of the patient's infertility:
  • ovulation dysfunction
  • tubal obstruction
  • varicocele	

Nursing Interventions

Provide information on the types of and rationale for diagnostic and therapeutic procedures that will be performed.

1. Diagnostic studies may include but are not limited to:
   - basal body temperatures to assess ovulatory function
   - serum progesterone to assess ovulatory function
   - endometrial biopsy to assess corpus luteum function
   - hormonal studies (follicle-stimulating hormone, luteinizing hormone, prostaglandin E_2) to assess pituitary and ovarian function as well as other endocrine studies to evaluate thyroid and adrenal function
   - postcoital test to evaluate cervical mucus and sperm presence in the mucus
   - hysterosalpingogram to evaluate the uterine cavity and tubal patency
   - hysteroscope to evaluate the uterine cavity
   - laparoscope to evaluate pelvic anatomy
   - immunological studies to document the presence of anti-sperm antibodies or autoimmune diseases
   - semen analysis to assess sperm count, motility, and morphology
   - sperm penetration assay to assess the sperm's penetrating ability
   - ultrasound follicle studies to assess follicular growth

Rationales

Adequate information is essential for patients to make their own assessment of the risks, benefits, and demands of treatment and to decide whether they want to undergo treatment. Information may help couples set realistic goals and expectations for treatment.

Nursing Interventions	**Rationales**
2. Therapeutic interventions may include: • ovulation induction with medications such as human menopausal gonadotropin (HMG), follicle-stimulating hormone (FSH), human chorionic gonadotropin, gonadotropin-releasing hormone (GnRH) agonist to correct ovulatory dysfunction • intrauterine inseminations to optimize the number of sperm close to the vicinity of the egg during the periovulatory period • sperm processing to optimize sperm performance • corrective surgeries to correct anatomical abnormalities (e.g., lysis of adhesions, tuboplasty, varicocelectomy) • in vitro fertilization to bypass abnormal/occluded fallopian tubes • gamete intrafallopian transfer or zygote intrafallopian transfer for women with normal fallopian tubes in whom conventional treatments have failed.	
Instruct patient regarding the correct way to perform procedures (e.g., basal body temperature, urine testing for luteinizing hormone surge, injections).	
Instruct patient on the proper use and administration of all medications. Allow her to perform a demonstration of the more difficult psychomotor skills (e.g., preparing and/or administering injections) before performing the procedure alone at home.	Immedite feedback allows learner to make corrections rather than practicing the skill incorrectly.

▼

NURSING DIAGNOSIS: PAIN

Related To diagnostic procedures, treatments, injections

Defining Characteristics
Pain or discomfort
Moaning, crying, grimacing, tensing muscles
Autonomic nervous system responses such as diaphoresis, changes in heart
rate, blood pressure and respiratory rate, and pupillary dilatation

Patient Outcomes
Patient will
- verbalize comfort and pain relief.
- use nonpharmacological pain-coping strategies.
- use pain-relieving medications that may interfere with conception or
  be harmful to a developing pregnancy.

Nursing Interventions	Rationales
Observe patient's verbal and non-verbal response to uncomfortable and potentially painful procedures, e.g.: 1. endometrial biopsy 2. hysterosalpingogram	
Ask the patient to describe her perception of the pain or discomfort.	
Eliminate factors that may contribute to her physical discomfort; make sure that: 1. the examination room is warm enough 2. the procedure table is as comfortable as possible with a pillow 3. her bladder is empty	Patients may experience a decreased ability to tolerate discomfort if environmental factors are stressing them.
Whenever possible, allow a significant other to accompany the patient if the patient desires company.	The company and support of a significant other may help alleviate anxiety and reduce perception of discomfort.

Nursing Interventions	Rationales
Teach nonpharmacological coping strategies, such as relaxation and slow chest breathing.	These strategies can reduce their perception of pain.
When appropriate, use pharmacological agents to reduce pain (e.g., many physicians will prescribe a nonsteroidal anti-inflammatory agent to be taken before a hysterosalpingogram).	In procedures that are timed so that there is no chance that the patient may be pregnant or close to ovulation, some physicians may prescribe nonsteroidal anti-inflammatory agents.
Evaluate the efficacy of pharmacological and nonpharmacological pain relieving strategies.	
Notify the physician of any significant postprocedure or postinjection pain.	This may indicate the presence of a complication such as an infection or injury caused by the procedure.
If the pain is related to injections, examine the injection sites for signs of inflammation and make sure that injections are being prepared and administered properly.	Injections of the medications commonly used in fertility treatment [e.g., human menopausal gonadotropin (Pergonal), follicle-stimulating hormone (Metrodin), human chorionic gonadotropin (HCG) and gonadotropin-releasing hormone (leuprolide acetate)] usually cause minimal discomfort if administered properly, using the appropriate gauge needle.
Teach the patient to gently massage the muscle after an injection to reduce discomfort.	

▼

NURSING DIAGNOSIS: ALTERED SEXUALITY PATTERNS

Related To
- Timing of diagnostic procedures
- Timing of treatments
- Scheduled intercourse
- Abstinence for specimens and during early pregnancy
- Producing semen specimens by masturbation

Defining Characteristics

Changes in sexual behaviors and activities

Patient Outcomes

Patient will

- resume spontaneous sexual activity during phases of the menstrual cycle when abstinence or intercourse is not required.
- verbalize knowledge of other methods of achieving intimacy and sexual satisfaction without having intercourse or orgasm.

Nursing Interventions	Rationales
Obtain a sexual history to determine previous sexual activity patterns.	This provides a baseline for care planning.
Determine whether the altered sexual pattern (e.g., engaging in intercourse at recommended times, producing semen by masturbation) is disruptive or distressing to the couple. Explain why sexual activity patterns may need to be altered for some diagnostic procedures and treatments.	
Determine whether any of the couple's personal or religious beliefs are in conflict with sexual practices required for diagnosis and treatment (e.g., abstinence, timed intercourse, masturbation).	Such beliefs will impact on their willingness to participate in further treatments.
Offer suggestions for activities that meet the couple's need for contact and intimacy without having intercourse or orgasm (e.g., hugging, kissing, massages, evenings out).	Restrictions on sexual activity should not deprive the couple of activities that convey the message that they are loved and desired nor should such restrictions deprive them of intimate physical contact.
Reassure the patient that other couples find altered sexuality patterns to be stressful. Remind them that such alteration is temporary.	

▼

NURSING DIAGNOSIS: HIGH RISK FOR SEXUAL DYSFUNCTION

Risk Factors

- Altered pattern of sexual activity
- Changes in self-esteem and body image

- Thinking of sexual activity as a means of reproduction instead of for pleasure.
- Performing procedures that may be in conflict with personal or religious beliefs
- Misinformation or lack of knowledge

Patient Outcomes

Patient will

- verbalize knowledge about how infertility treatment may affect sexual function.
- identify religious or personal beliefs that may be in conflict with infertility treatment.
- achieve sexual satisfaction.

Nursing Interventions	Rationales
Assess whether there is any history of sexual dysfunction.	
Determine whether there are other factors that can disrupt sexual function (e.g., stress, marital difficulty, substance abuse, illness).	
Determine whether any of the couple's personal or religious beliefs are in conflict with sexual practices required for diagnosis and treatment (e.g., abstinence, timed intercourse, masturbation).	Such beliefs will impact on their willingness to participate in treatment regimen.
Offer suggestions to help enhance sexual pleasure (exercises such as the partner examination, sensate-focus).	These strategies are commonly used in sex therapy to help couples learn the types of stimulation and the areas of the body that produce pleasurable sensations without having intercourse or orgasm.
Offer suggestions that may help the couple separate sexual activity from fertility treatment (e.g., engaging in spontaneous sexual activity in the days of the cycle when abstinence or timed intercourse are not required).	Giving permission to the couple to participate in sex for pleasure instead of focusing on sex for reproduction may help increase sexual fulfillment and decrease the pressure to perform sexually.

Nursing Interventions	Rationales
Offer suggestions that can help reduce anxiety relating to sexual performance, e.g.: 1. When possible, allow the couple to produce semen specimens at home. 2. Try to schedule procedures so that the couple can have intercourse at a time that is part of their sexual routine (e.g., postcoital tests can frequently be scheduled so that the couple can have intercourse at night and the test can be performed the following morning).	
Avoid qualitative statements about test results that the couple may interpret as an evaluation of their sexual technique (e.g., a "poor" postcoital test, "inadequate" semen specimen).	
Refer the couple to a sex therapist if their problems are significant enough to cause problems in their relationship or interfere with treatment.	Sexual dysfunctions are often complex and require therapy beyond that which can be offered by a health care professional who does not have training in sex therapy.

▼

NURSING DIAGNOSIS: ANXIETY

Related To
- Knowledge deficit
- Threat to self-esteem and body image
- Concern that treatment will not be successful
- Concerns about discomfort and inconveniences of diagnosis and treatment
- Unresolved conflicts about undergoing infertility treatment

Defining Characteristics

Statements of increased tension, apprehension, fear, worry, anxiety, distress, excitability

Statements of helplessness, inadequacy, uncertainty

Increased alertness
Restlessness, jitteriness
Insomnia
Facial tension
Quivering voice
Aggressiveness
Withdrawal
Irritability
Decreased attention span
Sympathetic nervous system stimulation (cardiovascular alterations, superficial vasoconstriction, pupillary dilatation, perspiration)

Patient Outcomes

Patient will verbalize presence of reduced tension, fear, worry, excitability.

Nursing Interventions	Rationales
Assess level of anxiety. Determine whether anxiety is disrupting the couple's relationships, ability to work, and ability to perform activities of daily living.	
Allow the couple to verbalize their feelings of anxiety.	This should validate the existence of the feelings.
Inform the couple that many other men and women experience varying levels of anxiety when they undergo infertility treatment.	Knowing what others also experience may provide comfort to the couple "that they are not alone."
Help the couple identify the source of their anxiety, e.g.: 1. cost of treatment 2. pain, discomfort, and inconvenience of treatment 3. concern that they will not be able to follow all of the instructions and perform procedures correctly 4. fear of not having the opportunity to be a parent	Accurate assessment of contributing factors is the first step to resolution.
Provide the couple with written literature about the emotional crisis of infertility.	There are several excellent publications on the psychosocial aspects of infertility. These publications can help validate the couple's feelings and provide coping strategies for dealing with the feelings.

Nursing Interventions	Rationales
Explain the benefits of counseling to the couple, particularly if their emotional state is disrupting relationships or is interfering with their ability to work or perform the activities of daily living. Many programs suggest that all couples undergoing infertility treatment receive counseling.	Infertility is a crisis and patients should be offered appropriate psychosocial support and guidance. Because the psychosocial implications of infertility are complex, counseling should be done by a professional skilled in counseling techniques.
Teach the patient relaxation techniques or suggest the names of audiotapes or books that teach relaxation.	Relaxation can reduce the patient's perception of anxiety and can reduce the physical manifestations of anxiety.

▼

NURSING DIAGNOSIS: SITUATIONAL LOW SELF-ESTEEM

Related To patient's perception that his/her body is unable to perform a normal, expected function: reproduction

Defining Characteristics
Negative feelings about self
Negative feelings about body
Expressions of shame or guilt
Change in pattern of social involvement
Change in pattern of sexual activity

Patient Outcomes
Patient will
- verbalize positive statements of self-worth.
- maintain an appropriate level of social involvement.
- maintain a satisfying sexual relationship.

Nursing Interventions	Rationales
Assess the patient's feelings and perceptions about being infertile, and how being infertile affects how she/he views herself/himself.	
Allow the patient to express her feelings about herself and her body.	Validates the existence of the feelings.

Nursing Interventions	Rationales
Inform the patient that many other men and women experience negative feelings about their self and their body when they undergo infertility treatment.	
Assist the patient to develop an inventory of the positive aspects about herself and her body (e.g., a good employee, a wonderful cook, attractive, physically fit, funny, well organized).	

▼

DISCHARGE PLANNING/CONTINUITY OF CARE

- Refer couple to Resolve (organization providing information and support to infertile couples).
- Consider referral to psychologist/social worker/psychiatric nurse skilled in counseling couples with infertility.
- Refer to infertility support groups.
- Refer to sex therapist, if indicated.
- Provide information on adoption counseling when indicated.
- Provide information on relaxation tapes/classes/books.

REFERENCES

Abbey, A., Halman, L. J., & Andrews, F. M. (1992). Psychosocial, treatment, and demographic predictors of the stress associated with infertility. *Fertility and Sterility, 57,* 122–128.

American Fertility Society. (1991). *Investigation of the Infertile Couple.* Birmingham, AL: American Fertility Society.

Garner, C. (Ed.). (1991). *Principles of Infertility Nursing.* Boca Raton, FL: CRC Press.

Siebel, M. M. (Ed.) (1990). *Infertility: A Comprehensive Text.* E. Norwalk, CT: Appleton & Lange.

Speroff, L., Glass, R. H., & Kase, N.G. (1989) *Clinical Gynecologic Endocrinology and Infertility,* (4th ed). Baltimore, MD: Williams & Wilkins.

▼

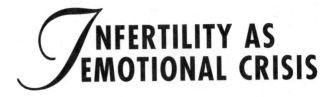

INFERTILITY AS EMOTIONAL CRISIS

Margaret Hixson, RN, BSN

Infertility as emotional crisis is an affective disturbance characterized by feelings of failure, alienation, anger, and grief related to infertility. The couple may or may not have participated in an infertility diagnostic and treatment program.

ETIOLOGIES

- Inability to conceive a child
- Inability to meet normal role expectations

CLINICAL MANIFESTATIONS

- Feelings of inadequacy, shame, guilt
- Anger, alienation
- Grief, sorrow
- Crying
- Withdrawn

▼

NURSING DIAGNOSIS: SELF-ESTEEM/BODY IMAGE DISTURBANCE

Related To
- Belief that pregnancy is critical to personal/social fulfillment as woman
- Psychosocial pressures to conceive
- Biophysical imperativeness to conceive while pregnancy is physically possible
- Cultural/religious mandates that make pregnancy imperative

Defining Characteristics
Self-negating verbalizations
Expressions of shame/guilt

Rejects positive feedback
Hypersensitive to criticism
Change in social involvement
Negative feelings about body
Inappropriate blaming of personal inadequacies for infertility
Feelings of loss of identity; not feeling totally "female"
Distorted perception: "everyone is pregnant except me"

Patient Outcomes

Patient will

- express positive statements about self/body image.
- maintain an appropriate level of social involvement.

Nursing Interventions	Rationales
Assess the patient's feelings and perceptions about being infertile, and how infertility affects how she values herself.	Patients often fail to recognize the "normalness" of having difficulty coping with a problem such as infertility. They may put unreasonable expectations on themselves without being aware of it.
Discuss the "usual" emotional reactions to childlessness.	This allows patient/couple to see that their feelings are not uncommon.
Note statements about work, social, sexual, family withdrawal/incompetent performance.	Poor job performance, poor sexual performance, poor hygiene, and reduced social contacts are signs of decreased self esteem.
Assess level of social/family acceptance.	Often family/friends put uncalculated pressures and expectations on couple to have children. Knowledge of such factors aids in designing an appropriate coping plan.
Observe for isolation or statements of need to withdraw from family/friends/environments that have children.	
Note religious/cultural background and potential conflicts.	Cultural/religious mandates that make pregnancy imperative need to be identified and discussed if patient is to work through problem.

Nursing Interventions	Rationales
Note descriptions reflecting secrecy about infertility/inability to discuss.	
Observe for statements that project psychological inability to be good parent. ("I cannot conceive because God knows I will be a poor parent.")	
Advise patient to give minimal significance to the negative responses of others.	Patient must realize that some disagree with choices for family building/parenting; they are entitled to their personal decisions.
Stress importance of spouse support.	Expressing acceptance of one another can be helpful to both. Patient/spouse will need other's support during difficult waiting and testing of fertility treatment and afterward when infertility is diagnosed.
Reinforce positive emotional responses; redirect negative responses.	
Emphasize patient's value as an individual. Assist patient to develop an inventory of the positive aspects about herself and her body (physically fit, attractive, wonderful cook, etc.).	Focusing on positive attributes increases self-acceptance.
When indicated, provide information/assistance about adoption as a possible alternative.	Patient must realize alternatives.

▼

NURSING DIAGNOSIS: HIGH RISK FOR DYSFUNCTIONAL GRIEVING

Risk Factors
- Thwarted grieving response to loss
- Actual/perceived loss of potential life-giving ability
- Obsession/preoccupation with infertility

Patient Outcomes

Patient will

- adapt to inability to conceive child, as evidenced by normal social/family interactions.
- begin to cope with stress of childlessness.

Nursing Interventions	Rationales
Assess patient's feelings regarding infertility.	Infertility is a crisis. The nurse needs to determine the scope and impact of the patient's feelings so that appropriate coping strategies can be designed.
Encourage description of anticipated problems related to childlessness.	
Assist patient in identifying her usual response pattern in coping. Encourage use of past adaptive coping mechanisms.	Patient often knows what works best.
Assist couple through grief; recognizing, working through, overcoming intense/painful loss feelings.	
Confront patient gently to focus attention on feelings/behavior.	Patient may try to avoid/hide feelings. Gentle confrontation by nurse may lead to productive dialogue.
Provide attention to concerns of each individual (husband/wife).	Infertility affects both; husband also needs attention.
Facilitate communication between partners by including both in all aspects of care.	Often one partner assumes that the other knows how he/she feels or hesitates to verbalize feelings. This may further strain the relationship.
Provide emotional support.	Emotional support allows patient to work through/resolve conflicts and provides them with a resource/support person.
Encourage crying as appropriate.	Expression of emotional pain serves to decrease or diffuse the emotional stress the patient is experiencing.

Nursing Interventions	Rationales
Explain the benefits of counseling.	Patients should be offered appropriate psychosocial support and guidance. Because the psychosocial implications of infertility are complex, counseling should be done by a professional skilled in counseling techniques.
Facilitate contact with other women/couples who have successfully adjusted to infertility.	Patients may find it easier to relate to/speak with someone with similar experience. Such interactions serve to validate the patient's feelings. Offer information/guidance for successful adjustment.

▼

DISCHARGE PLANNING/CONTINUITY OF CARE

- Refer to Infertility Clinics.
- Refer for sexual counseling.
- Provide information about adoption counseling when indicated.
- Refer couple to Resolve (organization providing information and support to infertile couples).

REFERENCES

Davis, C. & Dearmon, C. (1991). Coping strategies of infertile women. *Journal of Obstetrical, Gynecologic, and Neonatal Nursing, 20*(3), 221–228.

Harris, B., Sandelowski, M., & Holditch-Davis, D. (1991). Infertility . . . and new interpretations of pregnancy loss. *American Journal of Maternal/Child Nursing, 16*(4), 217–220.

Stanton, A., Tennen, H., Affleck, G., & Mendola, R. (1991). Cognitive appraisal and adjustment to infertility. *Women and Health, 17*(3), 1–15.

▼

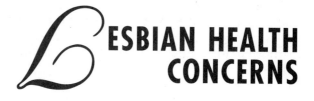

ESBIAN HEALTH CONCERNS

Lisa Hauser, RN, BSN

Lesbian health care addresses the unique psychosocial and physiological needs of women who self-identify as lesbians, whether sexually active or not. Complicating factors include homophobia, an irrational fear of homosexuals and homosexuality, which may hinder the ability of the individual to seek or provide appropriate health care, and heterosexism, an irrational belief in the inherent superiority of heterosexuality over homosexuality, giving rise to stereotyping and discrimination. Studies indicate that many lesbians who have access to health care do not seek such care because of actual and anticipated negative experiences with providers.

Lesbians may enter the health care system for routine care or as a result of trauma, concerns about sexually transmitted diseases, or the physical manifestations of dysfunctional grieving. If they encounter discrimination and judgment in these encounters, the quality of health care provided is seriously compromised.

ETIOLOGIES

N/A

CLINICAL MANIFESTATIONS

N/A

▼

NURSING DIAGNOSIS: ANXIETY

Related To potential for discriminatory behavior during gynecological exam

Defining Characteristics
Irritability/impatience
Withdrawal

Hyperattentiveness
Blocking of thoughts—inability to remember pertinent facts
Self-deprecation
Increased heart rate, respiratory rate, blood pressure
Dilated pupils
Restlessness

Patient Outcomes

Patient will
- describe her own anxiety.
- demonstrate a decrease in anxiety by speaking clearly, making eye contact, asking appropriate questions.

Nursing Interventions	Rationales
Assess for feelings of apprehension, rejection, or isolation.	
Assess for history of negative experiences with health care providers.	Assessment provides guidance/focus for ongoing care.
Obtain accurate sexual history by avoiding assumptions of heterosexuality: "Are you currently sexually active with men, women, or both? "Have you been sexually active with men in the past?"	This communicates that her perference is considered one of the normal expressions of human sexuality.
Obtain the patient's consent for documentation regarding her sexuality.	Homophobic and heterosexist cultural mores attach significant stigma to the terms "lesbian," "gay," and "homosexual." Lesbians may avoid disclosing their sexuality for fear of this stigma.
Document using terms such as: "Not sexually active with men;" "Sexually active—not in need of birth control."	
Acknowledge to yourself your beliefs about lesbianism.	Heterosexist and homophobic judgments impair nursing care and inhibit patient's health-seeking behaviors.
Encourage the patient to express her specific gynecological concerns.	Sharing feelings facilitates trust and reduces anxiety.

Nursing Interventions	Rationales
Encourage presence of significant other if so desired by the patient.	The presence of a significant other may be reassuring and indicates health care providers' non-judgmental acceptance of the patient's lifestyle.

▼

NURSING DIAGNOSIS: KNOWLEDGE DEFICIT

Related To limited understanding of modes of transmission of sexually transmitted diseases (STDs) between women

Defining Characteristics
Multiple questions
Lack of questions
Inaccurate perception of modes of transmission
Cannot correctly describe precautions to prevent transmission of infection to sexual partner

Patient Outcomes
The patient will
- verbalize understanding of modes of transmission of STDs between women.
- identify need for additional information regarding prevention of transmission of infection.
- describe precautions necessary to prevent transmission of STDs.

Nursing Interventions	Rationales
Assess understanding of etiology and modes of transmission of STDs.	This provides basis for further health teaching.
Provide information about infections that have been shown to be transmitted between women during oral-genital, genital-genital, or manual contact (when one partner touches her own vulva/vagina and then touches her partner's vulva/vagina (e.g., moniliasis, genital herpes, trichomonas, bacterial vaginosis, human immunodeficiency virus [HIV]).	Knowledge facilitates compliance with safe sex practices.

Nursing Interventions	Rationales
Instruct the patient that 1. female-to-female sexual transmission of HIV is rare, but has been reported. 2. most lesbians who are HIV-positive have contacted HIV by sharing needles during intravenous drug use. 3. presence of HIV in blood and vaginal secretions is clearly documented in the literature. 4. unprotected sexual contact puts the partners of lesbians who are HIV-positive at risk to contact HIV.	Focusing on current, accurate information will help dispel any misconceptions.
Provide information about safer sex techniques:	
1. Latex gloves and finger cots during manual-genital contact.	They prevent contact of vaginal secretions or menstrual blood with breaks in the integument on partner's hands.
2. Latex barriers (dental dam or a condom slit up the side and opened into a square of latex) during oral-genital contact.	They prevent contact of vaginal secretions or menstrual blood with partner's oral mucous membranes.
3. Not sharing sex toys, using condoms if sex toys are shared, washing sex toys with 1:10 solution of bleach and water after use.	
Encourage the patient to ask questions about the need to modify her specific sexual practices.	
Use clear, direct, descriptive language when teaching patient.	Such honest professional behavior by health professionals assists patients to maintain a positive self-image.
Involve significant other in teaching process if patient so desires.	

▼

NURSING DIAGNOSIS: POSTTRAUMA RESPONSE

Related To homophobic violence

Defining Characteristics

Expresses feelings of self-blame, shame, guilt, vulnerability, or helplessness
Reports flashbacks, intrusive thoughts, recurring nightmares
Reports episodes of rage or panic
Appears hyperalert or hypervigilant
Reports detachment from previously valued activities
Social isolation/withdrawal
Expresses inability to perform self-care activities
Reports or demonstrates self-destructive behavior (drug/alcohol abuse, reckless behavior, self-mutilation)

Patient Outcomes

Patient will

- acknowledge the traumatic event and begin to process it by expressing feelings such as anger, fear, and guilt.
- report a lessening of feelings of self-blame and shame.
- identify self-destructive behavior, and the need to seek help to control such impulses and improve coping mechanisms.

Nursing Interventions	Rationales
Determine if the patient has experienced a traumatic event related to her perceived sexuality.	Stereotyped perceptions of lesbian appearance and behavior place any woman who deviates from cultural norms of the female at risk for homophobic violence, (whether she is lesbian or not).
Assess the severity of response and its impact on her level of functioning.	
Evaluate her knowledge of and involvement with support people/services.	Support groups provide current and realistic picture of problems faced; they provide support for problem-solving.
Stay with patient and offer support during episodes of extreme anxiety.	Fear is decreased when thoughts and feelings are expressed.

Nursing Interventions	Rationales
Reassure patient that she is experiencing feelings and symptoms that are often experienced after a traumatic event.	
Explain that talking about and expressing feelings related to the traumatic event may intensify these feelings temporarily, including an increase in nightmares and flashbacks.	Sharing feelings may facilitate trust and reduce anxiety.
Help restore her dignity by reassuring her that she was not responsible for the violent act.	Homophobia is internalized by repeated exposure to cultural and societal homophobia; homophobic violence may reinforce the patient's internalized beliefs that lesbianism is "abnormal, and therefore she deserves to be ostracized and punished."
Assist in identifying patient's existing strengths and constructive coping mechanisms.	Focusing on positive attributes may increase self-image.
Assist her to develop a plan of action to cope with potentially disabled feelings (e.g., rage, anxiety, hopelessness), including self-care and support-seeking activities.	Creating a plan of action reinforces one's ability to seek help and diminishes her sense of helplessness related to the ongoing recovery process.
If the traumatic event included sexual assault, initiate Rape Trauma Syndrome care plan.	

▼

NURSING DIAGNOSIS: DYSFUNCTIONAL GRIEVING

Related To social invalidation of primary relationship

Defining Characteristics
Prolonged denial and loss
Depression (normal grief work involves beginning to break ties with the lost person after 6 to 12 months)
Social isolation and withdrawal
Inability to express the impact of the loss
Interference with life functioning
Sadness/crying

Patient Outcomes

The patient will

- acknowledge the loss and express feelings associated with the loss (the patient may elect to do this verbally, in writing, through art, or other methods significant to her).
- identify ongoing strategies for constructively coping with the loss.
- identify future-oriented goals and strategies for achieving them.

Nursing Interventions	Rationales
Determine if the client has experienced a significant loss.	Older lesbians may have experienced extensive discrimination and rejections in every aspect of their lives and may therefore be especially secretive about their same-sex relationships.
Assess the extent of the patient's support system (e.g.: "After the loss of your [friend, partner, spouse use terms the patient uses to refer to her significant other], who helped you most?").	
Support the patient's dignity by demonstrating respect for the limits she places on self-disclosure.	
Demonstrate respect for the patient' significant relationship.	Same-sex life partnerships are seldom acknowledged or supported by legal, religious, or social systems; fear of rejection and ostracism may compel a lesbian to disguise her life-partnership with another woman as a less significant friendship. Heterosexism and homophobia thereby invalidate same-sex life-partnerships and compromise functional grieving of the loss of a life-partner. Recognizing these relationships affirms each partner's humanity and dignity.

Nursing Interventions	Rationales
Assist the patient to identify her strengths. Encourage the patient to identify positive aspects of the relationship. Assist the patient to identify the strengths of her support system.	Lesbians may have experienced rejection by their families of origin and subsequently created a "chosen family" of friends.
Avoid attempts to force the patient to move beyond denial before she is emotionally ready.	
Encourage participation of surviving loved ones in the process of grief and resolution.	Interacting with friends can help reduce feelings of isolation.
Teach the patient and her support person(s) the signs of pathological grieving (prolonged depression, isolation, delusions, extreme hostility, self-destructive behavior).	
Teach the patient and her support person(s) the signs of resolution of grief (movement from past-oriented to present-oriented thinking, reinvolvement with her community, seeking new relationships, expression of future-oriented goals.)	This provides the patient with hope that she will be able to reach this stage.
Provide information about appropriate community-based support programs for gay men and lesbians.	Groups that come together for mutual support and information can be beneficial. However, be aware that many support groups for widows may compound dysfunctional grieving by not acknowledging life-partnerships between women.

▼

NURSING DIAGNOSIS: INEFFECTIVE FAMILY COPING— DISABLING

Related To domestic abuse/battering

Defining Characteristics

The patient relates experiences of physical, spiritual, emotional, financial, or sexual abuse.

Expresses concerns that suggest abuse has occurred: "It's not safe to go home." "I need help."

Relates a history of domestic abuse or coercion: physical assaults/threats

Control of one partner's finances or ability to work by another partner

Deprivation of food, heat, sleep, or medical care

Threats against children, friends, pets

Emotional abuse: humiliation, isolation

Homophobic abuse: threatening to tell employers, family, landlord, police, etc. that the patient is a lesbian, threatening her that no one will believe she is battered because no one believes that lesbians batter each other

Exhibits signs of trauma inconsistent with normal injuries, or inconsistent with history given (e.g., bruises, welts, scars, burns, fractures, dislocations, genital trauma)

Reports chronic somatic complaints (e.g., insomnia, headaches, gastrointestinal distress, dyspnea, fatigue, depression, pelvic, back, or chest pain)

Patient Outcomes

Patient will

- acknowledge the fact of coercion and abuse in her relationship.
- identify resources available when help is desired.
- formulate a plan of action to follow when help is desired (a safety plan).

Nursing Interventions	Rationales
Evaluate actual or potential danger to the patient (e.g., Is the batterer with her in the office or waiting room?). Evaluate actual or potential danger to the patient's children or to the batterer's children.	Professional help may be required to protect patient and significant other.
Determine what the patient identifies as her primary need at this time.	Such knowledge guides/prioritizes action plan.
Assess for factors that inhibit the patient from seeking help (e.g., knowledge deficit regarding legal options and services available, fear of reprisal by the batterer, fear of homophobic response from service providers, hopelessness).	Depending on the cause, a variety of strategies may be required.

Nursing Interventions	Rationales
Assess the extent to which drugs and alcohol compromise the patient's coping mechanisms.	Many battered women experience problems with substance abuse, which may include prescription drugs as well as alcohol and illicit drugs. The batterer's use of drugs and alcohol further complicates the problem and increases the danger.
Assess for thoughts of hurting or killing herself or another person.	Patients with suicidal/homicidal thoughts must be assessed for potential risk, and referred for professional help if the risk is high.
Assess for history of victimization (e.g., child abuse, incest, rape, assault by strangers, previous battering relationships).	Information guides development of treatment plan.
Assess knowledge of personal and community resources.	
Be aware of any personal and cultural homophobia staff may bring to their work as health care providers. Educate staff about the realities of battering in lesbian relationships.	Homophobic and heterosexist judgments and stereotypes, when enacted by health care providers, constitute a form of abuse and perpetuate the cycle of oppression and violence. Research indicates that the incidence of domestic abuse in same-sex relationships is proportionate per population to that of domestic abuse in opposite-sex relationships.
Obtain the caller's name, if contact is made by telephone, as well as the phone number and address from which she is calling, and be prepared to call the police to intervene if she is assaulted during the phone call.	The act of calling for help may increase the possibility of assault.
If the batterer has accompanied the patient to the office, attempt to see the victim alone (such attempts may involve accompanying to the bathroom to "obtain a urine specimen").	Private setting facilitates disclosure.

Nursing Interventions	Rationales
Carefully document, with diagrams, the nature and extent of physical harm inflicted.	This information is needed for legal purposes and to guide medical treatment.
Obtain information about the history of abuse. If time constraints keep you from obtaining a full history, obtain information about the first, last, and worst episodes of abuse.	This provides information about the pattern of abuse.
Inform the patient clearly and directly why you are seeking this information—that it can be used to help her plan for her safety.	
Respect the patient's right to refuse to answer certain questions, explaining the ways in which specific information may be used to help her.	
Avoid questioning that perpetuates blaming the victim.	Domestic abuse is not a relationship problem and cannot be addressed in terms of codependency; it is always an act of coercion and violence by the batterer.
Reinforce the realities: 1. Violence is not normal. 2. The victim is not responsible for the violence, no matter what her actions were prior to or during the episode of abuse. 3. Violence in relationships usually escalates.	
Encourage decision-making, informing the patient of options, but respecting her own process of decision-making.	Most battered women have made many attempts to improve their situation; as violence escalates, they may become discouraged and despair of being able to help themselves. The patient may not feel capable of using resources at the time they are presented. Remember that the act of seeking help is significant and pattern-breaking in itself.

Nursing Interventions	**Rationales**
Help the patient to create a safety plan, including what she can do to protect herself and her children when she feels a violent episode is imminent and during a violent episode, and a detailed plan of escape, including a list of the items she will need to be safe and comfortable and a safe location to keep them so they will be accessible to her during an escape. Encourage the client to record information about shelters carefully.	The discovery of information about shelters, etc. may endanger the victim. She may need to record this information under headings that are innocuous, but meaningful to her.
Maintain confidentiality at all times. Never disclose information without her permission.	

▼

DISCHARGE PLANNING/CONTINUITY OF CARE

- Provide information on organizations that offer support and advocacy services for lesbians and gay men.
- Provide resources for both emergency and long-term assistance, including one that is available 24 hours a day.
- Provide information on community resources, support groups, information networks for people with herpes and for women with acquired immunodeficiency syndrome (AIDS).
- For additional information and support write to:
  - National Clearinghouse on Domestic Violence, Post Office Box 2309, Rockville, Maryland 28052.
  - National Organization for Victim Assistance (NOCA), 717 D Street, NW, Suite 200, Washington, D.C. 20004.

REFERENCES

Devey, S. (1990). Assessing patient's special needs: Lesbian women. *Journal of Gerontological Nursing, 16*(5), 38.

Hitchcock, J. M. & Wilson, H. S. (1992). Personal risking: Lesbian self-disclosure of sexual orientation to professional health care providers. *Nursing Research, 41*(3), 178–183.

Lynch, M. (1993). When the patient is also a lesbian. *AWHONN's Clinical Issues in Perinatal and Women's Health Nursing, 4*(2), 196–202.

Trippet, S. E. & Bain, J. (1992). Reasons American lesbians fail to seek traditional health care. *Health Care for Women International, 13*(2), 145–153.

Zeidenstein, L. (1990). Gynecological and childbearing needs of lesbians. *Journal of Nurse-Midwifery, 35*(1), 10–18.

$\mathcal{M}$ASTECTOMY

Mary Ann Krol, RN, MSN

$\mathbf{M}$astectomy is the surgical removal of the breast. The standard intervention has been the modified radical, in which the entire breast, axillary nodes, and pectoralis minor muscle is removed. Recent clinical trials in patients with early breast cancer have demonstrated similar survival with breast-conserving procedures (i.e., tylectomy, lumpectomy, partial mastectomy, quandrantectomy, and segmented mastectomy) with axillary node dissection and follow-up radiation therapy.

INDICATION

Treatment of breast cancer

▼

NURSING DIAGNOSIS: HIGH RISK FOR INJURY—IMMEDIATE POSTOPERATIVE COMPLICATIONS

Risk Factors
- Breast amputation
- Surgical technique

Patient Outcomes
Postoperative complications will be recognized and reported for appropriate intervention.

Nursing Interventions	Rationales
Hemorrhage Observe wound for hematoma, ecchymosis in skin flaps, and bloody drainage from suction catheters.	Bleeding may occur in the first few hours if a vessel is left untied.

Nursing Interventions	Rationales
Notify surgeon of signs of hemorrhage.	
Prepare patient for wound exploration.	
Seroma formation Assess for seroma formation: fluid collection under the skin flap.	Seroma formation is the most common complication following mastectomy. Anatomic factors favoring fluid collection include large potential dead space, transection of lymphatic channels, respiratory movement in operative site.
Maintain proper suction on catheter; milk catheters as ordered.	
Document amount and character of drainage; report plugging of catheters to surgeon.	
Restrict excessive use of arm until drains are removed.	Suction tubes are usually removed in 3–5 days or when drainage is less than 25 ml in 24 hours.
Instruct patient to report any bulging under the skin flaps to surgeon.	
Skin flap necrosis Observe wound for darkened edges, drainage.	Skin flap necrosis may occur in 10–61% of mastectomy patients. It occurs more frequently in vertical incisions. It is caused by inadequate blood supply to the flap.
Report signs of flap necrosis to surgeon.	

▼

NURSING DIAGNOSIS: HIGH RISK FOR INFECTION

Risk Factors
- Inadequate primary defenses:
  - (broken skin
  - traumatized tissue
  - presence of lymph fluid under skin flaps
- Invasive procedure

Patient Outcomes

Infection potential will be reduced through good aseptic technique and patient teaching.

Nursing Interventions	Rationales
Observe for signs of infection in immediate postoperative period.	Wound infections occur in 5–14% of mastectomy patients.
Use sterile technique in dressing changes and emptying suction apparatus.	
Instruct patients being discharged with catheters of sterile technique in emptying the vacuum apparatus.	
Instruct patient to observe wound for signs of infection.	

NURSING DIAGNOSIS: ACUTE PAIN

Related To
- Breast amputation
- Surgical incision
- Limited mobility of arm

Defining Characteristics

Verbal pain report
Nonverbal cues

Patient Outcomes

Patient will
- verbalize relief or ability to cope with existing level.
- appear relaxed and comfortable.

Nursing Interventions	Rationales
Assess pain characteristics.	
Assess for signs of wound complications that may be contributing to pain.	Hematoma, skin flap necrosis, and infection can result in pain/discomfort.

Nursing Interventions	Rationales
Administer pain medications as required.	Postoperative pain is generally controlled by oral analgesics after the first or second postoperative day.
Position affected arm for comfort: elevate on pillows with hand higher than elbow.	This prevents tension on suture line and promotes lymph drainage.
Splint chest and support arm during coughing and deep breathing.	

NURSING DIAGNOSIS: CHRONIC PAIN

Related To
- Neuroma formation
- Nerve compression
- Phantom sensations

Defining Characteristics

Verbal report of pain

Pain described as tight, constricting, burning in the posterior aspect of the arm/axilla and radiating across the anterior chest wall.

Sensations of numbness, paresthesia, weakness in the affected arm.

Phantom pain: sensations in the area of amputated breast.

Patient Outcomes

Patient will
- express pain relief or ability to cope with pain/discomfort.
- express understanding concerning phantom breast sensations.
- utilize effective pain interventions/or will have appropriate referrals for treatment of pain.

Nursing Interventions	Rationales
Assess for painful sensations in the posterior arm, axilla, and anterior chest wall.	Postmastectomy pain syndrome, which occurs in 4–6% of patients, is caused by traumatic neuroma formation at the site of the sectioned intercostobrachial nerve. The pain may occur immediately or as late as 6 months following surgery. Pain may be exacerbated by movement and relieved by immobilization.

Nursing Interventions	Rationales
Instruct patient of diminished axillary sweating and numbness in the posterior aspect of the upper arm.	These changes are secondary to dissection of nerves during the surgical procedure.
Warn patient to use any heat applications cautiously.	Diminished sensation in area can easily result in burns when heat is applied.
Refer patient to physician for appropriate therapy.	Physical therapy, local trigger point injections, and medication may be required to control pain.
Assess for symptoms of numbness, parasthesias, and weakness in affected arm.	Mastectomy patients may develop brachial plexus compression and carpal tunnel syndrome in the presence of lymphedema and/or following radiation.
Refer to physician for appropriate diagnostic studies and interventions.	Differentiating the cause of nerve compression, e.g., lymphedema, radiation fibrosis, or tumor recurrence, may be difficult and require a neurological examination, scans, electromyography, and/or x-rays. Surgical release of compressed nerves may be considered.
Assess for phantom breast pain, e.g., pins and needles, twinges, itches, heaviness sensation in area of amputated breast.	Phantom breast sensations are largely unreported. Most are noticed in the first few weeks of surgery. Phantom breast syndrome may be painful for some women. It occurs more often in younger women who experienced pain prior to surgery. Pain can be provoked by environmental stimuli, e.g., touch, clothes, weather. It is not related to postoperative complications.
Reassure the patient that phantom sensations are not uncommon and do not indicate tumor recurrence or psychological abnormality.	Phantom breast sensations occur in 10–94% of mastectomy patients.
Instruct patient to use rest, touch, or heat to relieve the phantom breast pain.	

▼

NURSING DIAGNOSIS: IMPAIRED PHYSICAL MOBILITY IN AFFECTED SHOULDER

Related To
- Surgical procedure
- Radiation fibrosis
- Axillary contracture secondary to wound infection, necrosis, or seroma
- Postoperative pain
- Nerve damage secondary to operative procedure
- Formation of adhesions in skin flap

Defining Characteristics
Inability to move shoulder through preoperative range of motion

Patient Outcomes
Patient will
- demonstrate pain-free range of motion with affected arm and shoulder.
- regain preoperative level of function in affected arm/shoulder.

Nursing Interventions	Rationales
Assess range of motion in abduction, forward flexion, extension, and rotation of affected shoulder at each postoperative visit.	
Assess for factors that impair shoulder mobility.	Nerve damage to the medial and lateral pectoral nerves produce pectoral denervation and muscular atrophy, causing a chest depression similar to a radical mastectomy. Injury to the thoracordorsal nerve causes weakness in abduction and internal rotation. Injury to the long thoracic nerve causes weakness in the serratus anterior muscle, resulting in a winged scapula and functional impairment in reaching.
Encourage the patient to perform simple activities of daily living immediately postoperatively.	

Nursing Interventions	Rationales
Consult with the surgeon as to when range of motion exercises should begin.	Patients with skin grafts, wound necrosis, infection, or seromas may be delayed in starting exercises. A controversy exists whether to start exercises on the first or seventh postoperative day.

Teach the patient the following exercises to improve affected shoulder motion.
1. Forward Flexion
    • Bring affected arm forward and raise overhead.
2. Abduction/External Rotation
    • Raise arm sideways to shoulder level. Place hand on back of head and move elbow back as far as possible.
3. Extension/Internal Rotation
    • Bring arm backward, touch lower aspect of opposite scapula with fingers.
4. Wall Climbing
    • Stand with affected arm facing wall. Slowly move the fingertips up the wall until the highest point is reached. (The wall mark should be made doing the same exercise with the unaffected arm.)
	Range of motion exercises relax the muscles and promote joint motion.

Encourage the patient to do the exercises diligently 4–6 times a day.	
Add additional exercises as indicated (See Reach to Recovery booklet).	Patients generally can recover preoperative range of motion in 4–6 weeks).
Refer patients complaining of unusual pain to the physician to be evaluated for muscle spasms or myositis.	
Inform patients to continue exercises through their lifetime, especially those who have had radiation therapy.	

▼

NURSING DIAGNOSIS: HIGH RISK FOR INJURY— LYMPHEDEMA/INFECTION

Risk Factors
- Mastectomy
- Axillary dissection
- Scar formation secondary to radiation treatment
- Infection
- Delayed wound healing
- Obesity

Patient Outcomes
Patient will verbalize understanding of the rationale for
- prevention of infection
- treatment of minor injuries to the affected arm
- lifetime risk related to infection in the affected arm

Nursing Interventions	Rationales
Measure both arms at 3 points and record at each follow-up visit. Measure at 6 cm below and above the olecranon process, and 6 cm above ulnar wrist styloid. Record increase in arm measurements as: mild: 1.5–3 cm; moderate: 3–5 cm; or severe: >5 cm.	Excision of the axillary lymph nodes and channels cause edema formation in the first 4–6 weeks after surgery. Resolution of this edema occurs as new lymphatic channels are formed.
Instruct patient to report any arm swelling for possible antibiotic treatment.	The presence of lymphedema predisposes the patient to further infection because lymph is an ideal culture medium in the edematous arm; slight injury produces a serious risk for infection.
Anticipate additional treatment: arm elevation, isometric exercise, diuretics, compression sleeves, and pneumatic massage or surgical procedures.	

Nursing Interventions	Rationales
Teach patient to prevent infection in the affected arm. 1. Avoid pulling on nail cuticles, use liquid cuticle remover. 2. Avoid underarm shaving with a razor, use depilatory or electric razor. 3. Avoid cuts, burns, and insect bites, use gloves when using tools or working in the garden, use a thimble for sewing. 4. Avoid venipuncture or injections. 5. Avoid sunburn.	Since intact skin is the primary defense mechanism against entry of bacteria, all activities that may cause breakage in the skin continuity should be avoided.
Teach patient to prevent unnecessary constriction on the affected arm. Avoid tight wrist bands, carrying heavy objects, purses, packages. Avoid blood pressure measurement on the affected arm.	Constriction can facilitate lymphedema.
Teach patient to cleanse any skin breaks with soap and water, and to observe for signs of infection. If signs of infection appear, the physician should be notified.	
Teach patient that the risk of infection extends through the patient's lifetime.	It is generally believed that infection is a major factor in the development of lymphedema.

▼

NURSING DIAGNOSIS: KNOWLEDGE DEFICIT REGARDING BREAST HEALTH AND CANCER SURVEILLANCE

Related To lack of previous experience

Defining Characteristics
Many questions
Misconceptions
Lack of questions

Patient Outcome

Patient will verbalize knowledge of follow-up care guidelines.

Nursing Interventions	Rationales
Assess patient's knowledge regarding breast health and follow-up care.	
Instruct patient regarding:	
1. breast self-examination on remaining breast and palpation of mastectomy scar 2. lifetime medical follow-up for breast examination and mammogram 3. importance of female family members to follow guidelines for breast self-examination and mammography 4. follow-up with medical and radiation oncology, depending on nodal status	Early detection can facilitate early treatment and—it is hoped—improved prognosis.

▼

NURSING DIAGNOSIS: BODY IMAGE DISTURBANCE

Related To
• Breast amputation
• Psychosocial and cultural factors related to breast and femininity

Defining Characteristics

Verbal identification
Refusal to look at incision
Preoccupation with loss of breast
Expressed fears of intimacy and rejection by sexual partner
Verbalization of sexual concerns

Patient Outcomes

Patient will utilize appropriate resources to cope with body image change and sexuality issues.

Nursing Interventions	Rationales
Assess perceived impact of change on relationships and roles.	
Encourage verbalization of feelings.	
Acknowledge normalcy of responses.	
Help patient identify specific concerns and methods of coping with body image.	Anxiety and depressive moods are found in approximately 25% of women following modified radical mastectomy. Social support has been found to favorably influence a woman's adjustment to breast cancer.
Assess perception of impact of breast amputation on sexual functioning.	Negative feelings about surgery, incision, and loss of femininity can significantly affect one's interest in sexual relationships.
Provide information on resumption of sexual activity.	Physically, patients should be able to achieve sexual satisfaction. If psychological barriers exist, appropriate professional referral should be discussed.
Advise patient regarding prosthesis. 1. Soft prosthesis can be worn immediately. 2. Weighted (silicone) prosthesis can be worn 4–6 weeks after wound is healed. 3. List shops where prosthesis can be purchased. 4. Shop with a friend and compare prices and goods.	Women gain both psychological and physical benefits from wearing of prosthesis. Health professionals and cancer consultants can guide patient in appropriate selection.
Encourage patient to talk to the surgeon about breast reconstruction if she is interested.	Reconstructive surgery may improve patient's self-image and assist her in coping with the deformity of mastectomy.

▼

DISCHARGE PLANNING/CONTINUITY OF CARE

- Refer to Reach for Recovery for information and emotional support.
- Refer patients who are noncompliant or having difficulty with range of motion exercises to physical therapy before they develop a frozen shoulder.
- Inform patients of any available exercise programs in the community for mastectomy patients.
- Refer for sexual counseling if appropriate.
- Refer for counseling or psychiatric service if appropriate.

REFERENCES

Colley, M. E. & Erickson, B. (1991). Rehabilitation. In Fowble, B., Goodman, R. L., Glick, J. H., Rosato, E. F. (Eds.). *Breast Cancer Treatment: A Comprehensive Guide to Management.* St. Louis, MO: Mosby-Year Book.

Ganz, P. A., Schag, A. C., Lee, J. J., Polinsky, M. L., & Tan, S. J. (1992). Breast conservation versus mastectomy: Is there a difference in psychological adjustment or quality of life in the year after surgery? *Cancer*, 69(7), 1729–1738.

Nelson, J. P. (1991). Perceived health, self-esteem, health habits, and perceived benefits and barriers to exercise in women who have and who have not experienced stage I breast cancer. *Oncology Nursing Forum*, 18(7), 1191–1197.

Pozo, C., Carver, C., Noriega, V., Harris, S., Robinson D., et al. (1992). Effects of mastectomy versus lumpectomy on emotional adjustment to breast cancer: A prospective study of the first year postsurgery. *Journal of Clinical Oncology*, 10(8), 1292–1298.

▼

$\mathcal{M}$ENOPAUSE

Meg Gulanick, RN, PhD

Menopause is the time in a woman's life when menstrual periods cease. The average age for menopause is 51 years. The way a woman responds physically and emotionally to menopause varies greatly.

ETIOLOGY

Reduced estrogen production

CLINICAL MANIFESTATIONS

- Cessation of menstrual periods
- Hot flushes/vasomotor symptoms
- Atrophy of vaginal epithelium
- Emotional lability

DIAGNOSTIC FINDINGS

- Increased FSH levels (follicle-stimulating hormone)
- Increased LH levels (luteinizing hormone)

▼

NURSING DIAGNOSIS: KNOWLEDGE DEFICIT

Related To unfamiliarity with process

Defining Characteristics
Many questions
Lack of questions
Verbalized misconceptions

216

Patient Outcomes

Patient will

- describe common clinical manifestations seen during menopause.
- discuss the benefits and disadvantages of hormone replacement therapy (HRT).
- explain dosing schedule and follow-up care associated with hormone replacement therapy, if prescribed for her.

Nursing Interventions	Rationales
Assess knowledge of menopause: physiology, clinical manifestations, management.	Most women have no current information about menopause. Myths and misconceptions abound. Knowledge may improve acceptance of change and compliance with treatment regimen.
Clarify terminology associated with menopause: 1. natural menopause 2. artificially induced menopause 3. climacteric (perimenopause) 4. amenorrhea 5. hormone replacement therapy.	
Provide information on tests for menopause: 1. follicle-stimulating hormone (FSH) 2. leuteinizing hormone (LH)	FSH and LH are responsible for ovulation. Elevated FSH and LH in the presence of low estrogen indicates menopause.
Describe clinical manifestations commonly experienced during menopause.	Type and duration of symptoms vary greatly among women. Usually symptoms are more pronounced if menopause occurred suddenly, as with surgical removal of ovaries:

Nursing Interventions	Rationales
1. hot flushes • intense feeling of heat experienced above waist, especially head and neck • attributed to the effect changes in estrogen levels have on hypothalmus • usually last a few minutes, but can last an hour • may occur for a few months or years 2. dry vaginal tissue • decline in estrogen causes vaginal atrophy • vaginal tissue becomes thinner, easily irritated, and infected 3. change in sleep pattern (often related to hot flushes at night) 4. emotional lability (may include crying, depression, loss of libido)	
Explain use of hormone replacement therapy: HRT is the use of estrogen- and progesterone-containing drugs to replace the hormones which are no longer produced by the ovaries during and after menopause.	Enthusiasm for replacement therapy has undergone periodic shifts over the past 4 decades. Initially it was prescribed "to maintain youth." Then concerns over an increased risk of uterine cancer reduced its popularity. Today better dosing of estrogen with the addition of progesterone has reduced the risk for uterine cancer and provides menopausal symptom relief and protection against osteoporosis and heart disease.
Clarify the advantages and disadvantages of hormone replacement.	Women must make an informed decision regarding hormone replacement. The benefits and risks must be weighed against each woman's needs.

Nursing Interventions	**Rationales**
1. Advantages include • relief of hot flushes (estrogen may be used only short-term while symptoms are present • treatment for vaginal atrophy • strengthening of bones; protection against osteoporosis • reduction in coronary artery disease risk • protects against loss of breast tissue, muscle tone (especially vaginal support of the bladder) • improves memory, reduces mood swings and insomnia	 Women have one chance in four of developing osteoporosis without hormone replacement. Some women are at even higher risk. Heart disease is responsible for 10 times more deaths in postmenopausal women than breast cancer. Estrogen decreases atherogenic low-density lipoproteins (LDLs) and increases the protective high-density lipoproteins (HDLs). Research is ongoing to determine the optimal dose/combination to achieve best effect.
2. Disadvantages/side effects of hormone replacement therapy: • breast tenderness • bloating/fluid retention • nausea • acne • increased blood pressure • blood clotting disorder (through not common since estrogen dose is less than that of birth control pills) • stimulates breast cancer that is already present. • increases risk of uterine cancer if high-dose estrogen is given alone (unopposed by progesterone)	

Nursing Interventions	Rationales
Describe types of hormone therapy available:	
1. estrogen plus progesterone • drugs prescribed separately, not combined as in birth control pills	Progesterone provides protection against uterine cancer; however, it does *lower* the protective HDL cholesterol, thereby negating some of the positive effects of estrogen on reducing coronary artery disease risk.
• used for women with intact uterus.	
• have breakthrough bleeding 2–3 days after last dose of progesterone (mimics period)	The addition of progestin during the last part of the estrogen cycle causes shedding of the endometrius, thereby preventing endometrial hyperplasia.
2. estrogen alone • oral—several doses/schedules exist. • cream—approved only for vaginal atrophy • transdermal patch—has reduced side effects; helps prevent osteoporosis, but may not have cardioprotective effect, since it bypasses the liver • estrogen implant—newest technique being researched.	Low-dose estrogen is used to relieve assorted symptoms. Indicated for women post-hysterectomy who do not need progesterone protective effect on uterus:
Describe length of time hormone replacement therapy is indicated. 1. short-term to only relieve symptoms 2. long-term/lifetime to protect against osteoporosis and heart disease.	Length of time for HRT is still controversial. Research needs to continue.

Nursing Interventions	Rationales
Provide information on necessary follow-up if on replacement therapy:	
1. endometrial biopsy	Vaginal bleeding may also be caused by endometrial cancer.
2. cholesterol screening	Women postmenopause are at greater risk of heart disease.
3. mammogram	This is necessary to screen for breast cancer.
Clarify when estrogen therapy is contraindicated: 1. history of breast or uterine cancer 2. estrogen-dependent neoplasia 3. positive family history 4. hypertension (estrogen may increase blood pressure) 5. unexplained or abnormal vaginal bleeding 6. liver dysfunction 7. history of blood clots related to birth control pills NOTE: History of thrombus formation without use of birth control pills is *not* an absolute contraindication and needs to be discussed.	
Instruct patient in self-help measures to reduce problems associated with menopause: 1. aerobic exercise routine for 30 minutes three times a week 2. diet that includes 1500 mg/day of calcium or calcium supplements	

▼

NURSING DIAGNOSIS: BODY IMAGE DISTURBANCE

Related To
- Permanent alteration in body function
- Side effects of hormone replacement therapy

Defining Characteristics

Changes in reproductive ability
Negative feelings about body
Preoccupation with change
Frustration with symptoms, such as hot flushes, fluid retention, vaginal
    dryness, increased facial hair growth
Changes in social behaviors

Patient Outcomes

Patient will
- verbalize beginning acceptance of bodily changes.
- speak of self in positive way, noting the strong qualities she has as a
  mature women.

Nursing Interventions	Rationales
Assess perception of change in body function.	The extent of the response is more related to the value the woman puts on her reproductive ability or body function than to the *actual* value or importance.
Assist patient to identify specific concerns regarding her body changes.	Loss of reproductive ability is directly related to menopause. However, much apprehension about menopause is related to fear of *aging*. Other body changes such as graying of hair, weight gain, and facial hair may signify signs of aging.
Acknowledge the normalcy of the patient's emotional response to menopause.	Women are used to being in control of their environments; it is difficult to cope with the loss of control that menopause poses. Also, cultural stereotypes have often characterized menopausal women as incapacitated by "raging hormones," or no longer being a "functional woman." This image certainly would not be one to look forward to. In addition, aging itself is accompanied by negative images.
Emphasize that menopause is an important physical and emotional life transition, which can lead to a very satisfying period of life.	Most women live one-third of their life postmenopause. The quality of life is important.

Nursing Interventions	Rationales
Encourage the use of support groups.	Networks of women support groups can provide important emotional support as well as valuable personal information about body change.

▼

NURSING DIAGNOSIS: HIGH RISK FOR ALTERED SEXUALITY PATTERNS

Risk Factors
- Painful intercourse
- Depression
- Body image disturbances
- Change in hormone levels
- Aging

Patient Outcomes
Patient will
- verbalize contentment/satisfaction with social/sexual relationships.
- list resources available to help her cope with any sexual difficulties she may experience, as well as menopause and aging.

Nursing Interventions	Rationales
Assess premenopausal pattern of sexual functioning.	Determination provides baseline for evaluating change.
Inquire as to woman's current interest in sexual activity.	Women live one-third of their lives after menopause; some can be sexually active in their 70s and 80s. Many women are more interested in sex at this time because they no longer fear pregnancy, have more time for their own interests and pleasures, may be newly married in later years. In contrast, some women experience pain during intercourse and lose interest.
Assess for presence of spouse/male significant other in woman's life.	Many women would like to be sexually active; however, as women age there are fewer men in their age group.

Nursing Interventions	Rationales
If sexually active, determine whether she needs to use a form of birth control.	Birth control is recommended until one year has passed since the last period. Birth control pills and IUDs are not recommended for midlife women.
Determine if the sexually active patient is experiencing pain/discomfort during intercourse. If so, provide information on water-soluble jelly or estrogen creams that can provide lubrication. Reassure her that frequent sexual activity will also increase lubrication.	Dyspareunia is caused by dry vaginal tissues secondary to estrogen depletion.
Discuss both physiological and emotional influences on sexual functioning.	Changes in a woman's reproductive ability frequently challenges her concept of her femininity. Common stereotypes devalue postmenopausal women.
Explain that the usual functions can continue unchanged for most women.	
Evaluate woman's/couple's interest in/conflict with other means of sexual expression besides intercourse.	Alternate approaches for intimacy such as touching, closeness, warmth, and sensitivity can be romantic and sexually satisfying for many.

▼

DISCHARGE PLANNING/CONTINUITY OF CARE

- Refer to gynecologist.
- Refer to psychiatric/women's health professional.
- Refer to single/widowed/seniors' group.
- Provide written materials on menopause.
- Refer to dietitian for calcium-rich diet planning.
- Refer to exercise program.

REFERENCES

Cook, M. (1993). Perimenopause: An opportunity for health promotion. *Journal of Obstetric Gynecologic and Neonatal Nursing, 22*(3), 223–228.

Dickson, G. (1990). A feminist poststructural analysis of the knowledge of menopause. *Advances in Nursing Science, 12*(3), 15–31.

Holm, K., Penckofer, S., Keresztes, P., Biordi, D., & Chandler, P. (1993). Coronary artery disease in women: assessment, diagnosis, intervention, and strategies for life style changes. *AWHONN's Clinical Issues in Perinatal and Women's Health Nursing, 4*(2), 272–285.

Lichtman, R. (1991). Perimenopausal hormone replacement therapy: Review of the literature. *Journal of Nurse-Midwifery, 36*(1), 30–48.

MacPherson, K. (1993). Cardiovascular disease prevention in women and the human debate. *AWHONN's Clinical Issues in Perinatal and Women's Health Nursing, 4*(2), 244–249

McCraw, R. K. (1991). Psychosexual changes associated with the perimenopausal period. *Journal of Nurse-Midwifery, 36*(1), 17–24.

Philosophe, R. & Seibel, M. M. (1991). Menopause and cardiovascular disease. *NAACOG's Clinical Issues in Perinatal and Women's Health Nursing, 2*(4), 441–451.

Quinn, A. A. (1991). A theoretical model of the perimenopausal process. *Journal of Nurse-Midwifery, 36*(1) 25–29.

Rickert, B. (1992). Estrogen replacement, Making informed choices. *R.N., 55*(9), 26–32.

Sheehy, G. (1992). *Silent Passage: Menopause.* New York: Random House.

▼

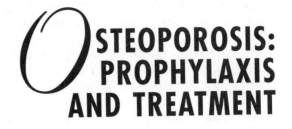

OSTEOPOROSIS: PROPHYLAXIS AND TREATMENT

Meg Gulanick, RN, PhD

Osteoporosis is a disease characterized by low bone mass, deterioration of bone tissue, and a consequent increased risk of fracture.

ETIOLOGIES

- Female gender
- Increasing age
- White and Asian races
- Estrogen deficiency
- Inadequate calcium intake
- Early menopause
- Family history
- Excessive exercise, when accompanied by amenorrhea
- Prolonged immobility
- Cigarette smoking
- Excessive alcohol/caffeine use
- Sedentary lifestyle
- Diseases such as
  - increased exposure to or use of glucocorticoids
  - hyperthyroidism
  - primary hyperparathyroidism
  - multiple myeloma

CLINICAL MANIFESTATIONS

- Back pain
- Spontaneous fractures

DIAGNOSTIC FINDINGS

Positive bone mass studies

▼

NURSING DIAGNOSIS: KNOWLEDGE DEFICIT REGARDING CAUSES OF AND DIAGNOSTIC PROCEDURE FOR OSTEOPOROSIS

Related To unfamiliarity with disease process

Defining Characteristics
Many questions
Lack of questions
Misconceptions

Patient Outcomes
Patient will state causes/diagnostic process for osteoporosis.

Nursing Interventions	Rationales
Assess knowledge of causes and diagnostic process for osteoporosis.	
Provide information on osteoporosis statistics: 1. major cause of fractures in postmenopausal women 2. more prevalent today because people are living longer	
Provide information on causes/risk factors for osteoporosis: 1. Estrogen deficiency is main cause of rapid bone loss in postmenopausal women. 2. An early menopause will aggravate the condition. 3. Premenopausal estrogen deficiency contributes to bone loss. 4. Risk factors also include • inadequate calcium intake • Caucasian and Asian females • lack of physical activity • cigarette and alcohol use	Genetic, endocrine, and lifestyle factors contribute to osteoporosis—but further research is needed.

Nursing Interventions

Inform patient that diagnosis is difficult:
1. undetectable on x-rays before >25–40% of bone calcium is lost
2. bone density measurement more accurate:
   - single photon absorptiometry (SPA): uses low-dose radiation scanner, useful to assess bone mass in peripheral skeleton
   - dual photon absorptiometry (DPA): allows scanning of thicker body parts (spine/hip)
   - computerized tomography scan (CT): used for total bone density, especially spine
3. biochemical assessment.

Explain that, although osteoporosis occurs throughout skeletal body, fractures/problems are more evident in the spine, hips, and wrists.

Rationales

Bone mass measurements are required for accurate evaluation of fracture risk. Biochemical assessments, such as serum osteocalcin, are sensitive markers of osteoblastic activity.

NURSING DIAGNOSIS: HEALTH-SEEKING BEHAVIORS

Related To understanding of high incidence of disease in women

Defining Characteristics
Desire for information
Unfamiliarity with information resources
Desire for increased control of health practice

Patient Outcomes
Patient will describe
- why women have higher incidence of disease.
- prevention/treatment regimen for osteoporosis, which may include calcium supplements, medication, physical activity.

Nursing Interventions	Rationales
Provide information on why osteoporosis is more prevalent among women: 1. Women have less bone mass due to smaller physical size. 2. Women usually have lower calcium intake. 3. Reabsorption occurs at an earlier age; it accelerates during menopause. 4. Conditions such as breast-feeding and pregnancy can easily deplete calcium. 5. Women live longer than men.	Osteoporosis is eight times more common in women.
Provide information on sources of dietary calcium: 1. whole and skim milk 2. yogurt 3. ice cream 4. sardines with bones 5. salmon 6. spinach/mustard greens/turnip greens/broccoli 7. almonds/hazelnuts	Calcium supplements inhibit bone loss.
Provide information on medications that affect calcium supply/metabolism: 1. corticosteroids 2. caffeine 3. nicotine 4. tetracycline	These medications increase calcium excretion and bone wasting
Discuss need for calcium supplements (calcium tablets, calcium-rich antacids).	Adequate calcium intake is 1000 mg/day in premenopausal women, and 1500 mg/day postmenopause. However, a high calcium intake is not enough to counteract the effects of estrogen loss postmenopause.

Nursing Interventions	Rationales
Discuss standard therapies to prevent and treat osteoporosis.	
1. estrogen, as drug of choice	It reduces calcium excretion, thereby reducing bone loss to the whole skeleton. In postmenopausal osteoporosis, the results of estrogen therapy are most notable in the lumbar spine. The benefits persist as long as medication is taken.
2. estrogen combined with progesterone	This has the same effect on osteoporosis, but also reduces risk of endometrial cancer.
Discuss newer medical treatments for osteoporosis:	
1. inhibitors of bone resorption • calcitonin, given by injections or nasal sprays, an alternative to women who cannot/will not take estrogen • biphosphonates, given orally	
2. stimulators of bone formation • fluoride. • anabolic steroids • parathyroid hormone	This increases bone mass, but may decrease cortical bone density. It may not be effective in postmenstrual osteoporosis.
3. etidronate (Didronel) • newer agent under government investigation • not FDA-approved	
Explain the role of activity/exercise in preventing/treating osteoporosis:	
1. Weightbearing exercise, along with calcium intake, stimulates development and maintenance of bone mass.	
2. Physical activity helps prevent further bone loss.	Immobility contributes to bone loss.

Nursing Interventions	Rationales
3. Adaptive equipment such as a cane or a walker may be needed to support body weight for pain related to weightbearing. 4. Referral to physical therapy may be indicated.	
Explain need for protective steps for the elderly: 1. Remove environmental hazards to reduce risk of falls • remove throw rugs • use grab bars in bathroom 2. Wear corset to stabilize vertebral column. 3. Wear low, comfortable shoes.	Pathological fractures are a complication of osteoporosis. Hip fracture is the second most common factor in which women require long-term care.

▼

DISCHARGE PLANNING/CONTINUITY OF CARE

• Refer to dietitian for counseling as needed.
• Refer to physical therapist as needed.

REFERENCES

Ainsworth, B. (1993). Approaches to physical activity in women. *AWHONN's Clinical Issues in Perinatal and Women's Health Nursing*, 4(2), 302–310.

Bond, K. (1991). Osteoporosis. *NAACOG's Critical Issues in Perinatal and Women's Health Nursing*, 2(4), 497–508.

Christiansen, C. (1991). Consensus development conference: prophylaxis and treatment of osteoporosis. *American Journal of Medicine*, 90, 107–110.

Holm, K., Wilbur, J. E, Dan, A., Montgomery, A., Chandler, P., & Walker, J. (1993). Bone loss in mid-life women. *Journal of Women's Health*, 1(2), 131–135.

Ingram-Fogel, C. (1991). Nutrition and health patterns in midlife women. *NAACOG's Clinical Issues in Perinatal and Women's Health Nursing*, 2(4),509–525.

Lindsay, R. & Tohme, J. F. (1990). Estrogen treatment of patients with established postmenopausal osteoporosis. *Obstetrical Gynecology*, 76(2), 290–295.

Riggs, B. L., Hodgson, S. F., O'Fallon, W., Chao, E., Wohner, H., et al. (1990). Effect of fluoride treatment on the fracture rate in postmenopausal women with osteoporosis. *New England Journal of Medicine*, 322(12), 802–809.

Storm, T., Thamsborg, G., Steiniche, T., Genant, H. K., & Sorensen, O. H. (1990). Effect of intermittent cyclical etidronate therapy on bone mass and fracture rate in women with postmenopausal osteoporosis. *New England Journal of Medicine*, 322(18), 1265–1271.

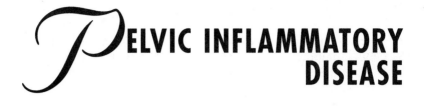

PELVIC INFLAMMATORY DISEASE

Janet L. Engstrom, RN, PhD, CNM

The term pelvic inflammatory disease (PID) is used to describe inflammation of the upper genital tract due to infection. The infection can occur in any or all of the organs of the upper genital tract (uterus, fallopian tubes, ovaries), and the infection can spread to the surrounding soft tissues and peritoneum as well as other abdominal organs.

ETIOLOGIES

Numerous anaerobic and aerobic organisms can infect the upper genital tract after exposure to the organism during intercourse, pelvic surgery, abortion, or childbirth. The infection is frequently a polymicrobial infection. Specific causative organisms are:
- *N. gonorrhoeae*
- *C. trachomatis*
- Streptococcus
- Group B Streptococcus
- Coagulase-negative Staphylococcus
- Bacteriodes
- Peptostreptococcus
- Peptococcus

CLINICAL MANIFESTATIONS

Symptoms vary according to the site of infection, the organism, and the stage of the infection.
- Fever
- Inflammation
- Lower abdominal tenderness or pain
- Vaginal discharge

DIAGNOSTIC FINDINGS

- Abdominal tenderness on exam
- Cervical motion tenderness and uterine tenderness on pelvic exam
- Temperature > 38°C
- Elevated white blood count (> 10,000 WBC/mm^3)
- Elevated erythrocyte sedimentation rate
- Elevated C-reactive protein
- Ultrasound evidence of pelvic abscess
- Laparoscopic evidence of purulent material or abscess
- Positive bacterial cultures

▼

NURSING DIAGNOSIS: HIGH RISK FOR INFECTION

Risk Factor
Exposure to pathogens

Patient Outcomes
Patient will
- manifest signs of treated/contained infection, as evidenced by absence of fever, inflammation, tenderness, pain, and vaginal discharge.
- verbalize precautionary measures to prevent spread of infection.

Nursing Interventions

Obtain a history of the patient's presenting symptoms:
1. pain
   - duration
   - intensity
   - location
   - character
2. urinary symptoms
   - dysuria
   - urgency
   - frequency
3. dysmenorrhea
4. dyspareunia
5. gastrointestinal disturbances
   - nausea
   - vomiting
6. rectal symptoms
   - pain
   - tenderness
   - burning
   - pressure
7. vaginal discharge
   - duration
   - color
   - amount
   - odor
8. genital lesions
   - location
   - color
   - size
   - exudate
   - pain
9. irregular vaginal bleeding
10. fever
11. chills

Obtain a sexual history; assess vital signs:
1. number of sexual partners
2. contraceptive methods used
3. history of any genitourinary infections in partner(s)

Rationales

This provides information as to the acuity and extent of the infection. Infection occurs in any part of the upper genital tract, which may spread to adjacent tissues and organs, the peritoneum, and the bloodstream. Infection of the upper genital tract, adjacent structures, and peritoneum could lead to long-term sequelae, such as tubal damage, tubal obstruction, and pelvic adhesions.

This provides information regarding behaviors that may increase the risk of a PID.

Nursing Interventions	Rationales
Obtain or assist with obtaining laboratory specimens as ordered: 1. cervical cultures for gonorrhea and chlamydia (if indicated) 2. cervical specimens for possible Gram stain 3. vaginal specimens for microscopic examination 4. blood specimens for white blood count with differential, erythrocyte sedimentation rate, and, possibly, C-reactive protein 5. blood specimen for quantitative beta-hCG if ectopic pregnancy is suspected 6. blood cultures if indicated	
Administer antibiotics as prescribed.	Immediate treatment reduces the possibility that the infection will spread to adjacent tissues and organs, the peritoneum, and the bloodstream.
Teach the patient how to use medication correctly including: 1. importance of completing the entire prescription 2. importance of taking medication on time 3. avoiding food products that may interfere with the absorption of the medications (e.g., if tetracycline is used, it should not be taken with dairy products)	The full course of antibiotic therapy should be completed correctly to reduce the possibility of inadequate treatment.
Teach the patient how to use and read a thermometer.	Temperature readings are important to evaluate response to treatment.

Nursing Interventions	Rationales
Teach the patient signs and symptoms of complicated PID and instruct the patient to call the health care provider immediately for: 1. pelvic pain 2. abdominal pain 3. elevated temperature 4. shaking chills 5. nausea 6. vomiting Provide the patient with a phone number for 24-hour emergency care.	Complicated cases of PID are managed on an inpatient basis with intravenous antibiotics.

▼

NURSING DIAGNOSIS: PAIN

Related To
- Inflammation and infection of the upper genital tract
- Examinations and diagnostic procedures

Defining Characteristics
Pain
Moaning/crying
Grimacing
Tensing muscles
Autonomic nervous system responses such as diaphoresis, changes in heart rate, blood pressure and respiratory rate, and pupillary dilatation

Patient Outcomes
Patient will
- verbalize comfort and pain relief.
- report any increase in the amount of pain to a healthcare provider.

Nursing Interventions	Rationales
Obtain and document vital signs.	
Ask the patient to describe any pain she was experiencing at home and at present.	Severe abdominal pain may require admission to the hospital.

Nursing Interventions	Rationales
Identify what coping strategies have been used, and determine whether these strategies are effective.	
Determine if the patient is able to learn new nonpharmacological coping strategies 1. relaxation 2. slow chest breathing	Learning new skills requires concentration, motivation, and energy. Factors such as pain or anxiety can impede learning.
Evaluate the efficacy of nonpharmacological pain-relieving strategies.	
Observe patient's verbal and non-verbal response to potentially painful procedures (e.g., pelvic examinations).	
Determine whether there are psychological factors that may contribute to her perception of pain (e.g., fear, anxiety, being alone during procedure). Whenever possible, allow a significant other to accompany the patient during the procedure if the patient desires company.	The company and support of a significant other may help alleviate loneliness, fear, and anxiety.
Eliminate factors that may contribute to her physical discomfort (e.g., make sure that the examination room is warm enough, the procedure table is as comfortable as possible with a pillow, her bladder is empty).	

▼

NURSING DIAGNOSIS: ALTERED SEXUALITY PATTERNS

Related To
- Recommendation for abstinence until the patient's symptoms have resolved and the patient and all of her sexual partners have completed treatment
- Recommendation to reduce the number of sexual partners for women who have multiple partners

- Recommendation to use condoms to prevent the transmission of sexually transmitted diseases

Defining Characteristics
Change in sexual behaviors and activities

Patient Outcomes
Patient will verbalize
- that she is abstaining from intercourse until her treatment is complete, her symptoms have resolved, and all sexual partners have been treated (if indicated).
- knowledge of other methods of achieving intimacy and sexual satisfaction without having intercourse or orgasm.
- knowledge of safe sex practices, including information about reducing the number of sexual partners and using condoms.

Nursing Interventions	Rationales
Obtain a sexual history to determine pretreatment sexual activity patterns, number of sexual partners, safe sex practices.	Multiple sex partners, or contact with untreated male partners increases risk of occurrence of PID.
Provide a private environment to discuss any aspect of sexual activity.	Most women are hesitant to discuss personal sexual matters. The proper setting may facilitate discussion.
Explain why sexual activity patterns need to be restricted during treatment for PID.	Prevent risk of reinfection from infected partner(s).
Offer suggestions for activities that meet the couple's need for contact and intimacy without having intercourse (e.g., hugging, kissing, massages).	Restrictions on sexual activity should not deprive the couple of other activities that convey the message that they are loved and desired nor should such restrictions deprive them of intimate physical contact.
Reassure the patient that the recommendation for abstinence is temporary.	Couples may find it easier to cope with restrictions if they see them as temporary.

Nursing Interventions	Rationales
Discuss the role of sexual activity in the transmission of PID and other sexually transmitted diseases. Offer information that can help the patient reduce her risk of PID (e.g., reduce the number of sexual partners, use condoms, have regular examinations for sexually transmitted diseases if she is not in a monogamous relationship).	

▼

NURSING DIAGNOSIS: KNOWLEDGE DEFICIT

Related To unfamiliarity with the causes, diagnostic procedures, treatment, and prevention of PID

Defining Characteristics
Need for more information
Multiple questions about the causes, diagnosis, treatment, and prevention
  of PID
Incorrect follow-through of instructions
Lack of compliance with treatment
Resistance to treatment
Statement of misconceptions and/or misunderstandings
Inappropriate or exaggerated behavior

Patient Outcomes
- Patient will describe how to obtain information and assistance from health care providers.
- Patient will verbalize correct information about the causes, diagnosis, treatment, and prevention of PID.
- Patient will describe signs and symptoms that need immediate evaluation by a health care professional.
- Patient's sexual partner(s) will receive appropriate treatment for sexually transmitted diseases.

Nursing Interventions	Rationales
Assess patient's knowledge of normal male and female reproductive anatomy and physiology.	

Nursing Interventions

Assess patient's knowledge of the causes, diagnosis, treatment, and prevention of PID.

Provide the following information:
1. normal reproductive anatomy and physiology
2. pathophysiology of PID
3. transmission of PID
4. types of diagnostic and therapeutic procedures that will be performed (e.g., pelvic examination, cultures, blood tests, and possibly ultrasound and laparoscopy.) Describe the types of sensations the patient will experience during those procedures
5. rationale for all diagnostic, therapeutic, and preventive procedures
6. instructions on the proper use of all medications and signs and symptoms of medication complications
7. signs and symptoms of complications of PID
8. sources of 24-hour emergency care for the patient if she has problems after she leaves the office
9. safe sex practices, including limiting the number of sexual partners, use of condoms
10. discontinue douching; place nothing into vagina

Include significant others in explanations and instructions if the patient desires their presence. Provide written materials that reinforce explanations and instructions.

Rationales

Gathering information facilitates development of appropriate teaching plan.

Written instructions can reinforce verbal teaching and can also be shared with sexual partners.

Nursing Interventions	**Rationales**
Use audiovisual teaching resources (e.g., videotapes, anatomic models).	Audiovisual materials reinforce explanations and instructions. Demonstrations (live or on video) are useful for acquiring psychomotor skills (e.g., condom use).

▼

DISCHARGE PLANNING/CONTINUITY OF CARE

- Schedule the appropriate follow-up appointments for patients who are being treated on an outpatient basis. The first appointment should be scheduled within 72 hours according to the Centers for Disease Control. Subsequent appointments will depend on the patient's response to treatment.
- Refer all sexual partners to a clinic or care provider that is familiar with the Centers for Disease Control's Treatment Guidelines for the partners of women with PID.
- Prepare the patient with complicated PID (i.e., peritonitis, gastrointestinal symptoms, abscess), pregnant patients, patients with an intrauterine device in place, and patients who cannot be compliant with outpatient management for admission to the hospital. *Complicated cases of PID are managed on an inpatient basis with intravenous antibiotics.*
- Prepare women with complicated cases of PID for possibility of additional diagnostic procedures such as ultrasound and laparoscopy

REFERENCES

Centers for Disease Control (1991). Pelvic inflammatory disease: Guidelines for prevention and management. *Morbidity & Mortality Weekly Report.* 40(RR-5):1–25.

Droegemueller, W. (1992). Upper genital tract infections. In A. L. Herbst, D. R. Mishell, M. A. Stenchever, & W. Droegemueller (Eds.). *Comprehensive Gynecology* (pp. 691–720). St. Louis, MO: Mosby Year Book.

Jossens, M. O. & Sweet, R. L. (1993). Pelvic inflammatory disease: Risk factors and microbial etiologies. *Journal of Obstetric, Gynecologic and Neonatal Nursing,* 22(2), 169–179.

McNeeley, S. G. (1992). Pelvic inflammatory disease. *Current Opinion of Obstetrics & Gynecology,* 4(5), 682–686.

Spencer, M. R. (1989). Pelvic inflammatory disease. *Journal of Reproductive Medicine,* 34(Suppl. 8), 605–609.

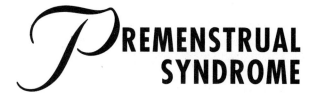

PREMENSTRUAL SYNDROME

Deborah Schy, RNC, MSN

In premenstrual syndrome (PMS) symptoms appear 10–14 days before the onset of menstruation. Symptoms may become progressively worse until the onset of menstruation, or symptoms may persist for several days after the onset of menses. There are over 150 symptoms associated with PMS, but the cyclical nature of the symptoms is the key to diagnosing PMS.

ETIOLOGIES

No one cause is attributed to PMS. Possible causes include:
- prostoglandin excess
- imbalances of ovarian hormones, prolactin, aldosterone.
- vitamin deficiency
- hypoglycemia
- psychological dysfunction

CLINICAL MANIFESTATIONS

- Symptoms may fall into several categories (as described by Dr. Guy Abraham):
- Type A:
  - anxiety
  - irritability
  - mood swings
- Type C:
  - sugar craving
  - fatigue
  - headaches
- Type H:
  - bloating
  - weight gain
  - breast tenderness

- Type D:
  - depression
  - confusion
  - memory loss
- Other symptoms include
  - dysmenorrhea
  - skin problems such as acne

▼

NURSING DIAGNOSIS: KNOWLEDGE DEFICIT

Related To unfamiliarity with disease process and treatment

Defining Characteristics
Expressed need for information
Multiple questions and repetition of questions
Lack of compliance with treatment regimen (exercise, proper diet)

Patient Outcomes
The patient will
- verbalize understanding of premenstrual syndrome and rationale for treatment.
- verbalize an understanding of the relationship between diet, exercise, and stress to PMS.
- verbalize understanding of PMS diet and integrate it into her life beginning with menu planning for one week.
- begin to integrate exercise into her life.
- verbalize positive steps to reduce stress in her life.

Nursing Interventions	Rationales
Assess patient's understanding of the menstrual cycle and symptomatology.	
Assess degree of discomfort with symptomatology and desire to change present status.	
Assess other factors contributing to PMS such as stress.	
Provide information on the menstrual cycle and its function. Instruct how to keep a monthly calendar documenting symptoms, temperature, and menstrual cycle (see Table 28.1).	The calendar will provide objective data for both the care provider and the patient and her significant other.

Nursing Interventions	**Rationales**
Include significant others in explanation of PMS.	PMS affects all members of a family and understanding of the true problem may help the patient and others to alleviate some contributing factors.
Assess patient's understanding of the effect of diet on PMS	
Assess knowledge of appropriate and inappropriate foods.	Helping the patient to understand foods that are appropriate and those which will make symptoms of PMS more severe will promote education and the ability to choose an appropriate diet. Changing of diet will help to alleviate symptoms of PMS.
Provide patient with dietary guidelines for reducing PMS. 1. foods to avoid: • coffee, black tea, soft drinks • cow's milk, cheese, butter, yogurt, eggs • chocolate, sugar • alcohol • beef, pork, lamb • wheat, white bread, white noodles, white rice, white flour pastries, added salt, bouillon • commercial salad dressings • ketchup • hot dogs	There are many items that increase the symptomatology of PMS.

Nursing Interventions	Rationales
2. foods that may be eaten in moderation: • oranges, papaya, pineapple • tomatoes • potatoes, egg plant • avocado • spinach 3. foods that are *high* in nutrient value and help to keep stress levels low; these foods should be encouraged: • beans, beets, broccoli, brussel sprouts • cabbage, lettuce, mustard greens • carrots, celery, collards, cucumbers • garlic, onions • horseradish, radishes • kale, okra • parsnips, peas, corn • rutabaga • squash, yams, turnips, turnip greens • brown rice, millet, oatmeal, buckwheat, barley, rye • sesame, sunflower, pumpkin seeds • almonds, peanuts • apples, berries, pears, seasonal fruits • corn, olive, sesame, safflower oil • poultry • fish	
Assess patient's knowledge of exercise and physical well-being on PMS.	

Nursing Interventions	Rationales
Take an exercise history to determine the number of times per week exercise is performed.	Exercise is an outlet for stress and can help to alleviate the symptoms of stress and PMS. An exercise regimen of active exercise for 30 minutes three times per week along with dietary changes has been shown to decrease PMS symptoms in 50% of the cases.
Assess patient's ability to identify stress and its effect on her body.	
Ask the patient to identify target organs/spots where stress tends to accumulate.	Each individual tends to experience stress in different areas of the body. Identification of tense areas will help so that stress reducing activities can be performed on those areas. Increased energy level from exercise may possibly prevent some of the PMS symptomatology.

▼

NURSING DIAGNOSIS: PAIN

Related To hormonal and dietary influences

Defining Characteristics
Breast tenderness, swelling

Patient Outcomes
The patient will verbalize a decrease in breast tenderness on a monthly basis.

Nursing Interventions	Rationales
Assess the degree of breast tenderness and swelling by reviewing symptomatology chart.	
Assess understanding of dietary influence on breast pain.	

Table 28.1 • PMS Symptom Log

Days in Month	1	2	3	4	5	6	7	8	9	10	11	12	13	14	15	16	17	18	19	20	21	22	23	24	25	26	27	28	29	30
Cycle Days (Day 1-onset of menses)																														
Temperature																														
Weight																														
*Symptoms ( )																														
*Symptoms ( )																														
*Symptoms ( )																														

*Symptoms Code: . Mild
/ Moderate
[] Severe

Nursing Interventions	Rationales
Instruct patient on the importance of the following dietary changes: elimination of caffeine in the diet, balanced foods, adequate vitamin and mineral intake, and elimination of added salt to diet.	These dietary changes will aid in reducing breast tenderness and swelling.
Encourage the use of a well-fitting bra that provides adequate support.	

▼

NURSING DIAGNOSIS: FLUID VOLUME EXCESS

Related To hormonal influences

Defining Characteristics

Weight gain of 2 pounds or more that begins in the premenstrual time and
disappears at the onset of menses
Edema noted in the 10–14 days before menses

Patient Outcomes

The patient will document less than 2-pound weight gain in the premenstrual period; no edema will be noted.

Nursing Interventions	Rationales
Assess any temporary water weight gain noted on a monthly basis. Encourage the documentation of daily weights for at least one month to document the timing of weight gain.	This will help to determine the proper reason for the water weight gain.
Encourage the use of foods that are natural diuretics.	
Instruct patient to cease the use of added salt and foods that have high salt content.	High salt content will only increase the water weight gain.
Reiterate any precautions if a diuretic has been prescribed. Reinforce need to continue with proper nutrition, and caution not to rely solely on diuretics to treat edema.	

▼

NURSING DIAGNOSIS: HIGH RISK FOR OR ACTUAL SITUATIONAL LOW SELF-ESTEEM

Risk Factors
Fluctuating hormonal levels

Defining Characteristics
Depression
Moodiness
Irritability
Verbalizes negative feelings about self (helplessness, uselessness)

Patient Outcomes
Patient will verbalize
- understanding of how hormonal changes affect mood state.
- an understanding of information presented and experience fewer symptoms of depression, moodiness and irritability.

Nursing Interventions	Rationales
Assess the frequency and occurrence of defining characteristics.	
Monitor estrogen and progesterone levels.	Estrogen and progesterone provide balance and promote moods and behavior patterns. Increased estrogen levels lead to anxiety while increased progesterone levels lead to depression.
Monitor vitamin intake.	With vitamin B deficiency there can be inadequate liver function leading to inappropriate estrogen/progesterone levels.
Promote abstinence from alcohol and tobacco products.	These substances can intensify feelings of low self-esteem.
Promote adequate exercise.	Exercise can help alleviate stress and promote physical and psychological well-being.
Encourage the use of therapeutic talking either to an individual, support group, or a therapist.	The ability to communicate openly in a therapeutic environment with others will help to alleviate some feelings that lead to low self-esteem.

▼

NURSING DIAGNOSIS: ALTERED NUTRITION—MORE THAN BODY REQUIREMENT FOR CARBOHYDRATES

Related To changes in appetite related to menstrual cycle/premenstrual syndrome

Defining Characteristics
Craving for sweets

Patient Outcomes
The patient will eat a well-balanced diet as evidenced by reduced intake of simple sugars.

Nursing Interventions	Rationales
Assess dietary intake for a one-month period, noting any change in carbohydrate intake.	
Determine the amount of a simple carbohydrate intake during the premenstrual period.	
Instruct patient to eat small, frequent meals.	This will help to maintain a more stable glucose level and prevent glucose swings.
Have patient identify simple carbohydrate foods. Instruct her to avoid them in her diet for the next month, replacing them with complex carbohydrates and proteins.	Reduction in simple sugars will help to avoid the glucose swings and help put the patient back in control. She can substitute foods that are high in protein or fruits with complex carbohydrates.

▼

DISCHARGE PLANNING/CONTINUITY OF CARE

- Refer to PMS support group.
- Refer to dietitian to aid in meal planning.
- Provide pamphlets.

REFERENCES

Abraham, G. E. (1977). The normal menstrual cycle. J. P. Givens (Ed.), *Endocrine Cause of Menstrual Disorders.* Chicago, IL: Year Book Medical Publishers.

Abraham, G. E. (1980). Premenstrual tension. *Current Problems in Obstetrics and Gynecology.* Chicago, IL: Year Book Medical Publishers.

Hsia, L. & Long, M. H. (1990). Premenstrual syndrome: Current concepts in diagnosis and management. *Journal of Nurse-Midwifery, 35*(6), 351–357.

Lindow, K. (1991). Premenstrual syndrome: Family impact and nursing implications. *Journal of Obstetrical, Gynecologic, and Neonatal Nursing, 20*(2), 135–138.

Mitchell, E. S. (1991). The elusive premenstrual syndrome. *NAACOG's Clinical Issues in Perinatal and Women's Health Nursing, 2*(3), 294–303.

Ornitz, A. & Broun, M. (1993). Family coping and premenstrual symptomatology. *Journal of Obstetrics and Neonatal Nursing, 22*(1), 49–55.

▼

$\mathcal{S}$YPHILIS

Jeffrey Zurlinden, RN, MS

$\mathcal{S}$yphilis is a sexually transmitted infection. If untreated, syphilis progresses over the remainder of the patient's lifetime through four stages: primary, secondary, latent, and tertiary. Screening blood tests are vital to detect syphilis; however, patients who are concurrently infected with HIV (human immunodeficiency virus) may remain falsely negative for syphilis serologies. This care plan does not describe the care of a patient with tertiary syphilis or a newborn with congenital syphilis.

ETIOLOGY

Bacterial infection with *Treponema pallidum*

CLINICAL MANIFESTATIONS

Infection is indicated by a fourfold increase in syphilis serology titer in a previously infected patient or any titer in patient without a previous infection.

Primary syphilis
- Chancre
  - solitary painless papule that eventually ulcerates at inoculation site
  - forms 21–90 days after infection
  - heals spontaneously in 1–6 weeks

Secondary syphilis
- Highly variable, nonpruritic skin rash with lymphadenopathy
  - begins in untreated infection 6 weeks after chancre heals
  - spontaneously resolves in 2–6 weeks

Latent syphilis
- Asymptomatic period after untreated infection that may last decades before progressing to last stage

Tertiary syphilis

- Degenerative changes in heart, central nervous system, and skeletal system
  - paresis
  - dementia
  - aortic insufficiency
  - tabes dorsalis

CLINICAL/DIAGNOSTIC FINDINGS

- Positive Venereal Disease Research Laboratory (VDRL)
- Positive rapid plasma reagin (RPR) test
- Positive fluorescent treponemal antibody (FTA) test

NURSING DIAGNOSIS: INFECTION

Related To presence of infectious organisms

Defining Characteristics

History of sexual contact with an infected person
Positive syphilis serology
Presence of chancre, condylomata lata, or rash

Patient Outcomes

Patient will exhibit no signs of infection, as evidenced by declining syphilis serology titers.

Nursing Interventions	Rationales
Determine date of last sexual contact, number of sexual partners, and description of recent sexual activities.	This provides information regarding behavior that increases risk of sexually transmitted diseases (STDs).
Assess syphilis serology results.	Low-titer biological false-positive results are possible during pregnancy, autoimmune disease, or other infections. Confirmatory test will exclude biological false-positive results in patients without previous syphilis infection. Because an infected person has a negative syphilis serology for the first 4–6 weeks after infection, contacts of infected people are treated as if they are infected.

Nursing Interventions	Rationales
Inspect skin, mouth, vagina, rectum, and perineum for chancre, condylomata lata, and rashes.	
Obtain history of previous sexually transmitted diseases (STDs).	
Screen for other STDs, hepatitis B, and HIV.	Patients with one STD are at higher risk for a concomitant STD.
Obtain menstrual history, including date of last period.	It can be difficult to get cultures during menstruation; results are less accurate, especially with tampon use, showing increased number of false negatives.
Determine method and compliance with birth control.	Contracting STDs suggests no use/improper use of condoms. Women may be at high risk for pregnancy. Nurse should use this opportunity for health screening/education.
Perform pregnancy test.	This is necessary for early detection of pregnancy. Some drugs used to treat syphilis have teratogenic effects. Fetal transmission and the development of congenital syphilis depends on the stage of the mother's infection. Fetal damage can be prevented if treated before the 16th week of gestation.
Administer antibiotics as ordered.	Treatment regimens change in response to the development of new antibiotics. Usually penicillin G is administered intramuscularly; however, the dose and length of treatment depend on the stage of syphilis. Follow the current guidelines from the Centers for Disease Control or your local Health Department.
Observe for possible anaphylactic reaction to intramuscularly administered antibiotics during clinic visit.	

Nursing Interventions	Rationales
Dispense condoms.	The use of latex condoms is the most effective means of preventing the spread of disease during sexual contact.
Instruct patient to inform all recent sexual partners of possible exposure to syphilis and need for treatment.	Untreated asymptomatic sexual partners are common source of reinfection.

▼

NURSING DIAGNOSIS: KNOWLEDGE DEFICIT

Related To new diagnosis

Defining Characteristics
Many questions
Few questions
History of repeated infections
Unable to state the causes, treatment, and prevention of syphilis

Patient Outcomes
Patient will state
- medication schedule
- medication side effects
- date of return visits
- how to use condoms to prevent future infections.

Nursing Interventions	Rationales
Assess patient's present level of understanding.	Misconceptions can increase anxiety/fear and foster spread of sexually transmitted disease.
Instruct patient about medication schedule and side effects of antibiotics.	Course of treatment depends on the stage of syphilis. Follow the current guidelines from the CDC or your local health department.
Instruct patient to refrain from vaginal, rectal, and pharyngeal sexual intercourse until patient and partners have completed treatment.	Patients with primary and secondary syphilis are contagious.

Nursing Interventions	Rationales
Instruct patient on mode of transmission: from chancre site to portion of patient's body that touches chancre. Chancres may be hidden in vagina, rectum, or mouth.	
Instruct patient to use latex condoms or use other nonintercourse sexual methods to prevent future infection.	Latex condoms are an effective barrier against contact with chancres.
Inform patient of signs and symptoms of Jarisch-Herxheimer reaction (fever, chills, malaise, myalgia, and sore throat 6–8 hours after antibiotic therapy; subsiding after 12–24 hours.) Patients may need aspirin for symptomatic relief.	This reaction occurs in 50% of patients with primary syphilis and 75% with secondary syphilis.

▼

NURSING DIAGNOSIS: INEFFECTIVE MANAGEMENT OF THERAPEUTIC REGIMEN

Related To
- Unwillingness to comply with treatment, prevention, or informing sexual partners
- Complexity of treatment regimen

Defining Characteristics
Titer of syphilis serology that does not decrease after treatment
Missed return visits
Incorrect pill count at return visit
Inadequate blood level of antibiotic

Patient Outcomes
Patient will
- complete course of treatment.
- notify sexual partners.
- keep return visits for follow-up serology.
- use condoms to prevent infection.

Nursing Interventions	Rationales
Compare actual effect and expected therapeutic effect.	

Nursing Interventions	Rationales
Plot patient's pattern of returning for tests of cure or follow-up visits.	
Determine social support system and presence of significant others.	Interpersonal influence can impact on compliance with treatment regimen.
Assess patient's and significant other's beliefs about current illness and treatment plan.	How one perceives susceptibility, severity, and threat of disease affects health behavior.
Assess quality of relationship between patient and health care workers and health care facility.	
Role-play to practice informing sexual partners of possible exposure to syphilis.	This gives patient the opportunity to rehearse the situation and allows nurse to provide feedback.
Suggest intramuscularly administered medications or short-term therapy, if patient has a history of not taking oral medication.	Medication administered intramuscularly eliminates the patient's need to participate in treatment.
Role-play to practice new behaviors in situations leading to reinfection (such as saying "no" or using condoms).	
Develop a positive relationship with the patient that encourages participation with treatment decisions.	The nurse-patient relationship is based on recognition of patient's right to self-determination and capacity for self-management with focus on decision-making and goal attainment.
Determine with the patient the plan of treatment she is most likely to complete.	Involving the patient in planning the regimen improves compliance.

▼

NURSING DIAGNOSIS: ALTERED SEXUALITY PATTERNS

Related To
- Imposed restrictions
- Fear
- Risk of spread of disease

Defining Characteristics

Patient or significant other expresses concern about the effects syphilis and its treatment has on their expressions of physical intimacy

Patient Outcomes

Patient will state ways of expressing physical intimacy during treatment.

Nursing Interventions	Rationales
Determine patient's or significant other's concerns.	
Determine if concerns are also related to fears about acquired immunodeficiency syndrome (AIDS).	An STD diagnosis may provoke fear of AIDS that alters sexual behavior.
Assess perception of meaning of syphilis infection.	Provides opportunity to clear up misconceptions.
Elicit patient's feeling about limits on sexual behavior.	
Explore ways to express physical intimacy during treatment excluding vaginal, rectal, and pharyngeal intercourse.	Restrictions on sexual activity should not deprive the couple of other activities that convey the message that they are loved and desired.
Explore ways to express physical intimacy that do not lead to reinfection.	Barrier contraception with latex condoms are effective.
Elicit patient's feeling about limits on sexual behavior.	

▼

DISCHARGE PLANNING/CONTINUITY OF CARE

- Schedule patient to return for repeat serology tests (usually performed at 1, 6, 12, 24 months after therapy).
- Instruct patient to return sooner for routine screening if high-risk sexual behavior continues.
- Refer for HIV counseling and testing. (Syphilis may be more difficult to detect and progress more rapidly in HIV-infected women.)
- Refer to family planning clinic.
- Refer to support group.

REFERENCES

Buckley, H. (1992). Syphilis: A review and update of the "new" infection of the '90s. *Nurse Practitioner, 17*(8), 25–32.

Crane, M. J. (1992). Clinical update: The diagnosis and management of maternal and congenital syphilis. *Journal of Nurse-Midwifery, 37*(1), 4–16.

Handsfield, H. H. (1991). Recent developments in STDs: I. Bacterial diseases. *Hospital Practice, 26,* 35–44.

Libbus, M. K. (1992). Condoms as primary prevention in sexually active women. *American Journal of Maternal-Child Nursing, 17*(5), 256–260.

Nettina, S. L. & Kaufman, F. H. (1990). Diagnosis and management of sexually transmitted genital lesions. *Nurse Practitioner, 15*(1), 20–26, 31, 34–39.

Sharts-Engel, N. C. (1990). Syphilis in pregnancy: Centers for Disease Control Guidelines. *American Journal of Maternal-Child Nursing, 15*(6), 355.

Talashek, M. L., Tichy, A. M., & Epping, H. (1990). Sexually-transmitted diseases in the elderly. *Journal of Gerontological Nursing, 16*(4), 33–40.

Tillman, J. (1992). Syphilis: An old disease, a contemporary perinatal problem. *Journal of Obstetrical, Gynecologic, and Neonatal Nursing, 21*(3), 209–13.

▼

Chapter adapted with permission from Gulanick, M. et al. (Eds). (1990). *Nursing Care Plans: Nursing Diagnosis and Intervention*, (2nd ed). St. Louis, MO: C. V. Mosby Company.

URINARY TRACT INFECTIONS

Peggy Cowling, RNC, MSN

Urinary tract infections are an invasion of bacteria in any part of the urinary tract system, which includes the bladder (cystitis), the urethra (urethritis), or kidney (pyelonephritis).

ETIOLOGIES

- Renal scarring, due to previous infections
- Urinary retention/calculi
- Relaxation of urethral peristalsis due to pregnancy hormones
- Introduction of bacteria during urinary catheterization/procedure
- Females: shorter urethra and close proximity of the vagina and rectum to the urinary meatus

CLINICAL MANIFESTATIONS

- Pain on urination
- Frequency
- Suprapubic pain
- Malaise
- Malodorous urine
- Hematuria
- Pyuria
- May be asymptomatic

CLINICAL/DIAGNOSTIC FINDINGS

- Increased leukocyte count
- Positive urine culture

▼

NURSING DIAGNOSIS: KNOWLEDGE DEFICIT REGARDING DISEASE PROCESS, METHODS OF PREVENTION, HOME CARE, AND FOLLOW-UP CARE

Related To
- Unfamiliarity/misconception regarding etiology and treatment
- Lack of exposure to disease process

Defining Characteristics

Frequent or lack of questions
Verbalizes misinterpretation of information or lack of recall
Noncompliance with personal hygiene measures.

Patient Outcomes

- The patient will verbalize understanding of and compliance with treatment regimen.
- Patient will verbalize prevention techniques to avoid future urinary tract infection.
- Patient's follow-up urine cultures will be negative.

Nursing Interventions	Rationales
Assess knowledge of treatment regimens and prevention techniques.	Education can help prevent the recurrence of urinary tract infections (UTIs) through understanding and compliance with treatment regimen and self-care.
Provide information on 1. diagnostic procedures (collection of urine specimen) 2. follow-up (possible repeat urine cultures, sign/symptoms of recurrence)	Recurrent UTIs are termed relapses when the same bacteria are identified within 1–2 weeks after completing antibiotic treatment. Reinfections are UTIs caused by a new bacterial strain.
Inform patient of methods of prevention: 1. Empty bladder every 2–3 hours. 2. Empty bladder before and after sexual intercourse. 3. Wipe perineum front to back.	*Escherichia coli* is the most common organism implicated in UTIs.

▼

NURSING DIAGNOSIS: PAIN
Related To inflammation of urinary tract

Defining Characteristics
Suprapubic pain
Lower back pain
Bladder spasms
Burning on urination
Urinary frequency
Urinary hesitancy
Urinary urgency
May be asymptomatic

Patient Outcomes
Patient will
• verbalize a decrease in symptoms.
• demonstrate a relaxed facial expression and comfortable body
  position.

Nursing Interventions	Rationales
Assess nature, location, duration, precipitating factors, and alleviating factors of pain.	Symptomology provides a clinical picture upon which diagnosis and treatment will be based.
Provide information on comfort techniques: 1. sitz baths	Sitz baths will provide comfort for pain and itching.
2. heating pad	Heat will promote muscular relaxation, decreasing perception of pain.
3. increased fluid intakes	Increased fluids will dilute urine, increasing comfort when voiding.
4. avoidance of coffee, tea, cola, and alcoholic beverages	These beverages are irritating to the bladder.
5. medications: • antibiotics • antispasmodics • analgesics	

▼

NURSING DIAGNOSIS: INFECTION

Related To presence of bacteria in urinary tract

Defining Characteristics

Pyuria
Malodorous urine
Fever, chills, malaise
Increased leukocyte count
Positive urine culture

Patient Outcomes

Patient will
- exhibit no signs of infection after treatment regimen as evidenced by a negative urine culture.
- have a normal temperature within normal limits.

Nursing Interventions	Rationales
Note character of urine.	Collect midstream, clean-catch urine for culture and sensitivity.
Collection of urine culture and sensitivity ensures proper antibiotic therapy.	Improper technique in collection of urine will produce inaccurate results.
Instruct patient on urine-acidifying agents, as ordered.	Urine-acidifying agents will change the environment to one less suitable for bacterial growth.
Encourage patient to consume oral fluids of 2000–3000 ml/day unless contraindicated.	
Instruct patient to complete entire course of antibiotics, even if symptoms subside.	This reinforces knowledge on use of antibiotics as an effective form of treatment. Antibiotics must be given on schedule to maintain blood levels and the course completed to ensure sterilization of the urine.
Instruct patient to monitor temperature until stable and report any elevation >101°F.	Reporting further signs of infection may prevent or provide early treatment of polynephritis.

▼

DISCHARGE PLANNING/CONTINUITY OF CARE

- Provide written information on prevention techniques.
- Inform of need for follow-up culture to assess efficacy of medications.

REFERENCES

Foxman, B. (1990). Recurring urinary tract infection: incidence and risk factors. *American Journal of Public Health, 80*(3), 331–333.

Howes, D. S. (1992). UTI: Advances and controversies. *Emergency Medicine, 24*(11), 218–220, 223–224, 226–227.

Pinkerman, M. L. (1992). Myths and facts . . . about urinary tract infections. *Nursing '92, 22*(9), 86.

Richardson, D. (1990). Dysuria and urinary tract infections. *Obstetrics and Gynecology Clinics of North America, 17*(4), 881–888.

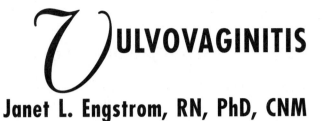

VULVOVAGINITIS

Janet L. Engstrom, RN, PhD, CNM

Vulvovaginitis is defined as inflammation of the vulva and vagina.

ETIOLOGIES

- An infection resulting from any of a number of bacteria, viruses, fungi, or protozoa
- Chemical or mechanical irritants

CLINICAL MANIFESTATIONS

Vary according to the cause of the inflammation:
- swelling
- redness
- pain
- vaginal discharge
- foul odor

CLINICAL/DIAGNOSTIC FINDINGS

- Positive cervical cultures for gonorrhea and chlamydia
- Positive cultures for herpes
- Positive Gram stain
- Microscopic evidence of yeast, trichomonas vaginalis, or findings consistent with bacterial vaginosis

▼

NURSING DIAGNOSIS: HIGH RISK FOR INFECTION

Related To exposure to pathogens

Defining Characteristics

Vaginal discharge

Abnormal odor

Edema, erythema, pain or discomfort, or pruritus of the vulva and vagina

Patient Outcomes

Patient will

- verbalize precautionary measures to prevent spread of infection.
- manifest signs of treated/contained infection, as evidenced by absence of pain, redness, swelling, discharge, and odor of the upper genital tract.

Nursing Interventions	Rationales

Obtain a history of the patient's presenting symptoms:
1. pain
  • duration
  • intensity
  • location
  • character
2. urinary symptoms
  • dysuria
  • urgency
  • frequency
3. pruritis
  • location
  • intensity
  • duration
4. dyspareunia
5. vaginal discharge
  • duration
  • color
  • amount
  • odor
6. genital lesions
  • location
  • color
  • size
  • exudate
  • pain
	This provides information as to the acuity and extent of the infection. Inflammation of the vulva and vagina may cause impaired tissue integrity, which predisposes the patient to infection or superinfection. Infection of the lower genital tract may predispose the patient to pelvic inflammatory disease.

Obtain a sexual history: 1. number of sexual partners 2. contraceptive methods used 3. history of any genitourinary infections in partner(s)	This provides information regarding behavior that may increase the risk of a sexually transmitted disease

Nursing Interventions	Rationales
Obtain or assist with obtaining laboratory specimens as ordered: 1. cervical cultures for gonorrhea and chlamydia (if indicated) 2. cervical, vaginal, and vulvar cultures for herpes (if indicated) 3. cervical specimens for Gram stain 4. vaginal specimens for microscopic examination 5. culture of vulvar and vaginal lesions (if indicated)	
Administer medication as prescribed.	Immediate treatment with the appropriate antimicrobial therapy reduces the possibility that the infection will spread to adjacent tissues and will reduce further inflammation.
Teach the patient how to use medication correctly, including: 1. importance of completing the entire prescription 2. importance of taking/applying/inserting medication on time 3. how to insert vaginal and apply topical medications correctly	The full course of medication should be completed correctly to reduce the possibility of inadequate treatment.
Teach the patient signs and symptoms of pelvic inflammatory disease (e.g., pelvic pain, abdominal pain, elevated temperature, shaking chills, nausea and vomiting) and instruct the patient to call the health care provider immediately. Provide the patient with a phone number for 24-hour emergency care.	Some vaginal discharges are associated with infection of the upper genital tract.
Inform the patient about the need for following appointments.	Scheduling of follow-ups will depend on the cause of the vaginitis and the treatment. Some infections require test of cure to assure adequate treatment.

▼

NURSING DIAGNOSIS: PAIN

Related To
- Inflammation of the vulva and vagina
- Trauma due to scratching
- Examinations
- Treatments

Defining Characteristics

Discomfort or pain
Grimacing
Tensing muscles
Scratching

Patient Outcomes

Patient will verbalize comfort and pain relief.

Nursing Interventions	Rationales
Observe patient's verbal and non-verbal response to potentially painful procedures (e.g., pelvic examinations).	
Ask the patient to describe her perception of the discomfort or pain.	
Identify what comfort measures are being used to cope with the discomfort and determine whether these strategies are effective.	
Eliminate factors that may contribute to her physical discomfort during procedures (e.g., make sure that the examination room is warm enough, the procedure table is as comfortable as possible with a pillow, her bladder is empty).	Patient may experience a decreased ability to tolerate discomfort if environmental factors are stressful
Teach the patient comfort measures that may help her cope with the discomfort (e.g., cool sitz baths, loose clothing, cotton underwear).	These strategies can help reduce some of the inflammation.

▼

NURSING DIAGNOSIS: ALTERED SEXUALITY PATTERNS

Related To
- Recommendation for abstinence until the patient's symptoms have resolved and the patient and all of her sexual partners have completed treatment
- Recommendation to reduce the number of sexual partners for women who have multiple partners
- Recommendation to use condoms to prevent transmission of sexually transmitted diseases

Defining Characteristics
Reported change in sexual behaviors and activities

Patient Outcomes
Patient will verbalize
- that she is abstaining from intercourse until her treatment is complete, her symptoms have resolved, and all sexual partners have been treated (if indicated).
- knowledge of other methods of achieving intimacy and sexual satisfaction without having intercourse or orgasm.
- knowledge of safe sex practices including information about minimizing the number of sexual partners and using barrier contraception, preferably condoms.

Nursing Interventions	Rationales
Obtain a sexual history to determine pretreatment sexual activity patterns, number of sexual partners, safe sex practices.	This provides a baseline for care planning.
Provide a private environment to discuss any aspect of sexual activity.	Most women are hesitant to discuss personal sexual matters. The proper setting may facilitate discussion.
Explain why sexual activity patterns need to be restricted during treatment.	

Nursing Interventions	Rationales
Offer suggestions for activities that meet the couple's need for contact and intimacy without having intercourse (e.g., hugging, kissing, massages).	Restrictions on sexual activity should not deprive the couple of other activities that convey the message that they are loved and desired nor should such restrictions deprive them of intimate physical contact.
Reassure the patient that the recommendation for abstinence is temporary.	Couples may find it easier to cope with restrictions if they see the restrictions as temporary.
Discuss the role of sexual activity in the transmission of sexually transmitted diseases. Offer information that can help the patient reduce her risk of acquiring a sexually transmitted disease, e.g.: 1. reduce the number of sexual partners 2. use condoms 3. have regular examinations for sexually transmitted diseases if she is not in a monogamous relationship	

▼

NURSING DIAGNOSIS: KNOWLEDGE DEFICIT

Related To unfamiliarity with the causes, diagnostic procedures, treatment, and prevention of vulvovaginitis

Defining Characteristics
Expressed need for more information
Multiple questions about the causes, diagnosis, treatment, and prevention of vulvovaginitis
Statement of misconceptions and/or misunderstandings
Incorrect follow-through of instructions
Lack of compliance with treatment
Resistance to treatment
Inappropriate or exaggerated behavior

Patient Outcomes
- Patient will describe how to obtain information and assistance from health care providers.

- Patient will verbalize correct information about the causes, diagnosis, treatment, and prevention of vulvovaginitis.
- Patient will describe signs and symptoms that need immediate evaluation by a health care professional.
- Patient's sexual partner(s) will receive appropriate treatment for sexually transmitted diseases, if indicated.

Nursing Interventions	Rationales
Assess patient's knowledge of normal reproductive anatomy and physiology.	
Assess patient's knowledge of the causes, diagnosis, treatment, and prevention of sexually transmitted diseases.	Gathering information facilitates development of appropriate teaching plan.
Provide the following information: 1. normal reproductive anatomy and physiology 2. pathophysiology of vulvovaginitis 3. transmission of sexually transmitted diseases (when appropriate) 4. types of diagnostic and therapeutic procedures that will be performed (e.g., pelvic examinations, cultures, specimens) and describe the types of sensations the patient will experience during those procedures 5. rationale for all diagnostic, therapeutic, and preventive procedures 6. instructions on the proper use of all medications and signs and symptoms of medication complications 7. signs and symptoms of pelvic inflammatory disease 8. sources of 24-hour emergency care for the patient if she has problems after she leaves the office	

Nursing Interventions	Rationales
9. safe sex practices, including limiting the number of sexual partners, condom use 10. discontinue douching	
Include significant others in explanations and instructions if the patient desires their presence. Provide written materials that reinforce explanations and instructions.	Written instructions reinforce verbal teaching and can also be shared with sexual partners.
Use audiovisual teaching resources (e.g., videotapes, anatomic models, demonstrations) to reinforce explanations and instructions.	Demonstrations are useful for acquiring psychomotor skills (e.g., condom use, inserting vaginal medications).

▼

DISCHARGE PLANNING/CONTINUITY OF CARE

- Refer to clinic to evaluate the effectiveness of treatment if indicated.
- Refer sexual partner for evaluation and treatment if the woman has sexually transmitted infection (e.g., trichomonas). Refer to a clinic or care provider that is familiar with the Centers for Disease Control's Treatment Guidelines for sexually transmitted diseases.

REFERENCES

Barbone, F., Austin, H., Louv, W. C., & Alexander, W. J. (1990). A follow-up study of methods of contraception, sexual activity, and rates of trichomoniasis, candidiasis, and bacterial vaginosis. *American Journal of Obstetrics and Gynecology, 163*(2), 510–514.

Centers for Disease Control. (1989). 1989 sexually transmitted diseases treatment guidelines. *Morbidity and Mortality Weekly Report, 38*(S-8), 1–43.

Droegemueller, W. (1992). Infections of the lower genital tract. A. L. Herbst, D. R. Mishell, M. A. Stenchever, & W. Droegemueller (Eds.), *Comprehensive Gynecology*. St. Louis, MO: Mosby-Year Book.

Foxman, B. (1990). The epidemiology of vulvovaginal candidiasis: Risk factors. *American Journal of Public Health, 80*(3), 329–331.

Lichtman, R. & Duran, P. (1990). The vulva and vagina. R. Lichtman & S. Papera (Eds.), *Gynecology: Well-Woman Care*. E. Norwalk, CT: Appleton & Lange.

Pregnancy

▼

ABRUPTIO PLACENTAE

Deidra Gradishar, RNC, BS

Abruptio placentae is the separation of a normally implanted placenta before delivery of the fetus and after the 20th week of gestation.

ETIOLOGIES

Predisposing factors include
- Chronic and pregnancy-induced hypertension
- Trauma
- Short umbilical cord
- Hyperstimulation of the uterus, which may be caused by
  - oxytocin (used to induce labor)
  - abuse of drugs (such as cocaine)

CLINICAL MANIFESTATIONS

- Rigid boardlike uterus
- Tender uterus
- Increasing abdominal girth or rising fundal height
- Signs and symptoms of hypovolemic shock
- Failure of the uterus to relax between contractions
- Increasing uterine resting tone noted on fetal monitor strip
- Excessive pain with uterine contractions

CLINICAL/DIAGNOSTIC FINDINGS

- Falling hemoglobin and hematocrit values
- Derangements in clotting studies
- Abnormal sonogram (but many false positives and false negatives)

▼

NURSING DIAGNOSIS: PAIN

Related To tetonic uterine contractions

Defining Characteristics

Extreme tenderness of uterus
Excessive pain uncharacteristic of normal uterine contractions
Lack of relaxation periods between contractions
Rigid, boardlike uterus

Patient Outcomes

The patient will
• verbalize ability to cope with the contraction pain.
• notify staff of changes in the pain experienced.

Nursing Interventions	Rationales
Assess understanding of and explain (as needed) the difference between abruptio placentae discomfort and the pain of normal uterine contractions.	Premature separation of placenta from implantation site may cause extravasation of blood into myometrium. This produces irritability of the urine musculature and results in further placentae separation. Patient experiences extreme pain, failure of uterus to relax between contractions, and—at the time of separation—tearing pain, which may suddenly cease.
Solicit perception of discomfort: 1. length/frequency of contractions 2. quality/intensity of pain 3. presence/absence of uterine relaxation periods	
Evaluate mechanisms patient currently uses to manage discomfort, and observe for changes in her ability to cope with contractions.	
Reduce/eliminate, when possible, potential factors contributing to discomfort.	Fatigue, fear, loneliness, hunger, or distended bladder may increase pain experience.
Provide positive reinforcement and personal contact.	Patients who understand emergent, unpredictable conduct of this clinical condition may fear for baby's life. Contact may reduce sense of helplessness.

Nursing Interventions	Rationales
Teach nonpharmacological comfort measures when appropriate: 1. slow chest or pant-blow breathing modifications 2. progressive muscle relaxation 3. guided imagery 4. position changes	Pain medication may be contraindicated, as it may mask clinical signs of abruptio placentae. Distraction techniques shift concentration and awareness of painful stimuli; relaxation provides state of physical and mental tranquillity. Positioning should be aimed at supporting joints to decrease muscle/skeletal tension.

▼

NURSING DIAGNOSIS: HIGH RISK FOR FLUID VOLUME DEFICIT

Risk Factor
Hemorrhage

Patient Outcomes
Patient will maintain adequate fluid volume, as evidenced by
- stable hemoglobin and hematocrit
- urine output ≥50 ml/hr
- absence of symptoms of hypovolemic shock

Nursing Interventions	Rationales
Assess vital signs per unit routine.	
Inform physician of the following: 1. Uterus fails to relax between contractions. 2. Patient reports greater abdominal pain. 3. Patient's level of consciousness or behavior state changes. 4. Vaginal bleeding increases. 5. Fundal height or abdominal girth increases. 6. Urinary output falls below 50 mL/hr. 7. Changes in vital signs (central venous pressure (CVP) when indicated).	Abruptions are not always an immediate threat to maternal or fetal life. But changes in the parameters listed may reflect marked shift from stable condition to potentially lethal unstable condition.

Nursing Interventions	Rationales
Assess hemoglobin, hematocrit, prothrombin time, partial thromboplastin time, and fibrinogen as ordered.	These test are done to monitor extent of bleeding and effect on clotting system
Maintain complete bed rest.	In chronic abruptio placentae, a retroplacental clot may actually tamponade the portion of placenta detached from the uterine wall and control bleeding. Moving may dislodge the clot and escalate bleed. Each additional bleed provokes more placenta separation. Also, since patients have an electronic fetal monitor applied they are not able to ambulate.
Administer parenteral fluids, volume expanders, blood, and blood components as ordered.	
Institute intensive care flow sheet if applicable.	Patients may require more frequent assessments. In acute abruptio states or episodes of fetal stress patient may require 1:1 nursing care.
Prepare patient for emergency cesarean section as indicated.	

▼

NURSING DIAGNOSIS: HIGH RISK FOR INJURY TO FETUS

Risk Factors
- Maternal hemorrhage
- Resultant decreased perfusion to intervillous space

Patient Outcomes
- Injury to fetus will be reduced through early assessment of fetal stress and appropriate intervention.
- Fetus will maintain strong normal heart tones.

Nursing Interventions	**Rationales**
Monitor fetal heart tones electronically by internal or external devices: 1. baseline fetal heart rate (FHR) 2. presence or absence, increase or decrease in variability if internal monitor is used 3. presence and type of periodic patterns 4. late recovery time for decelerations.	
Notify physician immediately if signs of fetal stress are noted: 1. absent fetal heart tones 2. fetal bradycardia/tachycardia 3. hyperactive fetus 4. ominous periodic patterns 5. decrease/loss of variability 6. frank vaginal bleeding	Signs of fetal stress have been associated with poor outcomes. They may indicate the need for further evaluation or immediate surgical intervention.
Institute treatment if signs of fetal stress are noted: 1. Turn patient in an attempt to abolish the ominous pattern. 2. Increase the intravenous drip rate. 3. Apply O_2 per rebreather at 8–10 L.	 IV fluids increase circulating fluid volume.
Prepare for the delivery of a neonate who may be compromised: 1. Notify neonatologist of the imminent high-risk delivery. 2. Check emergency pediatric equipment. 3. Check transporter.	

▼

DISCHARGE PLANNING/CONTINUITY OF CARE

- Schedule routine postdelivery checkup.
- Refer family for support if patient experiences a fetal loss or an infant who must remain hospitalized for intensive treatment.

REFERENCES

Lowe, T. & Cunningham, G. (1990). Placental abruption. *Clinics in Obstetrics and Gynecology, 33*(3), 406–413.

Murphy, P. M. (1992). Problem pregnancies: Hemorrhagic complications in the third trimester. *Journal of Emergency Medical Services, 17*(9), 44–50, 52, 54–57.

Saller, D. N., Nagey, D. A., Pupkin, M. J., & Crenshaw, M. C. (1990). Tocalysis in the management of third trimester bleeding. *Journal of Perinatology, 10*(2), 125–128.

▼

AMNIOINFUSION, INTRAPARTUM CARE OF PATIENT RECEIVING

Patricia Douglas, RN

Amnioinfusion, is an infusion of a sterile isotonic solution into the uterine cavity to establish the cushioning effect that is lost when amniotic fluid decreases in volume. When the cord is no longer impinged, variable decelerations may be diminished or abolished. Amnioinfusion is also used to liquefy thick meconium-stained amniotic fluid, thereby decreasing the risk of meconium aspiration pneumonia.

INDICATIONS

- Treatment of variable decelerations
- Meconium-stained amniotic fluid

▼

NURSING DIAGNOSIS: KNOWLEDGE DEFICIT

Related To
- Unfamiliarity with condition/procedure
- Lack of experience/information relative to birth process
- Alteration in normal birthing process

Defining Characteristics
Need for more information
Lack of questions
Multiple questions
Noncompliance

Patient Outcomes
Patient will verbalize understanding of the rationale for and the manner in which an amnioinfusion is performed.

Nursing Interventions	Rationales
Assess patient's understanding of the rationale for and procedures associated with amnioinfusion.	
Provide information regarding the effects of decreased amniotic fluid on the fetus and its ability to tolerate the stress of labor.	Accurate information may decrease anxiety.

Explain the following regarding amnioinfusion:
1. Rationale
  • The procedure supplements lost amniotic fluid in an effort to "float the baby off the cord," which it has been compressing.
  • The procedure liquefies the meconium particulate matter.
2. Procedure
  • A special intrauterine pressure transducer is inserted into uterus.
  • The catheter is connected to intravenous fluid and a blood warmer.
  • There is an initial rapid infusion of warm fluid to "float baby" off the cord.
  • Continuous infusion replaces fluid lost once membranes have ruptured.
3. Discomfort
  • The sensation is the same as for any other vaginal examination.
4. Expected outcome (depends on purpose of procedure)
  • Variable decelerations from cord compression will decrease or cease.
  • Meconium secretions will liquefy.
	An understanding of what to expect may enhance the patient's ability to tolerate any discomfort and participate in the procedure.

Include significant others in information sessions.	Family support may be helpful to the patient.

▼

NURSING DIAGNOSIS: HIGH RISK FOR INJURY TO MOTHER

Risk Factors
- Insertion of intrauterine pressure catheter for amnioinfusion
- Amnioinfusion
- Polyhydramnios
- Abruptio placentae
- Amniotic fluid embolism

Patient Outcomes
Risk of maternal injury is reduced, as evidenced by
- early assessment of complications
- prompt intervention

Nursing Interventions	Rationales
Assess amount and character of vaginal bleeding during amnioinfusion.	Excessive vaginal bleeding may indicate perforation of uterus, cervical laceration, placentae abruptio, and hemorrhage.
Assess amount of amniotic fluid leakage during amnioinfusion.	Elevated temperature may indicate amnioitis. A change in blood pressure and heart rate could indicate hemorrhage or shock.
Monitor length and intensity of the contractions, as well as the relaxation between contractions.	Uterine resting tone normally increases 30–40 mmHg during amnioinfusion. Uterine hypertonicity could herald an abruption from polyhydramnios following infusion and fluid. Assessment of relaxation between contractions helps to rule out abruption.
Weigh underpads to approximate fluid leakage.	Continuous amnioinfusion in conjunction with minimal or no amniotic fluid leakage will result in uterine distention and polyhydramnios.
Measure abdominal girth every 2 hours.	A significant increase may indicate uterine overdistention, polyhydramnios, or abruptio placentae.

Nursing Interventions	Rationales
Assist physician with intrauterine pressure transducer insertion procedure. Document number of times the procedure was attempted and problems encountered. Document character of amniotic fluid at time of procedure.	
Infuse isotonic fluid (0.9 normal saline or lactated Ringer's solution) at room temperature or via a blood warmer per order. Use infusion pump. Suggested infusion:	
1. 500–1000 ml over 1 hr	This bolus replaces/restores the volume lost when the bag of water ruptured.
2. 150 to 200 ml/hr as continuous replacement	The continuous infusion is needed to replace ongoing fluid leaking from vagina.
Stop amnioinfusion if polyhydramnios occurs and notify physician.	Amnioinfusion is an essentially benign procedure and there have been very few reports in the literature of serious complications.

NURSING DIAGNOSIS: HIGH RISK FOR INJURY TO FETUS

Risk Factors
Unresolved fetal stress

Patient Outcomes
Fetal injury is reduced, as evidenced by
- strong fetal heart tones
- absence of meconium-stained fluid

Nursing Interventions	Rationales
Monitor fetal heart rate continuously by electronic means. Assess and document every 30 minutes. Monitor more closely in the presence of fetal stress.	Prompt identification and intervention for fetal stress can reduce the risk of further compromising the fetus and prevent fetal morbidity/mortality.

Nursing Interventions	Rationales
Assess and document: 1. baseline fetal heart rate 2. baseline variability 3. presence and type of periodic pattern 4. frequency, intensity, and duration of contractions	
Initiate the following procedure prior to amnioinfusion, if variable decelerations are present. 1. Maintain left lateral position.	Placental fetal perfusion is maximized by alleviating compression of the aorta and vena cava.
2. Administer O_2 via rebreather mask at 8–10 ml/min.	This increases maternal O_2 being presented to the intervillous space.
3. Increase intravenous fluid infusion rate.	This increases maternal circulation volume, which may result in increased blood flow to the intervillous space.
4. Lower the head of bed/change patient position.	This may relieve cord compressed by fetal parts.
Notify physician if periodic patterns are unresolved, or resolved after amnioinfusion is initiated.	
Start isotonic fluids at room temperature or warm by a blood warmer.	A cool solution has a chilling effect on the fetus, umbilical cord, and placenta, which can trigger fetal bradycardia.
Infuse only an isotonic solution such as 0.9 normal saline or lactated Ringer's solution.	The use of hypotonic or hypertonic solution for amnioinfusion can result in electrolyte imbalance in the neonate.
Monitor amnioinfusion rate closely.	
Prepare for delivery of potentially compromised fetus.	
Institute care plan for type of delivery anticipated.	

DISCHARGE PLANNING/CONTINUITY OF CARE

- Routine postpartum care
- Six-week postpartum checkup

REFERENCES

Haubrick, K. L. (1990). Amnioinfusions: A technique for the relief of variable decelerations. *Journal of Obstetrical, Gynecologic, and Neonatal Nursing, 19*(4), 299–303.

Stringer, M., Librizzi, R., & Weiner, S. (1990). Management of midtrimester oligohydramnios: A case for amnioinfusion. *Journal of Perinatology, 10*(2), 143–145.

Strong, T. & Phelan, J. (1991). Amnioinfusion for intrapartum management. *Contemporary OB/GYN, 37*(5), 15–24.

▼

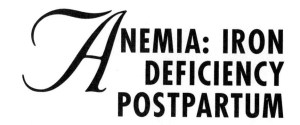

ANEMIA: IRON DEFICIENCY POSTPARTUM

Monalisa S. Bron, RN, BSN
Manie Omsin, RN, BSN

Hypochromic microcytic (iron-deficiency) anemia is commonly seen in the postpartum period.

ETIOLOGIES

- Excessive blood loss during delivery
- Deficient iron intake
- Poor iron absorption
- Increased iron requirement during pregnancy

CLINICAL MANIFESTATIONS

- Fatigue
- Pale conjunctivae
- Inflammation of tongue
- Headache
- Palpitations
- Dyspnea on exertion
- Smooth, sore tongue
- Pallor
- Pale mucous membranes

CLINICAL/DIAGNOSTIC FINDINGS

- Decreased hemoglobin
- Decreased mean corpuscular volume
- Decreased mean corpuscular hemoglobin

- Decreased mean corpuscular hemoglobin concentration
- Decreased serum iron
- Increased total iron-binding capacity
- Decreased serum ferritin

▼

NURSING DIAGNOSIS: ALTERED NUTRITION—LESS THAN BODY REQUIREMENTS

Related To
- Inadequate iron intake during pregnancy and low iron stores before pregnancy
- Iron malabsorption
- Poor dietary habits

Defining Characteristics

Documented inadequate intake of iron-rich foods
Observed dysfunctional eating patterns
Persistent low hemoglobin (<10.5 g/dl), hematocrit (<33%), serum ferritin (<15 µg/L)
Mean corpuscular volume $<80 \times 10^{-9}$ L

Patient Outcomes

Patient will
- verbalize understanding of role of iron-rich food in prevention/management of iron deficiency anemia.
- maintain normal hemoglobin levels.

Nursing Interventions	Rationales
Obtain nutritional history. Assess 1. understanding of nutritional iron requirements 2. ability to select well-balanced diet	Knowledge of previous dietary habits assists in care planning.
Assess for symptoms of iron deficiency and for blood loss during delivery and in postpartum period.	Accurate assessment provides guidance for treatment.
Monitor serum ferritin, hemoglobin, hematocrit, and mean corpuscular volume.	
Consult dietitian as needed to plan appropriate meals.	If nutrition has been inadequate, intake of iron-rich foods is indicated.

Nursing Interventions	Rationales
Administer prescribed iron medication between meals, on empty stomach. If gastrointestinal disturbances occur, administer iron with meals or juices.	Dietary supplements are usually indicated. Timing of medications is important, since food reduces absorption of iron.
Describe side effects of iron medication (e.g., dark green/black stool; possible loose stool or constipation).	Prepare patients for change in stool color due to excess iron excretion into GI tract.
Anticipate blood replacement if no response to diet/medications.	

▼

NURSING DIAGNOSIS: ACTIVITY INTOLERANCE

Related To
- Decreased O_2 supply to cells
- Decreased cellular ability to meet energy requirements

Defining Characteristics
Weakness
Fatigue
Dyspnea on exertion
Abnormal respiratory response to activity
Abnormal cardiac response to activity

Patient Outcomes
Patient will maintain activity within limits of ability.

Nursing Interventions	Rationales
Assess patient's ability to perform ADL and respiratory/cardiac status before and after activity.	Anemia results in decreased hemoglobin and subsequent imbalance between O_2 supply and demand.
Provide assistance for activities patient cannot perform.	This reduces oxygen demands.
Instruct patient to increase activity levels as tolerated.	
Reassure patient that anemia-associated fatigue is temporary.	Realistic understanding of time-limited problem facilitates coping.

Nursing Interventions	Rationales
Discuss ways to pace activities at home so infant's needs can be met.	Appropriate planning will allow mother to recover without compromising infant care.
Encourage patient to seek assistance with infant/household responsibilities after discharge. Inform significant other of patient's need for rest.	

▼

NURSING DIAGNOSIS: HIGH RISK FOR INFECTION

Risk Factors
- Decreased resistance
- Episiotomy/incision

Patient Outcomes
Patient will exhibit no signs of infection, as evidenced by
- no fever
- absence of foul-smelling lochia
- well-healing incision

Nursing Interventions	Rationales
Assess skin episiotomy/incision for signs of inflammation/drainage. Evaluate color, type, and amount of lochia and drainage.	Puerperal infection prolongs normal progression of involution and hospitalization.
Monitor serial hemoglobin.	
Culture incisional drainage as necessary.	
Send urine for culture and sensitivity.	Identification of the causative organism will allow for treatment with an antibiotic known to be specific and effective.
Administer antibiotics as ordered.	

▼

DISCHARGE PLANNING/CONTINUITY OF CARE

- Continue to monitor hemoglobin and hematocrit.
- Stress the importance of foods rich in iron.
- Stress importance of continuing to take iron supplement as ordered.

REFERENCES

Graf, L. A. & McPherson-Smith, L. (1991). Nongenetic perinatal anemias: Conventional, herbal, and homeopathic treatments. *NAACOG's Clinical Issues in Perinatal and Women's Health Nursing, 2*(3), 357–363.

Hytten, F. (1990a). Nutritional requirements in pregnancy: What should the pregnant woman be eating? *Midwifery, 6*(2), 93–98.

Hytten, F. C. (1990b). Nutritional requirements in pregnancy: What happens if they are not met? *Midwifery, 6*(3), 140–145.

Vogt, C. (1991). Iron requirements of pregnancy. *NAACOG's Clinical Issues in Perinatal and Women's Health Nursing, 2*(3), 364–367.

▼

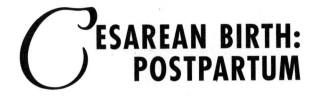

CESAREAN BIRTH: POSTPARTUM

Margaret Hixson, RN, BSN
Daria Lieber, RN

Nursing care for cesarean birth is aimed at promoting optimal recovery from a surgical delivery while facilitating bonding, family interaction, and patient teaching. This procedure is also called cesarean section, C-section, C/S.

INDICATIONS

- Fetopelvic disproportion
- Malpresentation
- Pregnancy-related/medical complications
- Placental abnormalities
- Previous operative delivery
- Fetal stress
- Fetal anomalies
- Cord accidents

▼

NURSING DIAGNOSIS: PAIN

Related To incisional or afterbirth pains

Defining Characteristics
Reports of pain at incisional site/abdomen
Facial mask of pain
Decreased mobility
Elevated blood pressure, pulse rate
Complaints of uterine cramping after breast-feeding or uterine Credé
    maneuver

Patient Outcomes
Patient will
- verbalize relief of pain, or ability to tolerate discomfort.
- appear comfortable and relaxed.

Nursing Interventions	Rationales
Assess pain. Assess effects of pain on activities of daily living (ADL), including ability to provide infant care.	
Offer pain medication before patient is very uncomfortable.	This will maximize the effect of analgesia.
Encourage patient to request pain relief before activity.	Patient more likely to move in bed and ambulate if comfortable. Premedication also eases afterbirth pains if used before nursing.
Provide other potentially helpful comfort measures (e.g., repositioning or changing environment, breathing/relaxation technique).	
Demonstrate various positions for breast-feeding and holding infant.	Patient may need more assistance in holding and positioning infant because of anxiety about incisional pain.

▼

NURSING DIAGNOSIS: HIGH RISK FOR FLUID VOLUME DEFICIT

Risk Factors
- Uterine atony
- Retained placental fragments/infection
- Unligated vessels

Patient Outcomes
Patient will maintain optimal fluid status as evidenced by
- blood pressure within normal limits
- no evidence of bleeding

Nursing Interventions	Rationales
Assess fundal height, tone, and position.	This will ensure that uterine involution is taking place.

Nursing Interventions	Rationales
Palpate and percuss urinary bladder for distention.	A full bladder may displace the uterus, resulting in uterine relaxation and increased bleeding. Patients who have had epidural/spinal anesthesia may be unable to spontaneously void until sensorium has returned.
Massage fundus if not firm.	Will cause uterus to contract; decreases bleeding from placental sinuses.
Instruct patient in fundal massage.	Allows patient to take part in care.
Evaluate vital signs for evidence of hemorrhage.	
Assess amount and color of bleeding, presence of blood clots. Observe perineal pad count.	
Maintain IV line for hydration, fluid replacement, and transfusion as needed.	IV infusion may be necessary to stabilize patient if hemorrhage/heavy blood loss results from uterine atony/retained placental fragments.

▼

NURSING DIAGNOSIS: HIGH RISK FOR INFECTION

Risk Factors
- Surgical incision
- Endometritis/peritonitis
- Urinary stasis
- Retained secretions in respiratory tract

Patient Outcomes
Patient will
- verbalize signs and symptoms of potential infections.
- demonstrate preventative safe care practices (perineal care; cough, deep breath; incentive spirometer).
- have normal temperature and white blood count.

Nursing Interventions	Rationales
Review patient's chart for medical history or prolonged rupture of membranes.	Rupture of membranes for greater than 24° has been associated with increased infection rate.
Monitor for signs of infection: 1. increased uterine tenderness 2. foul-smelling lochia 3. rigid abdomen (peritonitis) 4. separation of margins of incision 5. purulent incisional discharge 6. elevated white blood count 7. elevated temperature, heart rate	
Obtain wound, blood, and tissue cultures as needed.	
Assess for signs of cystitis: 1. elevated temperature, heart rate 2. increased urinary frequency, urgency, burning with urination 3. cloudy, foul-smelling urine 4. hematuria 5. suprapubic/flank pain, pressure	
Palpate and percuss bladder for distention. Assess patency of catheter.	Urinary stasis predisposes to infection.
Obtain clean urine specimen per order for urinalysis and culture.	
Administer intravenous fluids as ordered.	Diluted urine is associated with lower bacterial counts.
Instruct patient in perineal care.	Good perineal care will decrease risk of infection.
Assess for postanesthesia pneumonia: 1. difficult, painful respirations 2. presence of rales, rhonchi, unequal chest movement 3. chills, fever >101°F 4. productive cough with tenacious secretions 5. yellow or green sputum 6. cyanosis	
Obtain sputum cultures as ordered.	

Nursing Interventions	Rationales
Encourage turning, coughing, and deep breathing.	Helps mobilize fluids; prevents complication of positional pneumonia.
Demonstrate splinting as method to support incision during activity.	Splinting may decrease patient's anxiety/fear of pain/opening of incision with straining or with movement.
Encourage use of incentive spirometer.	Spirometry prevents atelectasis and optimizes lung expansion.
Administer antibiotics as ordered.	Careful timing of administration promotes maximum antibiotic effectiveness.

▼

NURSING DIAGNOSIS: HIGH RISK FOR URINARY RETENTION

Risk Factors
- Perineal edema
- Hyperemia of bladder
- Increased capacity and decreased sensation of bladder filling
- Paresthesia of perineum

Patient Outcomes
Patient will maintain urine output of at least 60 ml/hr.

Nursing Interventions	Rationales
Gently palpate bladder for distention.	
Assess patient for dysuria.	
Encourage voiding after removal of indwelling catheter. If patient is unable to void, straight catheterize per order as necessary.	Catheterization prevents bladder distention if patient has decreased sensation.
Assist patient in voiding by pushing fluids, running water, spraying warm water on perineum.	Techniques may aid in relaxing perineal muscles; promote urination.
Encourage ambulation and voiding in bathroom.	Patient may void more easily in bathroom.

Nursing Interventions	Rationales
Measure urinary output as indicated.	
Instruct patient on perineal care: 1. Spray perineum with one full bottle of warm water after elimination. 2. Wipe perineum front to back. 3. Change peripad every 2 hours.	

▼

NURSING DIAGNOSIS: HIGH RISK FOR CONSTIPATION

Risk Factors
- Decreased peristaltic activity
- Manipulation of intestines during surgery

Patient Outcomes
Patient will maintain preoperative pattern of bowel elimination.

Nursing Interventions	Rationales
Assess for presence of bowel sounds until bowel function is established.	
Ask patient about belching and passing flatus.	Bowel sounds and intestinal motility will be reduced as a result of intraoperative medications. As these effects wear off, bowel sounds will return (sometimes with rebound effect) as intestinal motility returns.
Increase hydration (2000–3000 ml/ day) when permitted.	Pushing fluids increases amount of water in intestines; promotes softer stool that is passed more easily.
Encourage patient to ambulate as tolerated.	Ambulation facilitates return of peristalsis.
Monitor dietary intake.	

Nursing Interventions	Rationales
Give stool softener/laxative as ordered; monitor effectiveness.	Many patients fear pain associated with straining to move bowels; stool softener may facilitate good elimination pattern.

▼

NURSING DIAGNOSIS: HIGH RISK FOR ALTERED CIRCULATION

Risk Factors
- Increased coagulation tendency during pregnancy
- Decreased mobility
- Previous history of deep vein thrombosis

Patient Outcomes
Patient will exhibit no signs of
- impaired peripheral circulation
- pulmonary embolism

Nursing Interventions	Rationales
Assess for signs of deep vein thrombosis: 1. localized tenderness 2. calf pain 3. redness 4. swelling 5. area warm to touch 6. positive Homans' sign	Patients who have had C-sections are three times more likely to experience thromboembolic problems than those who have had a vaginal delivery.
Assess for signs and symptoms of pulmonary embolism: 1. chest pain 2. dyspnea 3. tachycardia 4. change in blood pressure 5. change in mental status 6. hemoptysis	
Assess prothrombin, partial thromboplastin time, and fibrinogen.	Pregnancy is associated with hypercoagulation.
Assist with early ambulation.	This activity promotes improved circulation.

Nursing Interventions	Rationales
Provide appropriate teaching: 1. no leg crossing 2. elevate feet as needed	Modifying patient behavior may decrease risk of developing deep vein thrombosis caused by sluggish/impeded circulation.
Apply antiembolic support hose.	This promotes improved circulation.
Teach ankle-rolling exercises.	These exercises promote circulation and maintain range of motion.

▼

NURSING DIAGNOSIS: HIGH RISK FOR ALTERED PARENTING

Risk Factors
- Recovering from major abdominal surgery
- Pain related to surgery and complications
- Lack of confidence in ability to parent
- Unresolved conflict about operative delivery

Patient Outcomes
Patient will demonstrate positive attachment behavior:
- holding infant close.
- looking directly at baby.
- talking soothingly/playfully.

Nursing Interventions	Rationales
Provide opportunity for and observe maternal/infant interactions: 1. Holds infant close to body. 2. Establishes eye contact with infant. 3. Talks to infant soothingly or playfully.	
Provide support and encouragement as parents begin to interact with and care for infant.	Patient may be anxious/unsure about handling infant; support and encouragement may build confidence.
Assess mother/father's feelings about cesarean versus vaginal delivery. Affirm your confidence in patient's ability to parent.	Patient should not believe that failure to deliver vaginally means maternal failure or inability to care for infant.

Nursing Interventions	Rationales
Arrange for patient to view cesarean birth film.	Film may answer questions and allow patient to relive experience if unable to remember delivery.
Promote optimal comfort. Encourage mother to rest periodically throughout the day.	Recovery after surgical delivery requires more time. Rest periods and gradually increasing activity/responsibility facilitate optimal recovery.
Prepare patient for emotional ups and downs of postpartum period; explain that such changes are common.	"Postpartum blues" may exist to varying degrees. Patient should expect mood swings but should seek assistance if feeling unable to care for infant or likely to harm infant.
See also: Promoting Parent-Infant Attachment, p. 47.	

DISCHARGE PLANNING/CONTINUITY OF CARE

- Provide infant care hotline number to give patient resource beyond hospital.
- Encourage patient to arrange for support services to assist with household/family responsibilities during recovery.
- Instruct to return to care provider for removal of sutures/staples.
- Instruct in incision care techniques.
- Instruct to notify health care provider if signs of infection are observed.

REFERENCES

Baruffi, G., Strobino, M., & Paine, L. L. (1990). Investigation of institutional differences in primary cesarean birth rates. *Journal of Nurse-Midwifery, 35*(5), 274–281.

Pridjian, G., Hibbard, J. U., & Moawad, A. H. (1991). Cesarean: Changing the trends. *Obstetrics and Gynecology, 77*(2), 195–200.

Reichert, J., Baron, M., & Fawcett, J. (1993). Changes in attitudes toward cesarean birth. *Journal of Obstetrics Gynecologic and Neonatal Nursing, 22*(2), 159–167.

Rosen, M. G., Dickinson, J. C., & Westhoff, C. L. (1991). Vaginal birth after cesarean: A meta-analysis of morbidity and mortality. *Obstetrics and Gynecology, 77*(3), 465–470.

Tighe, D. & Sweezy, S. R. (1990). The perioperative experience of cesarean birth: Preparation, considerations, and complications. *Journal of Perinatal and Neonatal Nursing, 3*(3), 14–30.

CHEMICAL ADDICTION DURING PREGNANCY

Sharon Broderick, RN, MS
Marleen Mrozek, RN, BSN

Addiction is a chronic disease that, without intervention, will progress to death. Addiction does not relent during pregnancy. Denial, rationalization, and minimization hallmark the addiction process. These defense mechanisms were originally activated in an effort to explain behaviors and preserve self-esteem. Now, integrated into the unconscious, they become primary deterrents to recognizing the scope of the addiction and the potential for recovery.

Access of health care services during pregnancy offers an opportunity for promotion of perinatal health as well as interruption of the addiction process. The following plan of care will outline the needs of the woman who is pregnant and chemically addicted.

ETIOLOGY

No single etiology or cause of addiction has been identified.

CLINICAL MANIFESTATIONS

- Alcohol
  - loss of control
  - disorganized thought processes
  - decreased coordination
  - unclear/slurred speech
  - Korsakoff's syndrome (severe recent memory loss, confusion, confabulation)
  - Wernicke's syndrome (neurological problems, ataxia, nystagmus, paralysis of certain eye muscles)
- Marijuana
  - impairment of specific psychomotor tasks
  - loss of perspective

  – interference with transfer of data to long-term memory storage
  – paranoia
- Cocaine
  – elevated blood pressure
  – tachycardia
  – increased physical activity
  – increased temperature
  – seizures
  – decreased appetite
- Opiates
  – analgesia
  – drowsiness
  – euphoria
  – respiratory depression

DIAGNOSTIC FINDING

Positive urine and blood toxicology

▼

NURSING DIAGNOSIS: ALTERED HEALTH MAINTENANCE

Related To
- Ineffective coping
- Lack of support systems
- Knowledge deficit
- Lack of ability to make thoughtful judgments

Defining Characteristics
Lack of knowledge regarding basic health practices
Observed inability to take responsibility for meeting maternal/fetal needs
Desire for more information
Rationalization and minimizing effects of drugs on self and fetus

Patient Outcomes
Patient will
- verbalize effects of chemical dependence on self and developing fetus.
- enter treatment program/participate in support group.
- discontinue or decrease use of alcohol or chemical substance.

Nursing Interventions	Rationales
Utilize disease concept framework in providing education on addiction.	The chronic disease framework recognizes addiction as a lifelong illness in which ongoing support of abstinence is required to prevent death. This disease model allows the individual, family, and health care providers to focus on the illness rather than the moral weaknesses of the individual. It also recognizes relapse, or the resumption of alcohol or drug use, as part of the disease.
Reinforce that addiction is a chronic, progressive disease that will end in death without intervention.	This reinforces the need for ongoing treatment and intervention.
Review Jellinek chart and ask the individual to identify where she sees herself in relationship to this chart.	The Jellinek chart is a schematic diagram of lifestyle changes that occur with progression of an addictive disease. Visual representation and self-reflection will facilitate decreased denial and rationalization.
Identify drug-seeking behaviors and activities (e.g., sharing needles, promiscuity, decreased nutrition).	Activities that are involved in acquisition and use of drugs are often detrimental to the individual's health and can further complicate pregnancy.
Discuss changes and care needs of pregnancy and identify how current lifestyle characteristics interfere with acquisition of health care needs.	Emphasis on maternal health and care needs encourages self-care, communicates interest in patient, acknowledges the woman as separate from her child and promotes problem-solving within the individual.
Review placental physiology and the ability for alcohol and drugs to cross this barrier.	Many women believe that the fetus is protected from drugs and alcohol. Knowledge that the fetus may also become addicted may cause patient to seek treatment.

Nursing Interventions	Rationales
Review risks to fetus relative to intrauterine drug exposure. Also, emphasize positive neonatal outcomes associated with discontinued drug exposure during pregnancy.	Decreasing or quitting drugs at any time during pregnancy improves obstetrical and neonatal outcomes. Defense mechanisms of denial, minimizing, and rationalization decrease the woman's ability to internalize information on potential harm of drugs to her fetus. Focusing on negative consequences also increases guilt and anxiety which may lead to increased drug intake. Emphasizing benefits of abstinence instills hope without reinforcing guilt and shame and is a more effective motivator for decreased or discontinuation of drug intake.
Encourage involvement in treatment programs that include pregnancy and parenting components.	Contact with other individuals with similar experiences will facilitate recovery and help confront denial, rationalizations, and minimalization.

▼

NURSING DIAGNOSIS: HIGH RISK FOR INJURY TO MOTHER

Risk Factors
- Systemic effects of abused drugs
- Pregnancy complications related to drug use

Patient Outcomes
Patient will remain free of injury secondary to close monitoring and early intervention as needed.

Nursing Interventions	Rationales
Assess blood pressure, pulse, and respiratory rate every 30 minutes until stable.	Changes may reflect respiratory depression, cardiomyopathies, cardiac arrhythmias, dehydration.

Nursing Interventions	Rationales
Assess for signs/symptoms of abruption: 1. vaginal bleeding 2. boardlike uterus 3. uterine tetany 4. constant sharp uterine pain 5. increased abdominal girth 6. increased fundal height	Cocaine is a powerful vasoconstrictor and places the woman at increased risk of placental abruption.
Institute peripad count if vaginal bleeding is present.	Counting/weighing of pads is necessary to assess blood loss.
Type and cross-match for blood as ordered.	Blood replacement may be indicated if bleeding persists.
Initiate intravenous access and titrate fluids.	This facilitates circulatory support.
Encourage side-lying positioning.	Side-lying positioning removes weight of gravid uterus from aorta and vena cava and maximizes blood flow to and from placental unit.
Implement seizure precautions: 1. Pad side rails. 2. Provide calm/quiet environment. 3. Ensure that anticonvulsive medications are available.	Cocaine may precipitate grand mal seizures. Continued use can sensitize the individual to seizures.

▼

NURSING DIAGNOSIS: HIGH RISK FOR MATERNAL INJURY

Risk Factors
Withdrawal from addictive substance

Patient Outcomes
Patient will not exhibit harm to self or fetus during withdrawal process.

Nursing Interventions	Rationales
Ask patient what signs/symptoms she normally experiences during withdrawal.	Patient's previous experiences may help alert health care provider to signs/symptoms of withdrawal.

Nursing Interventions

Assess for signs/symptoms of drug withdrawal:
1. alcohol
   - 4–6 hours since last drink:
     - tremors
     - irritability
     - retching
     - nausea/vomiting
     - diaphoresis
     - increased body temperature
     - increased respirations and increased blood pressure
   - 48 hours since last drink:
     - hallucinations
     - seizures
     - delirium tremors (tremors, agitation, fever, rapid pulse)
2. cocaine
   - depression
   - irritability
   - social withdrawal
   - intense cravings for more cocaine
   - muscle pain
   - tremors
   - eating disturbances
   - changes in sleep pattern
3. marijuana withdrawal
   - anorexia
   - tremors
   - perspiration
   - cramps
   - diarrhea
   - nausea/vomiting
   - sleep disturbances

Rationales

Withdrawal is the appearance of physical symptoms when drug is stopped too quickly. The peak withdrawal from alcohol is 12–24 hours since last drink. Hallucinations occur in 25% of people withdrawing from alcohol. Visual and tactile hallucinations are more common than auditory. Audible hallucinations often reflect messages that promote self-harm. Delirium tremens are a result of increased excitation of the autonomic system and can occur between 24 hours and 2 weeks after last alcohol intake. Withdrawal symptoms associated with opiates usually occur 8–12 hours after last dose is taken. Symptoms subside over 7–10 days.

Nursing Interventions	Rationales

4. opiate withdrawal
  • 8–12 hours since last intake:
    – increased respiratory rate
    – diaphoresis
    – lacrimination
    – yawning
    – rhinorrhea
    – tremors
    – anorexia
    – irritability
    – anxiety
    – dilated pupils
  • 24–48 hours since last intake:
    – insomnia
    – nausea/vomiting
    – diarrhea
    – weakness
    – abdominal cramps
    – tachycardia
    – hypertension
    – involuntary muscle spasms
    – chills alternating with
      sweating/flushing.	

Explore coping techniques used in previous experiences with withdrawal.	Successful mechanisms need to be instituted.
Administer antidiarrheals, antiemetics, and antipyretics as ordered.	
Assess vital signs and physical status every 30 minutes until stable.	
Implement seizure precautions as needed.	Seizure activity can occur within 48 hours of last drink.
Prepare anticonvulsive therapy as indicated.	Valium (2–10 mg) may be administered if labor is not anticipated. Magnesium sulfate would be selected if delivery was imminent.
Promote calm, quiet, darkened environment.	Calm minimizes central nervous system irritability.

Nursing Interventions	Rationales
Institute continuous electronic fetal monitoring.	Electronic fetal monitoring allows for early recognition of signs/symptoms of fetal stress in utero.
Administer methadone as scheduled.	Methadone helps prevent withdrawal. Withholding the drug from the patient can likewise induce withdrawal.

NURSING DIAGNOSIS: HIGH RISK FOR INJURY TO FETUS

Risk Factor
Decreased placental blood flow

Patient Outcomes
Risk of injury is reduced through early assessment and immediate treatment.

Nursing Interventions	Rationales
Determine accurate expected date of delivery (EDD).	Menstrual irregularities are common effects of habit-forming drugs, making correct EDD difficult. Patients often seek no prenatal care, making following course of pregnancy difficult.
Palpate fundus to determine gestational age; check against ultrasound measurements.	Since mother usually has poor nutrition, anemia, and decreased blood flow to placenta, infant's size may be less than expected for gestational age.
Assess amniotic fluid for meconium staining.	
Assess fetal heart tones. Monitor fetal heart rate tracings.	Assessment of fetal heart rate pattern is necessary to assess for signs of abnormal fetal response.
If monitor tracing reveals fetal stress, initiate treatment: 1. Change mother's position. 2. Increase intravenous infusion rate. 3. Apply oxygen.	May increase oxygen blood flow to baby.

Nursing Interventions	Rationales
Prepare for emergency delivery of possibly compromised infant.	

NURSING DIAGNOSIS: HIGH RISK FOR INFECTION

Risk Factor
Lifestyle behaviors associated with acquisition/use of drugs

Patient Outcomes
Patient will
- identify high-risk behaviors.
- use adequate barrier protection when engaging in sexual activity.
- participate in antibiotic drug treatment as recommended.
- remain free of sexually transmitted diseases after treatment.

Nursing Interventions	Rationales
Obtain the following screening tests: 1. complete blood count 2. urinalysis 3. VDRL 4. cervical cultures for chlamydia and gonorrhea 5. Pap smear 6. hepatitis profile 7. tuberculin skin test	Behaviors and activities to obtain drugs or in drug use often increase risk of infections (e.g., sharing needles, unprotected intercourse, prostitution, multiple sex partners).
Assess for vaginal redness and edema.	Cocaine administered vaginally can lead to tissue trauma.
Counsel and obtain informed consent for HIV testing.	HIV transmission rate is increased in IV drug-using populations.
Assess for signs/symptoms of abscesses/cellulitis.	Abscesses/cellulitis can occur from repeated IV injection or infection.
Provide instruction and counseling on practices to minimize sexually transmitted diseases (STDs).	Exploration of lifestyle needs and comfort facilitates selection of protection aids.
Treat symptoms of STD. Encourage treatment of partner.	Treatment of partners is necessary to prevent reinfection.

Nursing Interventions	Rationales
Assess for signs/symptoms of premature labor.	Infections of uterus or urinary tract system are often associated with preterm labor.
Provide instructions on detection of and immediate actions for premature labor.	Early recognition and treatment of premature labor may prevent preterm delivery.

▼

NURSING DIAGNOSIS: HIGH RISK FOR ALTERED NUTITION—LESS THAN BODY REQUIREMENTS

Risk Factors
- Desire for food replaced by substance use
- Poor nutritional choices
- Altered gastrointestinal absorption.
- Social isolation

Patient Outcomes
- Patient will identify good nutritional food choices.
- Patient will gain adequate weight during pregnancy.
- Fetus will demonstrate appropriate growth during pregnancy.

Nursing Interventions	Rationales
Obtain nutritional history. Assess for eating patterns suggestive of pica.	Common during pregnancy in some ethnic and cultural groups.
Assess for signs of nutritional deficit: 1. inadequate weight gain/weight loss 2. anemia 3. fatigue 4. vitamin deficiency 5. poor skin turgor 6. pallor 7. fetal growth retardation	Pregnancy places increased dietary needs on the mother in order to support development and growth of the fetus.

Nursing Interventions	Rationales
Provide instruction on dietary needs during pregnancy and recovery period. Encourage high protein, low carbohydrate diet.	Both pregnant women and addicts have increased vitamin and iron needs. Additional vitamin and mineral supplementation is often required. Chronic low blood sugar is common and can trigger cravings for alcohol.
Assist with meal planning.	Educating patient regarding role of nutrition in health maintenance can facilitate self-care skills and enhance sense of well-being.
Assess resources and ability to obtain food. Consult social worker as needed for assistance.	Lifestyle patterns in addiction may have negated resources necessary to obtain food (loss of job/support systems).

▼

NURSING DIAGNOSIS: PAIN

Related To
- Labor pains
- Potential tolerance to analgesics
- Symptoms of withdrawal

Defining Characteristics
Frequent requests for pain medication
Attempts to self-medicate
Preoccupation with pain management
Restless, uncomfortable appearance

Patient Outcomes
- Patient maintains comfort as evidenced by controlled actions and behaviors, and resting/relaxing between contractions.
- Patient remains free of signs and symptoms of withdrawal during labor.

Nursing Interventions	Rationales
Assess need for analgesic on a regular schedule.	Patient may require an increased dose of narcotic due to increased tolerance levels.

Nursing Interventions	Rationales
Assess last use of self-medication prior to admission.	Patient may have self-medicated prior to coming to hospital.
Notify anesthesiologist of patient's drug history.	They will need the information for planning anesthesia during labor or for an emergency caesarean section.
Include patient in planning for pain management.	Inclusion of patient will decrease anxiety and foster feelings of control.
Encourage patient to verbalize fears related to reliance on the institution to provide pain management services.	Encouraging patient to verbalize feelings communicates understanding and willingness to listen to lay health care provider.
Institute nonpharmacological comfort measures: 1. massage 2. relaxation 3. breathing techniques 4. positioning	Though they may not eliminate discomfort, nonpharmacological methods may help distract patient from pain.
Provide analgesics as needed. Avoid medications that have narcotic antagonist properties (Talwin, Stadol, Nubain).	Antagonist properties can potentiate withdrawal symptoms. Regional anesthesia is often the medication of choice.
Maintain narcotic antagonist (Narcan) at bedside.	Narcan should be available for use in case of respiratory depression.
Evaluate effects of analgesics within 30 minutes of administration. Assess for relief and also for signs of respiratory or central nervous system depression.	

▼

NURSING DIAGNOSIS: HIGH RISK FOR ALTERED PARENTING

Risk Factors
- Lack of effective parenting skills
- Altered self-concept secondary to guilt and shame of addiction
- Absence of effective support systems
- Newborn experiencing irritability from withdrawal

Patient Outcomes

Patient will

- recognize infant needs as separate from maternal needs.
- continue participation in parenting/treatment program.
- demonstrate increasing responsibility for self and newborn care.

Nursing Interventions	Rationales
Assess patient's perception of pregnancy and of motherhood.	Acceptance of pregnancy and differentiating self from fetus are two developmental tasks of pregnancy. Failure to complete these tasks before delivery may decrease readiness for parenting role.
Assist patient in identifying support systems.	Family and support systems may have abandoned the woman during her period of active drug involvement.
Discuss newborn care techniques and comforting techniques for newborn experiencing withdrawal.	Newborns exposed to drugs in utero may have complications making them difficult to console, feed, and care for.
Review newborn "time-out signals" (e.g., yawning, sneezing, averting gaze).	Newborn time-out signals may be interpreted as rejection by the mother.
Encourage involvement in multidisciplinary treatment center that treats the mother and newborn together.	Group counseling and continued education will help decrease maternal guilt and reinforce care techniques.

▼

NURSING DIAGNOSIS: HIGH RISK FOR RELAPSE

Risk Factors

- Stresses of postpartum period
- Hormonal changes during postpartum period
- Inadequate support systems

Patient Outcomes

- Patient will verbalize an understanding that relapse is a component of addiction.
- Patient and family will identify factors that predispose the individual to relapse.

- Patient will develop a relapse prevention plan prior to discharge.
- Patient will remain free of relapse.
- Patient will resume abstinence following an episode of relapse.

Nursing Interventions	Rationales
Openly discuss potential for relapse during education related to addiction process.	Abstinence during pregnancy does not indicate a cure from addiction. Addiction is a chronic disease in which relapse is a characteristic.
Discuss potential triggers of drug-seeking/drug-use behaviors: 1. absence of pregnancy as a deterrent 2. hormonal changes of postpartum period 3. fatigue and stress inherent in incorporating newborn into family system 4. stress of comforting a newborn experiencing withdrawal 5. guilt related to newborn outcome or experiences of withdrawal	By openly discussing relapse, the care giver communicates willingness and openness to discuss feelings related to use.
Discuss signs of potential relapse with patient and family: 1. minimizing problems 2. unrealistic goals and expectations 3. denial 4. dishonesty with self and others 5. remorse, self-pity and guilt become pronounced 6. loss of self-confidence; loss of self-esteem 7. feelings of hopelessness and loneliness 8. avoiding others 9. infrequent utilization of AA meetings 10. placing self in situations where drug use/drinking is present 11. preoccupation with alcohol and drugs	Relapse is potentiated by excessive stress, improper diet, fatigue, and lack of exercise.

Nursing Interventions	Rationales
12. creating a series of crises 13. focusing on positive memories of drug use while minimizing, rationalizing, and blocking out negative memories 14. returning to use of drugs other than drug of choice 15. returning to use of drug of choice	
Develop a relapse prevention plan prior to discharge that includes strategies for minimizing potential for relapse and strategies to initiate if relapse does occur.	This plan allows for planning for resumption of treatment if relapse does occur and helps minimize guilt, shame, and remorse that occur following a relapse.
Encourage involvement in a comprehensive treatment program that includes both maternal and newborn issues.	

▼

DISCHARGE PLANNING/CONTINUITY OF CARE

- Refer to appropriate self-help group: Alcoholics Anonymous, Narcotics Anonymous.
- Refer to treatment program.
- Refer to nutritionist.
- Refer to social worker.
- Refer infant for follow-up at high-risk clinic.

REFERENCES

Barbour, B. G. (1990). Alcohol and pregnancy. *Journal of Nurse Midwifery, 35*(2), 78–85.

Byrne, M. W. & Lerner, H. M. (1992). Communicating with addicted women in labor. *American Journal of Maternal-Child Nursing, 17*, 22–26.

Chasnoff, I. J. (Ed.). (1986). *Drug Use in Pregnancy: Mother and Child.* Lancaster: MTP Press.

Janke, J. R. (1990). Prenatal cocaine use: Effects on perinatal outcome. *Journal of Nurse-Midwifery, 35*(2), 74–77.

Kenney, J. & Leaton, G. (1991). *Loosening the Grip.* St. Louis, MO: Mosby.

Lynch, M. & McKeon, V. A. (1990). Cocaine use during pregnancy: Research findings and clinical implications. *Journal of Obstetrical, Gynecologic, and Neonatal Nursing, 19*(4), 285–292.

Smith, J. (1988). The dangers of prenatal cocaine use. *American Journal of Maternal-Child Nursing, 13*, 174–179.

Starr, K. & Chisum, G. (1992). The chemically dependent pregnant woman. In L. Manderville & N. Troiano (Eds.). *High Risk Intrapartum Nursing.* Philadelphia, PA: Lippincott.

▼

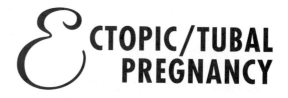

ECTOPIC/TUBAL PREGNANCY

Deidra Gradishar, RNC, BS
Denise Pang-Hong, RNC, MS

Ectopic pregnancy describes a gestation implanted anywhere outside of the uterus. Ectopic pregnancies occur in 1 of 200 pregnancies. The most common site for implantation—90% of all ectopics—is the fallopian tube. The fertilized ovum may also implant in the ovary, the cervix, or the abdomen.

ETIOLOGIES

- Adhesions in the tube from inflammatory/infectious process
- Tubal adhesions secondary to previous ectopic pregnancies or surgical procedures
- The presence of extrauterine endometrial tissue, which invites implantation.
- Migration of an ovum cross the peritoneum from one ovary to the opposite tube, thereby delaying implantation

CLINICAL MANIFESTATIONS

Symptoms vary depending upon the location of the ectopic:
- suspected/unruptured ectopic
  - suspected or confirmed pregnancy
  - severe lower abdominal pain
  - scant dark brown vaginal bleeding
- ruptured ectopic
  - suspected or confirmed pregnancy
  - vaginal bleeding: usually not more than a period or silent bleeding into the peritoneal cavity
  - recurrent attacks of dull abdominal pain
  - referred right shoulder pain

– fainting, weakness, and other associated symptoms of hypovolemic shock

▼

NURSING DIAGNOSIS: HIGH RISK FOR FLUID VOLUME DEFICIT

Risk Factors
Ruptured fallopian tube resulting in hemorrhage

Patient Outcomes
Patient will maintain normal fluid volume, as evidenced by
- normal blood pressure
- urine output of 50 ml/hr
- good skin turgor

Nursing Interventions	Rationales
Assess for pain.	Sharp, intense pain, which suddenly ceases, indicates ruptured fallopian tube.
Assess for evidence of bleeding: 1. tachycardia 2. decreased blood pressure 3. decreasing hemoglobin/ hematocrit 4. pale skin	Usually silent bleeding into the peritoneal cavity occurs.
Observe for any signs of vaginal bleeding.	
Maintain complete bed rest.	Reduced activity protects patient from sudden circulatory shifts, which may cause fainting.
If symptoms of shock occur, insert an additional intravenous line for administration of volume expanders, blood, and blood components.	It is necessary to replace blood lost during hemorrhage.
Prepare patient for surgical intervention.	Surgery is necessary to remove ectopic pregnancy and repair or remove damaged fallopian tube.

▼

NURSING DIAGNOSIS: PAIN

Related To tubal pregnancy

Defining Characteristics
- Recurrent, sharp fleeting pain in lower abdomen
- Progression to sudden, sharp abdominal pain, unilateral or bilateral
- Pain with movement of cervix during vaginal examination

Patient Outcomes
Patient will
- communicate any changes in pain experience which will aid in diagnosis and assist in predicting rupture.
- express ability to cope with pain experienced.

Nursing Interventions	Rationales
Elicit patient's description of discomfort or pain.	
Assess patient's present mechanisms to deal with discomfort/pain.	Supporting familiar effective methods may be more useful than learning new techniques.
Reduce/eliminate possible factors that may contribute to discomfort (e.g., patient may be more comfortable if bladder is kept empty through frequent voiding.	Full bladder may apply direct pressure to the fallopian tube.
Provide emotional support and explanation if analgesia is contraindicated at this time.	
Use nonpharmacologic comfort measures: 1. position change 2. relaxation techniques 3. distraction techniques	Analgesics may mask the symptoms of impending or actual rupture of the ectopic pregnancy and may be contraindicated until after surgical intervention.

▼

NURSING DIAGNOSIS: KNOWLEDGE DEFICIT

Related To
- Lack of familiarity with hospital environment and medical procedures
- Unfamiliarity with tubal pregnancy, its causes, treatment, and outcome

Defining Characteristics
Inability to comprehend or retain information
Multiple questions or lack of questions
Noncompliant with medical care
Overt confusion over events

Patient Outcomes
Patient will verbalize basic understanding of tubal pregnancy and nursing/medical interventions.

Nursing Interventions	Rationales
Assess knowledge of ectopic pregnancy.	
Provide information about 1. possible causes of tubal pregnancy 2. reasons for hospitalization and surgery.	When individuals experience a pregnancy loss, they search for reason. Patient may be inclined to blame self/partner unless this issue is addressed.
When applicable, explain procedures that aid in diagnosis:	
1. vaginal/speculum examination	This examination is performed to aid in localizing/assessing source of bleeding.
2. culdocentesis	The cul-de-sac is the lowest portion of the peritoneal cavity. Blood from a ruptured ectopic will pool here. It can be aspirated during a culdocentesis.
3. pregnancy test	This test is used to diagnose pregnancy and to determine if human chorionic gonadotropin levels are consistent with gestational age.
4. ultrasonography	This procedure is used to visualize the site of abnormally implanted pregnancy.
5. laparoscopy	The laparascope is used to directly visualize/rule out ectopic pregnancy.

▼

NURSING DIAGNOSIS: HIGH RISK FOR DYSFUNCTIONAL GRIEVING

Risk Factors
- Loss of pregnancy
- Possible loss of future reproductive potential

Patient Outcomes
Patient begins to verbalize acceptance of loss of pregnancy and reproductive potential.

Nursing Interventions	Rationales
Observe for verbal/nonverbal expression of grief.	
Assess pregnancy history for previous pregnancy loss or fertility problems.	A previous history of pregnancy loss may heighten the patient's sense of helplessness.
Accept all expressions of grief except those that threaten someone's safety.	People's expression of grief differ widely as individuals, and as cultural and religious experiences.
Acknowledge that surgery will result in ultimate loss of pregnancy.	People tend to focus on imperativeness of surgical procedure rather than loss of pregnancy.
Promote physical contact between family members and care providers.	This communicates concern when verbal messages cannot be taken in and integrated because of overwhelming grief.
Avoid attempts to reassure patient that she "can have another baby."	This approach denies real and present loss and natural accompanying grief. Also it is unknown at this time what effect the ectopic pregnancy, rupture of the fallopian tube, and surgery will have on the potential reproductive potential.

▼

DISCHARGE PLANNING/CONTINUITY OF CARE

- Refer to support groups for families experiencing perinatal loss.
- Instruct patient on postoperative recovery regimens:
  - pain management
  - work/activity
  - postoperative checkup

REFERENCES

Hauswald, M. & Kerr, N. L. (1989). Gynecologic causes of abdominal pain. *Emergency Care Quarterly, 5*(3), 37–48.

Jacobson, S. (1990). More than clinical . . . ectopic pregnancy. *Emergency Medicine, 22*(8), 96.

Joesoef, M., Westrom, L., Reynolds, G., Marchbanks, P. & Cates, W. (1991). Reoccurance of ectopic pregnancy: The role of salpingitis. *American Journal of Obstetrics and Gynecology, 165*(1), 46–50.

Nederlof, K, Lawson, H., Saftlas, A., Atrash, H., & Finch, E. (1990). Ectopic pregnancy surveillance: United States 1970–1987. *Morbidity and Mortality Weekly Report, 39*(SS-4), 9–17.

Nolan, T. & Gallup, D. (1989). Shock in ectopic pregnancy. *Female Patient, 14*(10), 66–72.

Shapiro, P. (1990). Pelviscopy for ectopic pregnancy: A safer and quicker alternative. *Today's OR Nurse, 12*(6), 6–10.

Shartz-Engel, N. (1991). Methotrexate in ectopic pregnancy. *Journal of Maternal-Child Nursing, 16,* 346.

▼

$\mathcal{E}$PIDURAL ANESTHESIA DURING LABOR AND DELIVERY

Sarah Cohen, RN

During labor and delivery anesthetics may be injected into the epidural space to block neurological pathways. This results in temporary interruption of the conduction of nerve impulses, eliminating pain sensation, and sometimes impairing leg movement. Continuous epidural anesthesia extends the duration of anesthesia. This procedure is also termed regional anesthesia and lumbar epidural anesthesia.

INDICATIONS

- To reduce the pain associated with labor and birth
- Intraoperative anesthesia during cesarean birth

▼

NURSING DIAGNOSIS: KNOWLEDGE DEFICIT

Related To
No previous experience with epidural anesthesia

Defining Characteristics
Apparent confusion
Need for more information
Misconceptions
Many questions

Patient Outcomes
Patient will
- make informed decision about anesthesia.
- describe benefits and disadvantages of epidural anesthesia.

Nursing Interventions	**Rationales**
Assess to what degree anxiety/level of discomfort compromises ability to understand information.	
Discuss advantages and disadvantages of epidural anesthesia.	Information is necessary for informed decision-making.

1. Advantages
  • Mother remains alert and able to participate in childbirth.
  • Continuous epidural used in delivery may be modified for cesarean section if necessary.
  • Absence of pain may help mother with bonding.
  • Can be used with medical complications.
  • After an operative delivery, epidural morphine can be administered.
	There is virtual absence of operative pain for nearly 24 hours after surgery.

2. Disadvantages
  • Normal variations in anatomy may result in uneven/incomplete pain relief; some patients have no relief.
  • Maternal hypotension may occur.
  • Fetal bradycardia may result from maternal hypotension.
  • Bearing-down efforts may be partially or completely eliminated; may necessitate use of outlet forceps.
  • Temporary loss of ability to evacuate bladder may occur.
  • Temporary loss of sensation and motion in legs may occur.
  • Suppression of respirations may occur with total spinal.	

Explain necessity for anesthesiologist to evaluate patient and the fetus' physical condition, during and following the infusion.	

Nursing Interventions

Describe the procedure for epidural anesthesia:

1. A fluid load of 500–2000 mL lactated Ringer's solution is given.

2. Baseline vital signs are obtained at the beginning and at 2- to 5-minute intervals throughout procedure.

3. Patient is positioned either:
   - dangling at bedside with back arched
   - in side-lying position with knees drawn up and head bowed to present curved back to anesthesiologist.

4. The area is draped and an antiseptic solution is applied to the skin.

5. The anesthesiologist locates the site for the introduction of the needle/catheter.

6. A local anesthetic is injected over this site.

7. A spinal needle is used to locate the epidural space and a test dose of anesthetic agent is given. The patient is instructed to observe for signs and symptoms of toxicity:
   - metallic taste in mouth
   - ringing in ears
   - anxiety or abnormal behavior
   - convulsion due to intravascular injection of anesthetic agent

8. If no untoward effects are observed, a small catheter is inserted into the epidural space. The needle is withdrawn and the catheter is taped in place.

Rationales

This reduces likelihood of hypotension secondary to sympathetic blockade.

These positions allow for easy palpation of the intravertebral space.

Nursing Interventions	Rationales
9. The patient is dosed with the anesthetic agent and placed in supine position with a wedge under the hip.	This displaces the uterus off the vena cava.
10. Serial blood pressures and assessments of anesthesia level/effectiveness are made.	
11. Anesthetic is usually progressively more effective with loss of painful sensation within 20 minutes after injection of the agent.	
12. Either serial injections of anesthetic agent or a continuous infusion can be administered through the epidural catheter.	
13. At the time of delivery the patient may be able to sit up and be given a "perineal or final" dose.	This ensures particularly good anesthesia in the area where the episiotomy will be given. In this case, no local infiltration of anesthetic agent will be required.

▼

NURSING DIAGNOSIS: HIGH RISK FOR IMPAIRED PHYSICAL MOBILITY

Risk Factors
Epidural anesthesia effects

Patient Outcomes
Patient will
- move extremities if able.
- be protected from injury if she exhibits loss of sensation.
- be able to participate in delivery process as instructed.

Nursing Interventions	Rationales
Assess level of anesthesia.	
Assess role patient's position in bed may play in level of anesthesia.	Anesthesia level rises if patient's head is in dependent position. Never place patient with epidural anesthesia in Trendelenburg's position.
Assess ability to move/feel sensation in legs.	Patient may have normal, reduced, or absent ability to move extremities. Protective measures are needed if she is unable to feel/move legs.
Ensure patient's safety: protect legs from compression against side rails; wrap sheet around feet/legs.	This prevents feet/legs from falling off bed. Patient may have no motor control/sensory awareness of limbs.
Monitor respiratory status. Have equipment for ventilatory support available.	
Assess ability to bear down voluntarily in the second stage.	Patients may complain of "pressure" when they have completely dilated.
Facilitate delivery when patient is completely dilated; the care provider may:	
1. Place gloved fingers in vagina; apply pressure toward rectum. Instruct patient to push toward pressure sensation.	Patient may not feel pain but most feel pressure and push more effectively given this impetus.
2. Place mirror in position that allows patient to view perineum.	Patient can gauge efforts if she can visualize labia opening during pushing.

▼

NURSING DIAGNOSIS: HIGH RISK FOR PAIN/DISCOMFORT

Risk Factors
Leaking of cerebrospinal fluid from puncture/cannula site

Patient Outcome
Patient will verbalize relief from or absence of headache.

Nursing Interventions	Rationales
Assess severity of headache when changing position from lying to sitting or standing.	Headache is caused by accidental puncture of dura and leakage of cerebrospinal fluids; this depletion causes brain to sag in the cranium when patient is in upright position.
Encourage patient to lie flat in bed.	Headache is usually absent in this position.
Encourage oral intake. Provide intravenous hydration as indicated.	Fluids replace cerebrospinal fluid losses.
Assist anesthesiologist in administering blood patch.	A plasma sample of the patient's own blood is injected into the epidural space. It contains the factors necessary to seal the opening and prevent further leaking.

NURSING DIAGNOSIS: HIGH RISK FOR INJURY TO FETUS

Risk Factor
Maternal hypotension

Patient Outcome
Patient will maintain adequate blood pressure and perfusion to fetus.

Nursing Interventions	Rationales
Assess for decreased or late decelerations, or fetal bradycardia.	
Take measures to alleviate maternal hypotension: 1. Infuse intravenous fluids at rapid rate. 2. Place patient in lateral position or place wedge under hip. 3. Give oxygen to patient. 4. Notify anesthesiologist. 5. Have ephedrine on hand to support blood pressure.	Maternal hypotension results in decreased blood perfusion to fetal/placental unit; may produce fetal hypoxia. Fetus may also be depressed by direct action of anesthetic that crosses placenta.
Allow for intrauterine resuscitation whenever possible.	This reduces likelihood of infant's being born acidotic and requiring intensive medical resuscitation.

Nursing Interventions	Rationales
Prepare for delivery of compromised infant when factors causing maternal/fetal decline cannot be reversed.	

NURSING DIAGNOSIS: HIGH RISK FOR INJURY TO MOTHER

Risk Factors
- Allergic response to anesthetic agent
- High drug concentration
- Increased absorption rate (caused by rich vascularity)
- Intravenous or intra-arterial infiltration of anesthetic
- Hypotension from sympathetic blockade

Patient Outcomes
Patient will demonstrate no untoward effects from anesthesia, as evidenced by
- normal blood pressure
- absence of nausea/vomiting
- muscle twitching
- headache

Nursing Interventions	Rationales
Assess patient throughout procedure for signs of untoward responses.	Responses may range from mild reactions (headache, palpitations, vertigo), to moderate reactions (hypotension, muscle twitching, nausea/vomiting), to severe reactions (loss of consciousness, severe hypotension, death).
Have emergency equipment/drugs readily available in case of severe untoward effects.	
Infuse 1.5–2 L of lactated Ringer's solution over 30–45 minutes before beginning procedure.	Fluid loading may prevent hypotension.
Assess blood pressure every 2 minutes for 15 minutes after epidural anesthesia administration.	

Nursing Interventions	Rationales
Institute treatment measures for any signs of maternal hypotension: 1. Administer O_2 by rebreather at 10 L/min. 2. Increase intravenous drip rate; administer bolus of at least 300 ml rapidly. 3. Place patient in left lateral position. 4. Anticipate administration of ephedrine.	
Place wedge under right hip to displace uterus from vena cava and provide for optimal blood return and placental perfusion.	

▼

NURSING DIAGNOSIS: HIGH RISK FOR URINARY RETENTION

Risk Factor
Effect of anesthesia

Patient Outcome
Patient will maintain adequate urine output, as evidenced by ability to empty bladder.

Nursing Interventions	Rationales
Have patient empty bladder after fluid loading but before epidural.	
Assess ability to urinate spontaneously by determining amount of sensation remaining in perineum after epidural.	
Assess for distended bladder.	
Allow patient to sit upright on bedpan to void. Provide assistance/stimulation to precipitate urination.	
1. Let warm water trickle over perineum.	

Nursing Interventions	Rationales
2. Run water in bathroom.	Running water sometimes provides auditory impetus to void.
3. Place patient's hands in warm water.	
Catheterize patient if these measures fail	During second stage of labor, a full bladder can be traumatized/injured by descending fetus.

▼

DISCHARGE PLANNING/CONTINUITY OF CARE

- When epidural catheter is removed, ensure that distal part is intact.
- Provide for routine postpartum care and postdischarge follow-up.

REFERENCES

Endler, G. C. (1990). The risk of anesthesia in obese parturients. *Journal of Perinatology, 10*(2), 175–179.

Martin, J., Hudson-Goodman, P., & Herman, N. (1991). New aspects in lumbar epidural analgesia for labor. *CRNA-Clinical Forum for Nurse Anesthetists, 2*(4), 142–147.

Stampone, D. (1990). The history of obstetrical anesthesia. *Journal of Perinatal and Neonatal Nursing, 4*(1), 1–13.

Thorp, J., McNitt, D., & Lippert, P. (1990). Effects of epidural analgesia: Some questions and answers. *Birth: Issues in Perinatal Care and Education, 17*(3), 157–162.

▼

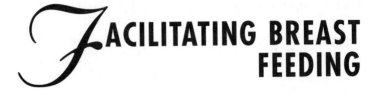

FACILITATING BREAST FEEDING

Catherine Folker-Maglaya, RN, MSN, IBCLC

The nurse will provide assistance/instruction to a mother/family to facilitate successful breast feeding (i.e., the synthesis and secretion of milk from the breast in the nourishment of an infant or child).

ETIOLOGIES

N/A

CLINICAL MANIFESTATIONS

N/A

▼

NURSING DIAGNOSIS: KNOWLEDGE DEFICIT

Related To
- Few role models
- New experience
- Unfamiliarity with process

Defining Characteristics
- Need for more information
- Multiple questions or lack of questions

Patient Outcomes
The mother/family will verbalize knowledge enabling them to successfully manage their breast-feeding experience.

Nursing Interventions	**Rationales**

Discuss feeding choice as early as possible postconception. Include advantages of breast versus bottle feeding:
1. Benefits of breast feeding:
  • complete nourishment for first 6 months of infant's life
  • easily digested
  • provides passive immunity to baby (for the duration of breast feeding); decreases the incidence of diarrhea, upper respiratory infections, otitis media, and some allergies
  • convenient, readily available at the right temperature, in the correct amounts
  • infant regulation of own intake
  • encourages optimal jaw, teeth, and speech development
  • decreases postpartum bleeding in mother (enhances uterine involution)
  • minimal financial cost (only cost is for foods to supply adequate maternal diet)
  • maternal weight loss (energy for lactation obtained from fat stores produced in pregnancy)
  • *very important:* promotes unique closeness between mother and infant
2. benefits of bottle feeding:
  • anyone may feed the infant	

Assist mother/family with decision-making.	
Assess the mother's educational needs and support her right to breast-feed, if she has made this decision. Data should include review of maternal breast-feeding experiences, support systems, etc.	

Nursing Interventions	Rationales
Provide mother with information about resources.	Factual information provides a firm base for proper breast-feeding management.
Explain changes that occur to the breasts during pregnancy in preparation for nourishing the baby: 1. increased size, caused by development of milk producing structures 2. visible veins due to increased blood flow 3. darkened areola, which serve as visual cue for the baby 4. colostrum (premilk) may leak as early as the fifth or sixth month of pregnancy	
Assure the mother that the size and shape of the breasts have no relation to the ability to breastfeed.	
Stress importance of breast examination and assessment: 1. Identify any potential problems early in pregnancy (e.g., inverted nipples, breast reduction surgery). 2. Refer problems to her health care provider or Lactation Consultant. 3. Explain that few conditions interfere with the ability to breast-feed.	
Teach mother about nipple preparation:	
1. Wash breasts with clear warm water during daily bath or shower, avoiding soap (as it is drying), and expose breasts to air whenever possible.	Studies have shown that nipple toughening techniques (i.e., brisk rubbing or pulling) do little to prevent soreness during early breast feeding.

Nursing Interventions

2. Flat or inverted nipples require early intervention and can be identified by pressing the areola between the thumb and forefinger and pulling back toward the chest ("pinch test"). A protractile nipple will protrude; the inverted nipple will retract.

3. Wear plastic milk cups (also known as shells) inside bra; these should be worn as soon as a problem is identified.

4. Select support nursing bra approximately one month prior to delivery, approximately one cup size larger.

Discuss selection of a health care provider for the baby, one who is knowledgeable and supportive of breast feeding. Encourage prenatal visit by expectant parents.

Rationales

Milk cups exert steady but gentle pressure on the areola causing the nipple to extend outward through the opening in the cup (not to be confused with a nipple shield).

Patient must accommodate increased size of breasts with breast pads.

These discussions provide opportunities to ask questions regarding breast-feeding support and other areas of infant care.

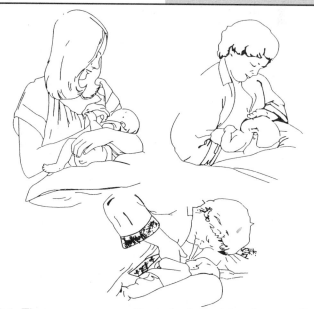

Figure 39.1 Three common positions for breast feeding: cradle, football hold, lying down position. Reprinted by permission from the Illinois Department of Public Health.

Postpartum—"Getting off to a good start"

Nursing Interventions	Rationales
Stress importance of early initiation of breast feeding.	Initiation within the first hour of life has been shown to increase success. Immediately after birth the infant is in a quiet alert state and apt to suckle with minimal assistance.
Provide information on the following:	
1. Breast milk is produced by "supply and demand."	The more often the baby suckles, the more milk produced.
2. Although mature milk may not appear for 3 to 5 days postpartum, colostrum is present, full of nutrients and antibodies, and is all the baby needs for the first few days of life.	
3. Breast-feed on demand (most babies breast-feed every 1½ to 3 hours) for the first several weeks.	
4. Avoid introducing a bottle until the baby is 3 to 4 weeks old.	This allows time to establish an adequate milk supply and prevents nipple confusion.
5. Rest and fluids aid in increasing milk supply.	
Explain that "letdown" (milk release) is encouraged by allowing the baby plenty of time to complete each feeding. Women can experience several "letdowns" during a breast-feeding session. Signs of "letdown:" 1. uterine cramping and increased vaginal flow for first few days postpartum 2. leaking of the breasts: as the baby breast-feeds on one, the other nipple may leak 3. tingling in the breasts 4. *best indicator:* "audible/visible" swallowing of the baby	Letdown can be stimulated by applying moist heat and gentle massaging of the breast before and as the baby breast-feeds.

Nursing Interventions	**Rationales**
Discuss growth spurts: 1. Babies experience periods of rapid growth throughout the first year; their demands for breast milk increase. 2. During these periods, the baby may be fussy and want to breast-feed more often. Encourage the mother to do so. After a few days of frequent breast feedings, her milk supply will increase to meet the baby's new demands. The baby will then return to his normal breast-feeding pattern.	
Discuss supplementation: 1. Breast milk fulfills all the baby's fluid and nutritional needs for the first 6 months of life. 2. Supplements can interfere with the baby's interest in later breast feedings and can result in a decreased milk supply. 3. The introduction of solids is not recommended until the baby is 4 to 6 months old. Generally, an iron-fortified infant cereal is the first solid introduced and is offered *after* breast feeding.	
Provide supportive information on "How To Get Started." 1. Explain that breast feeding is a learned process for both the mother and baby and requires practice. 2. Instruct mother to wash hands prior to each feeding. 3. Help mother to assume a comfortable position in bed or in an armchair using pillows for support.	

Nursing Interventions	**Rationales**
4. Demonstrate cradle, football, and side-lying positions. See p. 337.	
5. Using the cradle hold, place the infant in correct position in mother's arms so that the infant's chest, abdomen, and knees face the mother.	
6. Instruct the mother to • support her breast throughout the feeding, by placing her fingers under the breast and thumb on top.	
• gently stroke or tickle the baby's lower lip with her nipple until the baby opens his mouth widely with his tongue down, forming a large O.	This elicits the rooting reflex.
• guide the baby onto her breast, stressing the importance of the baby attaching or latching on the areola, not simply the nipple.	This facilitates compression of sinuses under the areola, which stimulates milk production and releases "letdown"; it is also a measure to prevent nipple soreness.
7. Remain with mother to ensure effective breast feeding.	Adequacy of the feeding is defined by the baby suckling in bursts with pauses; jaws should move rhythmically with visible and audible swallowing.
8. Encourage mother to offer both breasts at each feeding, although the baby may not always nurse at both breasts.	
9. Instruct the mother to: • burp the baby after the first breast and at the end of the feeding.	
• break the infant's suction on the areola by gently placing her finger between the infant's gums before removing him from the breast.	This helps prevent nipple trauma.

Nursing Interventions	**Rationales**
Instruct the mother that the baby is getting enough if he 1. is content. 2. receives 8 to 12 feedings in 24 hours. 3. wets 6 to 10 diapers in 24 hours (by the third day of life). 4. has at least one to two bowel movements in 24 hours (from birth).	Breast milk stools are generally mustard-colored, unformed, and may have a seedy appearance.
Provide mother instructions on whom to call for questions/difficulties.	
Discuss weaning: 1. Breast feeding is recommended for one year or longer by the American Academy of Pediatrics. 2. If weaning prior to 1 year of age, an infant formula should be provided (should be discussed with baby's health care provider). 3. Mother-initiated weaning should occur gradually over several weeks, and can be accomplished by dropping one breast feeding at a time with several days between and offering an age appropriate substitute (e.g., formula, whole milk).	
Discuss collection and storage of breast milk: 1. Teach mother hand expression techniques, or use of breast pump if preferred.	There are a variety of pumps available: manual, battery-operated, hand-held electric, and "hospital-type" electric pumps. The mother should be assisted to choose one that best suits her needs.

Nursing Interventions	Rationales

2. Instruct her to
  • carefully wash her hands.
  • make herself comfortable.
  • manually express or pump each breast until the flow subsides, then return to each breast a second or third time for a few more minutes.
 	
3. Freshly expressed or pumped breast milk may be stored in the refrigerator for 48 hours in presterilized bottles or bottle bags. Although refrigeration is preferred, studies have shown that freshly expressed breast milk may be kept at room temperature for up to 10 hours.
 	
4. Breast milk may be stored in the freezer for 6 months at 0°F.
 	
5. Defrosted breast milk may be refrigerated for 24 hours.	

Explain that working and breast feeding are compatible: 1. This arrangement requires planning and preparation. Collecting breast milk in advance and "stockpiling" in the freezer is advisable. 2. When at home, breast-feed as much as possible, making certain to breast-feed in the morning before leaving for work and immediately upon arriving home. 3. While at work, attempt to express as often as the mother would breast-feed the baby. This means two to three expressions for an 8-hour working day. 4. If time simply does not allow, expressing once during work hours is advisable, and (depending on the baby's age) provide supplemental formula, etc., as needed.	

Nursing Interventions	Rationales
Discuss breast feeding in public: 1. Raise up a loose-fitting top with the infant covering exposed skin. 2. Unbutton the bottom buttons when wearing a button-down blouse. 3. Drape a receiving blanket over the shoulder.	It is important for the mother/family to feel comfortable with the woman breast-feeding in public.
Provide additional information on: 1. Diet • Instruct the mother to eat three well-balanced meals and two snacks/day, chosen from the four basic food groups.	Energy intake requirements during lactation are similar to that required during pregnancy (malnourished or very active women may require more). Intake of approximately 2200 calories/day should be adequate.
• Encourage to drink to thirst. • Limit caffeine intake to small amounts.	Excessive caffeine can cause the baby to become irritable and fussy.

• Refer to nutritionist or dietary counselor as needed.
2. Viruses
   • Cold, flu, and gastroenteritis-type viruses experienced by the mother should not preclude breast feeding.
3. Drugs, alcohol, and smoking
   • Any substance used by the mother can be passed through her milk and thus given to her baby.
 	
   • The presence of a drug in breast milk does not mean that an adverse effect will occur.
	The drug may not be absorbed by the infant, may be destroyed by the baby's gastrointestinal tract, or may be pharmacologically inactive upon reaching the infant.

Nursing Interventions

- Should the mother require a prescription medication, instruct her to remind her health care provider that she is breast-feeding and confirm the drug's advisability with the baby's health care provider or a lactation consultant.

- For information regarding the safety of drugs while breast-feeding, one can refer to: American Academy of Pediatrics Committee on Drugs, "Transfer of Drugs and Other Chemicals Into Human Milk" or call "drug information line" of most major medical centers/university hospitals.

- Mother should contact baby's health care provider prior to taking any over-the-counter medications.

- Use of illicit "street" drugs is contraindicated with breast feeding.

- Alcohol passes into breast milk quickly and is excreted in time. Although a safe alcohol consumption level has not yet been determined, an infrequent alcoholic beverage after breast feeding appears to cause no problem in the infant.

- A breast-feeding mother should cut down or consider low nicotine cigarettes if she is unable to completely stop smoking.

Rationales

If there is a conflict, it may be possible to prescribe a different medication.

These drugs are released in breast milk and can have extremely harmful effects on baby.

Excessive alcohol intake has produced serious adverse effects in the infant.

Heavy smoking can diminish a mother's milk production and decreases the vitamin C available to the infant. The infant may be at greater risk for nausea and vomiting and incidence of respiratory infections.

Nursing Interventions

4. Sex/contraception
    - Explain that when intercourse is resumed in postpartum (4 to 6 weeks after delivery is advisable) the mother may experience vaginal dryness.

    - Breast stimulation and orgasm may cause the milk to "let-down" and leak. If leaking is bothersome, breast-feeding shortly before lovemaking or wearing a bra during lovemaking can be helpful.

    - Breast feeding delays the onset of ovulation and menstruation, thus tending to postpone pregnancy, but should not be depended upon to prevent pregnancy. Barrier methods of birth control (e.g., condoms and foam, intrauterine devices, diaphragm) are recommended. Low-dose estrogen oral contraceptives are listed as safe by the American Academy of Pediatrics Committee on Drugs. (Although some physicians remain reluctant to prescribe them during the breast-feeding period for fear of possible long-term effects on the baby).

Rationales

This is due to hormonal changes; a commercial lubricant can make intercourse more comfortable and pleasurable.

Nursing Interventions	**Rationales**
Assist the mother to initiate expressing her breasts within 24 hours postdelivery if circumstances (for reasons of maternal or infant health) warrant that the mother and baby be separated:	
1. Instruct her to express as often as she would be breast-feeding, ideally no less than six to eight times per day. The use of hospital-type electric breast pump (with double pump attachment) is recommended for long-term pumping.	The most efficient expression next to the baby, simultaneous breast expression increases prolactin levels, thus increasing milk production.
2. Preterm/sick infants can receive expressed breast milk via a nasogastric tube and assisted to breast as soon as stable.	
3. Refer to Lactation Consultant as recommended.	

▼

NURSING DIAGNOSIS: PAIN/DISCOMFORT

Related To
- Engorged breasts
- Improper positioning and latching of infant
- Impaired skin integrity

Defining Characteristics
Grimacing/moaning during breast-feeding session
Guarding behavior
Reluctance to initiate breast feeding
Pain

Patient Outcomes
- Nipple integrity will be maintained.
- Breasts will remain engorgement-free.

Nursing Interventions	**Rationales**
Nipple soreness	
1. Assess whether mother is experiencing any discomfort during the feeding.	A common cause of nipple soreness is improper positioning.
2. Observe breast-feeding technique, noting positioning and attachment of the baby.	
3. Instruct mother in steps to prevent nipple soreness:	
• Wash or shower breasts daily with clear warm water. Soap is drying.	
• Keep nipples free of moisture; change pads as needed.	
• Air-dry breasts for 10 minutes postfeedings. Apply colostrum/breast milk to the areola.	Breast milk serves as antibacterial and lubricating agent.
• Rotate nursing positions.	
• Ensure that baby grasps the areola correctly.	
• Break the baby's suction with her finger before removing him from the breast.	
4. Should nipple soreness occur, instruct mother in how to alleviate this condition:	
• Promote the "let-down" reflex prior to putting the baby to breast by using moist heat to the breasts, gentle massaging the breasts toward the nipple, briefly pressing breasts either by hand or using a pump, and/or participating in a relaxing activity (nap, shower, warm fluids).	
• Breast-feed more frequently (every 2 hours), but for shorter periods.	
• Air-dry breasts after each feeding.	A blow-dryer on the lowest setting may be used.

Nursing Interventions	Rationales
• Breast-feed on the least sore side first. • Use acetaminophen for pain (compatible with breast feeding/American Academy of Pediatrics Committee on Drugs). 5. If soreness persists or worsens in spite of these measures, instruct mother to consult her health care provider or Lactation Consultant.	

Engorgement
1. Assess for signs of engorgement:
   • feeling of heaviness, fullness, or tightness of the breasts
   • breasts may feel hard, warm, and tender
   • baby may have difficulty latching on to the areola due to the fullness
2. Instruct patient about engorgement:
   • occurs 3–5 days postdelivery when the transitional milk comes in and breasts become overfilled
   • later, when the breasts are insufficiently emptied (increased breast size and fullness are combination of interstitial and lymph fluid as well as colostrum/milk)

3. Instruct that the best treatment is prevention.	Babies should be breast-fed on demand around-the-clock (every 1½ to 3 hours). Engorgement is often secondary to infrequent feedings, skipping feedings, or excessive supplementation.

Nursing Interventions	**Rationales**

4. Should engorgement occur, instruct patient to
  • breast-feed frequently.
  • apply moist heat and gently massage breasts prior to breast feeding.
  • apply cold packs between feedings.
  • wear well-fitting supportive bra.
  • hand-express or pump enough to soften the areola so baby can latch-on.
  • use acetaminophen for pain.
5. If breasts remain full and uncomfortable after breast-feeding, it may be necessary to express the breasts to soften until comfortable. Avoid excessive expression/pumping (may lead to increased milk production). Emphasize that the baby is the best pump.	

▼

NURSING DIAGNOSIS: HIGH RISK FOR INFECTION

Risk Factors
• Bacteria passed from baby
• Entry of bacteria via cracked nipple
• Failure to remove plug
• Inadequate emptying of breasts
• Lowered resistance, stress, and fatigue

Patient Outcome
Risk of infection will be reduced by early assessment and prompt treatment.

Nursing Interventions

Plugged milk duct

1. Assess for signs/symptoms of plugged milk duct (most common during early weeks of breast feeding):
   - hard "pealike" area
   - localized redness and tenderness
   - large part of breast feels overly full and does not soften with breast feeding.
2. Provide instructions regarding management:
   - Remove bra if too tight or applies pressure to any area of breast.
   - Breast-feed frequently, at least every 2 hours, beginning each feeding on the affected breast.
   - Increase fluid intake.
   - Apply moist heat to the breast 15 minutes prior to feeding the baby.
   - Gently massage the breast just above the tender area prior to and while feeding the baby.
   - Be alert to signs that infection may be developing. Notify health care provider.

Mastitis

1. Assess for mastitis (symptoms usually subside within 24 hours with proper treatment):
   - usually affects one breast
   - localized area of redness, pain, and swelling
   - flulike symptoms: achiness, fever, chills, headache, and occasionally nausea and vomiting.
   - notify health care provider.

Rationales

Usually antibiotic therapy is indicated.

Nursing Interventions	Rationales
2. Instruct on management (same as for plugged duct, plus): • Get plenty of rest. • Take antibiotics for entire time prescribed regardless of disappearance of symptoms. • Apply moist heat to affected area before and between feedings. • Monitor temperature every 4 hours.	
3. Assure the mother that the baby will not become ill.	The infection involves the breast tissue not the milk. Temporarily discontinuing breast feeding may delay healing and lead to breast abscess.
4. If symptoms persist beyond a couple of days, suspect a breast abscess and call the health care provider.	An abscess requires draining. Breast feeding is temporarily discontinued on the affected side for a few days postdrainage with frequent emptying of the breast using an electric pump during that period.

▼

NURSING DIAGNOSIS: INEFFECTIVE BREAST FEEDING

Related To
• Infant anomaly
• Infant receiving supplemental feedings with artificial nipple
• Knowledge deficit
• Maternal anxiety
• Nonsupportive partner
• Poor infant suck
• Prematurity

Defining Characteristics
Actual or perceived inadequate milk supply
Infant arching and crying at the breast
Infant's inability to attach on to maternal breast correctly
Insufficient emptying of each breast per feeding
Non-sustained suckling at the breast
No observable signs of "letdown"

Observable signs of inadequate infant intake
Persistence of sore nipples beyond the first week of breast feeding
Unsatisfactory breast feeding process

Patient Outcomes

Mother/family will have successful breast-feeding experience, as evidenced by
- baby gaining weight.
- baby appearing satisfied.
- mother appearing relaxed.
- emptied mother's breast.

Nursing Interventions	Rationales
Determine mother's concerns/explanation of the breast-feeding problem.	
Assess mother's general state of health: Is she resting? Is she eating properly and drinking fluids adequately? Condition of breasts and nipples?	
Assess baby's general health: 1. activity level, contentness 2. weight gain 3. skin color and turgor 4. sucking reflex (strong or weak?) 5. frequency of stools and voids (noting character)	
Assess breast-feeding pattern, noting frequency and duration of feedings.	
Observe breast-feeding session for effectiveness, noting if 1. mother and infant are positioned comfortably. 2. baby attaches (latches-on) areola correctly. 3. mother and baby look relaxed. 4. baby's cheeks remain well-rounded without dimpling or indenting (no smacking or clicking should be heard). 5. baby is suckling rhythmically in bursts with pauses with audible/visible swallowing.	This "suck-suck-suck-swallow" pattern may occur steadily over several minutes or come in surges.

Nursing Interventions	**Rationales**
6. "Letdown" is apparent.	
If there is no identifiable problem (i.e., the baby appears healthy and is steadily gaining weight/mother is physically well), the problem may be a *"perceived"* problem. Stress "positives" (i.e., weight gain, adequate output) with reinforcement of breast-feeding instruction/management as indicated (increases confidence, decreases anxiety).	Praising the mother/family is also indicated. Telephone follow-up is recommended.
If an *"actual"* problem exists and management is within the realm of the health care provider's knowledge and skills, begin intervention and follow up as needed. Should the problem persist, refer to a Lactation Consultant.	On occasion, situations will warrant expert assistance by a Lactation Consultant. Referral to a Lactation Consultant is recommended (but not limited to) the following: multiple births, preterm/sick infants, babies with congenital anomalies (e.g., cardiac), genetic defects (e.g., cleft-lip and palate, Down syndrome), and neurologically impaired infants. Slow weight gain infants/failure-to-thrive infants. Chronic nipple soreness/recurrent mastitis. Insufficient milk supply. Induced lactation (e.g., breast-feeding an adopted infant).
Share the breast-feeding mother's strengths and praise efforts. Depending on the situation, the mother/family may choose to pursue alternative modes of management or decide to discontinue breast feeding; support her/their decision.	

▼

DISCHARGE PLANNING/CONTINUITY OF CARE

- Provide listings of breast-feeding resource books, films, and prenatal classes offered in the community.
- Provide a list of community breast-feeding support services, such as:
  La Leche League International (LLLI)
  9616 Minneapolis Avenue
  Franklin Park, Illinois 60131
  (708) 455–7730.
- Provide information on Breastpump Rentals and Breastfeeding Supplies:

Medela	Egnell
Post Office Box 386	765 Industrial Drive
Crystal Lake, Illinois	Cary, Illinois
60014	60013
1-800-TELLYOU (24-hrs)	1-800-323-8750.

- Refer to healthcare provider/lactation consultant for follow-up appointment.
- Information on hospital-based and private-practice lactation consultants may be provided by:
  International Lactation Consultant Association (ILCA)
  201 Brown Avenue
  Evanston, Illinois 60202
  (708) 260–8874

REFERENCES

American Academy of Pediatrics Committee on Drugs (1989). Transfer of Drugs and Other Chemicals Into Human Milk. *Pediatrics, 84*(5), 924–931.

Bronner, Y.L. & Paige, D. M. (1992). Current concepts in infant nutrition. *Journal of Nurse-Midwifery, 37*(2) (Suppl.), 43S–58S

de Stuben, C. (1992). Breastfeeding and jaundice. *Journal of Nurse-Midwifery, 37*(2) (Suppl.), 59S–66S.

Heffern, D. (1990). Reminders for building confidence in breast-feeding moms. *American Journal of Maternal-Child Nursing, 15,* 267.

Hill, P. D. (1991). The enigma of insufficient milk supply. *American Journal of Maternal-Child Nursing, 16,* 312–316.

Huggins, K. (1991). *The Nursing Mothers' Companion.* Cambridge, MA: The Harvard Common Press.

Lauwers, J. & Woesner, C. (1990). *Counseling the Nursing Mother: A Reference Handbook for Health Care Providers and Lay Counselors.* New York: Avery Publishing Group.

Wrigley, E. A. & Hutchinson, S. A. (1990). Long-term breastfeeding: The secret bond. *Journal of Nurse-Midwifery, 35*(1), 35–41.

▼

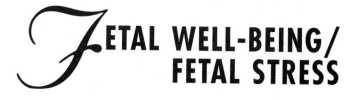

ETAL WELL-BEING/ FETAL STRESS

Paula Schipiour, RN, MS

Some of the more commonly ordered fetal screening tests available today are the non-stress test (NST), the contraction stress test (CST), the biophysical profile (BPP). These tests are typically performed in the last 10 weeks of pregnancy to assess fetal well-being. This care guide describes both testing parameters and the nursing actions indicated for the treatment of fetal stress

INDICATIONS FOR TESTING

Women with high-risk conditions such as
- Diabetes
- Hypertension
- Intrauterine growth retardation
- Multiple gestation
- Postdates pregnancy

CLINICAL MANIFESTATIONS OF FETUS STRESS

- Abnormal baseline fetal heart rate
- Decrease in variability
- Presence of worrisome/ominous periodic patterns
- Decreased fetal movement
- Failure to grow

▼

NURSING DIAGNOSIS: KNOWLEDGE DEFICIT

Related To unfamiliarity with procedure

Defining Characteristics
Misconceptions
Many questions
Lack of questions

Patient Outcomes

Patient will describe
- purpose of fetal testing
- general procedure

Nursing Interventions	Rationales
Assess for any past experience with fetal monitoring.	
Describe how fetal monitor produces recording of fetal activity, contractions, and heart rate.	
Relate how information on fetal activity provides assessment of fetal well-being.	
Describe procedures for common tests:	

1. Nonstress test
  • Fetal monitor is applied to maternal abdomen.
  • Recordings are observed for 20 minutes to assess fetal acceleration, fetal activity, and presence of spontaneous uterine contractions.
	In nonreactive test, fewer than two accelerations are noted in a 10 minute period of time.

2. Contraction stress test
  • Synthetic oxytocin is administered via fluid infusion pump to produce three contractions in a 10-minute period.
  • Contractions subside when infusion is discontinued.
	Absence of late decelerations denotes a negative test, which indicates favorable intrauterine environment. A positive contraction stress test can indicate poor placental perfusion and may necessitate delivery. False-positive rates of 25–40% have been reported in early gestational ages.

Nursing Interventions

Rationales

3. Breast-stimulation test: Intermittent nipple stimulation through the patient's clothes evokes release of endogenous oxytocin from posterior pituitary gland.
   - Nipples are stimulated for 2 minutes followed by a 2-minute rest period.
   - If contractions are inadequate by the time four cycles have been completed, then one nipple is stimulated for 10 minutes.
   - If contractions are still not adequate, then bilateral stimulation is done for 10 minutes.
   - After each contraction, nipple stimulation is stopped to determine if contractions will occur spontaneously or if more stimulation is required.
   - If the contractions are still not adequate after these measures are taken, synthetic oxytocin is used to stimulate contractions.
4. Biophysical profile (BPP): Real time ultrasonography performed evaluating four parameters:
   - fetal breathing motion
   - fetal tone
   - gross body motion
   - amniotic fluid volume
5. Fetal acoustical stimulation (FAS): FAS test is utilized if nonstress test is nonreactive. Sound is used to evoke a fetal acceleration:
   - fetal acoustical stimulation placed on maternal abdomen near fetal head after 5 minutes of nonreactivity
   - stimulation performed for 30 seconds

Nursing Interventions	Rationales
Adjust monitor for easy viewing by mother/significant others.	Review findings periodically to minimize apprehension.
6. Kick test: Explain method for monitoring and charting fetal activity. • Count fetal kicks for 30 minutes: twice a day at the same times every day, preferably after a meal. Record. • Three to five movements is considered normal. • Less than three movements should be reported.	Adequate fetal movement is an expression of fetal well-being.

▼

NURSING DIAGNOSIS: PAIN/DISCOMFORT

Related To
- Spontaneous or stimulated uterine contractions
- Discomforts associated with test procedure:
  - maintaining of same position because of external monitor application
  - maintenance of full bladder for ultrasound
  - intravenous lines
  - nipple tenderness from breast stimulation

Defining Characteristics
Facial expression of pain
Verbalized pain/discomfort
Frequent position changes

Patient Outcomes
Patient will
- verbalize relief of discomfort or ability to tolerate it.
- appear relaxed and comfortable.

Nursing Interventions	Rationales
Solicit patient's description of discomfort.	
Provide comfort measures, extra pillows, change in position, etc.	Increase patient comfort and acceptance of test procedures.

Nursing Interventions	Rationales
Assist patient to relax through: 1. breathing modifications 2. conscious release of muscle tension 3. concentrating on other stimulus than pain (e.g., music, reading, TV, touch)	These measures distract patient from pain.
Loosen or reposition monitor.	Increases patient's level of comfort.
Elevate head of bed.	Relieves compression of the vena cava by the gravid uterus.
Assess patient's perception of uterine contraction intensity.	
Assess resting uterine tonus.	Risk of hyperstimulating uterus exists while conducting contraction stress test (contraction activity than occurs more than every 2 minutes in frequency or a contraction duration of >90 seconds).

▼

NURSING DIAGNOSIS: HIGH RISK FOR INJURY TO MOTHER

Risk Factors
- Uterine rupture
- Dehiscence along previous cesarean section incision
- Hyperstimulation of uterine contractions
- Abruptio placentae

Patient Outcome
Potential complications to mother are reduced per early assessment and prompt intervention.

Nursing Interventions	Rationales
Assess for signs of uterine rupture or dehiscence: 1. failure of uterus to relax between contractions 2. intense pain that ceases suddenly 3. sudden tearing pain.	Patients at greatest risk of rupture are those who have had previous uterine surgery.

Nursing Interventions	Rationales
Assess for signs of hyperstimulation of uterus: 1. more than five contractions in 10 minutes 2. contractions lasting longer than 90 seconds	Hyperstimulation compromises blood flow to intervillous space.
Assess for signs of abruptio placentae: 1. rising fundal height 2. increasing abdominal girth 3. uterus that fails to relax 4. complaints of extreme relentless pain 5. frank bleeding 6. signs of shock	Hyperstimulation of the uterus may result in premature separation of the placenta.
Palpate abdomen to assess for proper placement of contraction transducer and presence of contractions. Compare findings with monitor.	
Assess patient's perception of uterine contractions and pain.	
In the event of hyperstimulation: 1. discontinue oxytocin infusion 2. flush distal intravenous tubing	 If oxytocin is not evacuated from the IV line before fluid loading to treat hyperstimulation, a bolus of oxytocin could be given, further compromising the situation.
3. Increase intravenous drip rate.	Increases perfusion to uterus and decreases uterine hypertonus.
4. Place patient in left lateral position.	
If hyperstimulation results from contractions produced through breast stimulation: 1. Stop breast stimulation. 2. Start intravenous infusion of normal saline, run at rapid rate until contractions subside.	
Prepare for emergency delivery if uterine rupture/dehiscence is noted.	These represent life-threatening problems to both mother and fetus.

NURSING DIAGNOSIS: HIGH RISK FOR INJURY: STRESS TO FETUS

Risk Factors
- Physiological stress of uterine contractions
- Umbilical cord compression
- Poor placental perfusion
- Premature delivery

Patient Outcomes
- The fetus will demonstrate no signs of stress, as evidenced by normal baseline heart rate, presence of short- and long-term variability and the absence of ominous periodic patterns.
- If signs of stress are noted, the fetus will receive prompt treatment.

Nursing Interventions	Rationales
Assess fetal monitor strip. Report and document: 1. fetal bradycardia: moderate, 110–100 beats per minute; severe, < 100 beats per minute 2. fetal tachycardia: moderate, 161–180 beats per minute; severe, 180–200 beats per minute 3. late decelerations 4. moderate to severe variable decelerations caused by cord compression. 5. alteration/decrease in fetal heart rate variability.	To determine severity of the variable deceleration use the 60 × 60 rule: decelerations < 60 beats per minute, lasts longer than 60 seconds, and a drop of > 60 beats below current baseline rate reflects severe variable decelerations.
Implement nursing measures to treat fetal stress: 1. Stop oxytocin infusion. 2. Reposition until pattern is improved or abolished. 3. Increase intravenous drip rate. 4. Administer O_2 per rebreather at 10 L/min. 5. Prepare for possible delivery of a premature/compromised newborn.	

Nursing Interventions	**Rationales**
Rule out supine hypotension as the cause of the fetal stress.	In supine position, gravid uterus compresses blood flow through maternal aorta and iliac artery, thereby reducing blood flow to and from the intervillous space.
Explain actions being initiated to reassure patient/significant others.	

▼

DISCHARGE PLANNING/CONTINUITY OF CARE

- Instruct patient to notify care provider if contractions increase in frequency or intensity, or if bag of water ruptures or leaks.
- Advise patient to return for ongoing evaluation.

REFERENCES

Daniels, S. M. & Boehm, N. (1991). Auscultated fetal heart rate accelerations: An alternative to the nonstress test. *Journal of Nurse-Midwifery*, 36(2), 88–94.

Gaffney, S. E., Salinger, L., & Vintzeleos, M. (1990). The biophysical profile for fetal surveillance. *American Journal of Maternal-Child Nursing*, 15(6), 356–360.

Gegor, C., Paine, L. L., & Johnson, T. (1991). Antepartum fetal assessment: A nurse midwifery perspective. *Journal of Nurse Midwifery*, 36(3), 153–167.

Gegor, C. & Paine, L. (1992). Antipartum fetal assessment techniques: An update for today's perinatal nurse. *Journal of Perinatal and Neonatal Nursing*, 5(4), 1–15.

Gibauer, C. & Lowe, N. (1993). The biophysical profile: Antipartal assessment of fetal well-being. *Journal of Obstetric, Gynecologic and Neonatal Nursing*, 22(2), 115–124.

▼

$\mathcal{F}$OURTH STAGE OF LABOR

Imelda Fahy, RN

The fourth stage of labor begins with the delivery of the placenta and continues for the first 1 to 2 hours of life. This period is marked by the mother's recovery from the physical process of birth and the fetus' transition to extrauterine life.

ETIOLOGIES

N/A

CLINICAL MANIFESTATIONS

- Uterine involution
- Lochia

▼

NURSING DIAGNOSIS: PAIN

Related To
- Involution of the uterus
- Episiotomy
- Distention and stretching of soft tissue (swelling)
- Bladder distention

Defining Characteristics

Discomfort
Moaning
Restlessness

Patient Outcomes

Patient will
- verbalize reduced or tolerable level of pain.
- appear calm and comfortable.

Nursing Interventions	Rationales
Assess patient's perception/description of discomfort.	
Apply ice packs to perineum if patient has discomfort due to episiotomy pain or swelling of perineum	Cold applications decrease swelling, ease discomfort.
Administer pain medications as ordered.	
Explain the reason for afterbirth pain.	Uterine contractions (much stronger than labor contractions), result from the uterus contracting down to control bleeding from the site where placenta was implanted. They begin the process of returning the uterus to its post-pregnancy size.
Palpate bladder for distention. Encourage patient to void. Catheterize if necessary.	A distended bladder may exaggerate discomfort, displace uterus, promote excessive bleeding, and prevent uterine involution.
Administer stool softener.	Straining for bowel movement could aggravate hemorrhoids, causing increased discomfort.

▼

NURSING DIAGNOSIS: HIGH RISK FOR FLUID VOLUME DEFICIT

Risk Factors
- Bleeding/hemorrhage
- Retained products of conception
- Hematoma
- Laceration
- Dehydration

Patient Outcomes
- Patient will maintain optimal fluid status as evidenced by fluid intake equal to or exceeding output.

- Risk of complications from fluid deficit is reduced through early assessment and intervention.

Nursing Interventions	Rationales
Assess for vaginal bleeding (amount, color). Assess for clots through uterine Credé maneuver.	If uterus is boggy/relaxed, clots or pooled blood will escape from the vagina when uterus is massaged.
Assess uterine status, including tone, fundal height, and position. Perform fundal massage.	Massage encourages uterus to maintain contracted state.
Monitor vital signs immediately following delivery and when needed as patient stabilizes.	
Palpate and percuss urinary bladder for distension.	
Encourage patient to void. Catheterize if necessary.	If bladder was damaged, patient might be unable to void freely. A distended bladder prevents normal uterine involution; it may cause increased vaginal bleeding/elevated blood pressure and fever.
Assess condition of perineum. Observe for swelling, ecchymosis, episiotomy. If no cause for excessive bleeding can be determined, rule out bleeding from other sites, including cervix, vagina, or perineal tears (firm uterus, but continued oozing of bright red blood).	
If hemorrhage continues: Assess blood loss on perineal pad. Institute a pad count. Weigh peripads/bedpad before and after use (1 g of weight is equal to 1 ml of blood).	Weighing pads is a good means to quantify amount of active bleeding.
Assess hemoglobin and hematocrit.	
If hemorrhage is related to retained products of conception, prepare to return to operating room for dilitation and curettage (D&C).	Retained placenta prevents the uterus from contracting. Bleeding from open sinuses may be profuse.

Nursing Interventions	Rationales
Assess for hematoma (often occurs beneath mucosa opposite the ischial spine), which palpate as full, crepitant, or fluctuant areas; may appear purple.	Hematoma results from an unligated vessel bleeding into interstitial tissues. If hematoma is visible, labia may appear edematous and shiny. The involved area may appear ecchymosed. With both visible and occult hematoma, pain will be severe. Silent bleeds are much more likely to result in hemorrhage. Patient may present with symptoms of shock.
If hematoma is cause of bleeding: Prepare for return to labor and delivery room or operating room. Anticipate surgical evacuation and ligation of vessel. Anticipate a drain being placed in the wound, and episiotomy site left open, packed, and allowed to heal by secondary intention.	
Assess for lacerations: 1. 1st degree: • involves mucosa and skin with some superficial muscle fibers • may not require suturing 2. 2nd degree: • includes deeper structures of the perineum • may or may not require suturing 3. 3rd degree: • involves the structures of the vaginal walls and the sphincter ani muscles 4. 4th degree: • the anus is laid open 5. Both 3rd and 4th degree lacerations will require suturing to achieve homeostasis and repair of structures.	These are classified by degree to aid in management.
Provide oral/IV fluids as indicated to maintain hydration.	

▼

NURSING DIAGNOSIS: HIGH RISK FOR URINARY RETENTION

Risk Factors
- Effects of anesthesia
- Trauma to urethra during delivery
- Local edema
- Discomfort
- Bladder distention

Patient Outcomes
- Patient will void in 150- to 400-ml amounts.
- Bladder will not be palpable after voiding.

Nursing Interventions	Rationales
Assess bladder every 15 minutes for 1st hour, then every 30 minutes.	
Assess level of sensation in perineal and lower extremities.	Decreased sensation is secondary to epidural/spinal anesthesia or to perineal analgesia, which may reduce the urge to void despite a full bladder.
Assist to bathroom or on bedpan as needed.	
Encourage patient to void: 1. Increase intravenous and/or oral fluids. 2. Run water within hearing distance.	
Straight catheterize as necessary.	

▼

NURSING DIAGNOSIS: HIGH RISK FOR SITUATIONAL LOW SELF-ESTEEM

Risk Factor
Negative feelings regarding role performance during labor

Patient Outcome
Patient will begin to verbalize some positive aspects of performance.

Nursing Interventions	Rationales
Assess patient's/couple's self-perceptions of delivery process/outcome.	
Encourage verbalization of feelings.	
Accept as normal any expressions of disappointment in her performance during delivery (need for medications, prolonged time, need for medical intervention).	Emphasizing the individual nature of each labor and the need to be flexible in how labor is managed will provide reassurance about performance anxiety.
Explain to mother/couple the normalcy of these feelings and behavior.	
Stress positive behavior displayed by patient and positive outcome of experience.	Emphasizing the things the patient managed well and the positive outcome will increase self-esteem.

▼

NURSING DIAGNOSIS: FAMILY COPING—POTENTIAL FOR GROWTH

Related To addition of new family member(s)

Defining Characteristics
Ability to see addition of new family member(s) as challenge and opportunity for growth
Expressions of caring and concern
Demonstration of interactions that suggest growth (appropriate bonding behavior; attempts at integrating child with other family members

Patient Outcome
Family will display positive growth behaviors, as evidenced by appropriate bonding behavior.

Nursing Interventions	Rationales
Assess mother's/significant other's feelings regarding their role in the birth process.	

Nursing Interventions

Encourage the integration of the whole family into the immediate postpartum activities by
1. encouraging family visiting
2. encouraging communication via phone
3. explaining activities/procedures and involving family in care
4. providing family with opportunity to review birth experience. Provide feedback/positive reinforcement when possible.

Rationales

Hospital procedures that are not family-centered can delay family consolidation and integration of the new family member.

▼

DISCHARGE PLANNING/CONTINUITY OF CARE

- Instruct patient to notify physician if
  - vaginal bleeding becomes excessive
  - lochia develops a foul-smelling odor
  - purulent drainage is noted
  - fever, or severe episiotomy or breast pain is experienced
  - profound depression is experienced.
- Instruct patient to make appointment for postpartum follow-up

REFERENCES

Andolsek, K. M. (1990). *Obstetric Care: Standards of Prenatal, Intrapartum and Postpartum Management.* Philadelphia, PA: Lea & Febiger.

Luegenbiehl, D. (1991). Postpartum bleeding. *NAACDG's Clinical Issues in Perinatal & Woman's Health Nursing, 2*(3), 402–409.

Luegenbiehl, D., Brophy, G., Artigne, S., Phillips, K. & Flak, R. (1990). Standardized assessment of blood loss. *American Journal of Maternal-Child Nursing, 15,* 241–244.

Morten, A., Kohl, M., O'Mahoney, P., & Pelosi, K. (1991). Certified nurse-midwifery care of the postpartum client: A descriptive study. *Journal of Nurse-Midwifery, 36*(5), 276–284.

▼

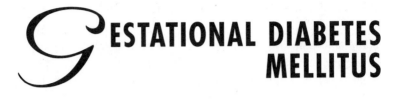

GESTATIONAL DIABETES MELLITUS

Charlotte Niznik, RN, MS, CDE

Gestational diabetes mellitus (GDM) is a carbohydrate intolerance of variable severity with onset or first recognition during pregnancy. The definition applies regardless of whether insulin is used for treatment or the condition persists after pregnancy. It does not exclude the possibility that unrecognized glucose intolerance may have antedated the pregnancy.

ETIOLOGIES

- Family history of Type II diabetes mellitus
- Previous obstetrical history of GDM
- Previous delivery of baby >9 lb
- Maternal obesity
- History of stillbirth, infant with anomalies or polyhydramnios

CLINICAL MANIFESTATIONS/DIAGNOSTIC FINDINGS

- Inappropriate or massive weight gain
- Polyhydramnios
- Polydypsia
- Blurred vision
- Inappropriate fetal growth for gestational age (LGA/SGA)
- Definitive diagnosis requires that two or more of the venous plasma glucose concentrations be met or exceeded on the glucose tolerance test (GTT):
  - fasting ≥105 mg/dl
  - 1 hour ≥190 mg/dl
  - 2 hours ≥165 mg/dl
  - 3 hours ≥145 mg/dl

▼

NURSING DIAGNOSIS: KNOWLEDGE DEFICIT REGARDING DIAGNOSIS, TREATMENT, FUTURE RISKS TO SELF AND FETUS

Related To new condition

Defining Characteristics

Confusion over events
Lack of questions
Need for information
Misconceptions

Patient Outcomes

Patient will verbalize understanding of
• screening tests for diagnosis.
• self-care practices to treat GDM.
• potential risks to self and fetus.

Nursing Interventions	Rationales
Assess knowledge about gestational diabetes	

Provide information on screening tests for gestational diabetes.
 1. Testing schedule
   • Pregnant women not identified as having glucose intolerance before 24th week should have a screening glucose load between the 24th and 28th week.
   • Women with history of a current glucose intolerance should be screened at initial presentation.
   • Rescreen women who had positive 1 hour glucose but negative glucose tolerance test (GTT) at 32 weeks.
	All pregnant women should be screened for glucose intolerance because selective screening based on clinical manifestations or past obstetric history has been shown to be inadequate.

Nursing Interventions	Rationales

2. Method:
   • A 50-g oral dose of glucose is given without regard to time of day.
   • Venous plasma glucose is measured 1 hour later.
   • A screening value of $\geq$140 mg/dl is recommended as a threshold to indicate the need for a full diagnostic glucose tolerance test.
   • Diagnosis is based on results of the 100-g oral glucose tolerance test.	

Educate patient on self-care skills for gestational diabetes
1. alteration in dietary meal plan to maintain normoglycemia:
   • carbohydrate intake maintained at no less than 4.3 g/kg of ideal body weight; protein no less than 1.5 g/kg body weight.
   • a weight gain of 9.9–10.4 kg recommended for normal pregnancy
   • total daily caloric requirement of 30–32 kcal/body weight prescribed for first trimester, and increased to 38 kcal in the second and third.
	The meal plan is designed to prevent fasting and postprandial hyperglycemia along with starvation ketosis. Three meals per day with an evening snack provide adequate calorie requirement and distribution to prevent hyperglycemia, ketonemia, and potential fetal complications.

2. self-monitoring of blood glucose:
   • fasting and premeal blood glucose levels between 70 and 90 mg/dl
   • 1-hour postprandial levels <140 mg/dl
	Glucose monitoring assists in evaluating the effects of metabolism and the need for insulin therapy.

3. daily activity and/or exercise maintenance.	Physical activity lowers blood glucose levels and potentiates the availability of endogenous insulin.
Monitor urine ketones.	Detects starvation ketosis during pregnancy.

Nursing Interventions	**Rationales**
Provide instruction on insulin therapy if prescribed. (Recommended if fasting plasma glucose consistently exceeds normal(≥105 mg/dl) and/or 1-hour postprandials are ≥140 mg/dl on two or more occasions.)	Insulin treatment is used to normalize blood glucoses and thus it is hoped, to reduce fetal morbidity from macrosomia, hyperbilirubinemia, polycythemia, hypoglycemia, hypothermia, and hypocalcemia.
Discuss blood glucose record-keeping while managing diabetes during pregnancy.	This assists health care team in evaluating home care and management as an outpatient.
Indicate when to call the health care team for help and when to review glucose control.	Frequent contact (such as a telephone call) with the health care providers may ensure glucose control and patient adherence to diabetes regimen.
Provide information about special care during labor and delivery: 1. monitoring blood glucose levels during labor and delivery 2. changes in insulin administration	Prolonged work and stress of labor decreases the need for exogenous insulin. Insulin may not be necessary during labor and delivery due to increased activity. Close/frequent monitoring of blood glucose levels must be done to determine the need for insulin. Blood glucoses should be maintained between 70 and 100 mg/dl.
Provide education/information on potential fetal complications.	Babies born to women with gestational diabetes may need to be observed in the special care nursery or follow specific protocols of care to detect hypoglycemia, hypocalcemia, hyperbilirubinemia, macrosomia, polycythemia, hypothermia, respiratory distress syndrome.

Nursing Interventions

Provide information on increased risk for later overt diabetes mellitus:

1. Explain the need to be assessed in the postpartum phase 6–12 weeks after delivery for glucose intolerance with a 2-hour 75-g glucose load.

2. Inform patient of signs and symptoms of diabetes mellitus:
   - increased thirst
   - frequent urination
   - fatigue
   - weight loss
   - increased appetite
   - blurred vision
   - lethargy
   - hyperglycemia

3. Educate patient about the risks of glucose intolerance in the future.

Rationales

Gestational diabetes is associated with an increased risk for overt diabetes mellitus (Type II).

Women should receive counseling by the health care provider concerning risks of glucose intolerance in future pregnancies. There is approximately a 50% chance of acquiring gestational diabetes in subsequent pregnancies. Women should also receive counseling on factors that adversely affect glucose metabolism such as oral contraceptives, thiazides, steroids, beta-blockers, increased weight gain. Low-dose oral contraceptives may be used safely in women with prior GDM whose postpartum glucose tolerance is normal. Yearly fasting blood glucose levels should be evaluated to determine glucose metabolism.

▼

NURSING DIAGNOSIS: HIGH RISK FOR INJURY TO FETUS

Risk Factor

Maternal hyperglycemia

Patient Outcome

Health risks to fetus will be reduced through early assessment of problem and appropriate intervention.

Nursing Interventions	Rationales
Assess maternal blood glucose control through: 1. diet 2. insulin management 3. self-monitoring of blood glucose results 4. hemoglobin A_1C values	These values reflect glucose control in the previous week. Elevated A_1C values are associated with fetal anomalies.
Assess fetal well-being: 1. nonstress tests at 32 weeks	Nonstress tests determine fetal heart rate, activity and uterine contractions in antepartum phase.
2. documentation of fetal movement by counting fetal kicks/activity for 15- to 20-minute period	Fetal movement has been correlated with fetal well-being.
3. ultrasounds	Ultrasounds assess fetal growth. Biophysical profiles may be used to identify infants who are decompensating in response to poor placental perfusion.
POSTPARTUM Assess neonate for physical/physiological complications: 1. macrosomia 2. hyperinsulinemia 3. potential birth trauma and morbidity from operative delivery 4. hypoglycemia, hypocalcemia, polycythemia, hyperbilirubinemia	

Nursing Interventions	**Rationales**
Determine glucose status of infant.	Elevated glucose levels of a woman with gestational diabetes during pregnancy creates fetal hyperinsulinemia. After delivery, hypoglycemia may occur in presence of fetal hyperinsulinism. Infants will require glucose either as oral feedings of breast milk or formula, or intravenous glucose to correct hypoglycemic state.

▼

DISCHARGE PLANNING/CONTINUITY OF CARE

- Evaluate 6–12 weeks postpartum with a 75-g 2-hour glucose tolerance test.
- Recommend yearly glucose evaluations with fasting blood glucose tests.
- Instruct women not to start oral contraceptives prior to the postpartum evaluation because these agents increase glucose levels.
- Instruct on barrier methods for contraception.
- Counsel women on the 50% risk of gestational diabetes mellitus that may occur in subsequent pregnancies.

REFERENCES

American Diabetes Association. (1992). Position statement on gestational diabetes mellitus. *Diabetes Care, 15* (Suppl. 2), 5–6.

Leff, E. W., Gange, M. P., & Jeffries, S. C. (1991). Type I diabetes and pregnancy: Are we hearing women's concerns? *American Journal of Maternal-Child Nursing, 16,* 83–87.

Mandeville, L. K. (1992). Diabetic ketoacidosis. *NAACOG's Clinical Issues in Perinatal and Women's Health Nursing, 3*(3), 514–520.

Metzger, B. E. (1991). Summary and recommendations of the third international conference on gestational diabetes mellitus. *Diabetes, 40,* (Suppl. 2), 197–201.

Phelps, R. L., Metzger, B. E. (1992). Caloric restriction in gestational diabetes millitus: When and how much? *Journal of American College of Nutritionists, 11*(3), 259–262.

▼

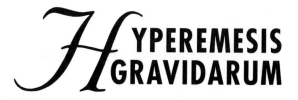

HYPEREMESIS GRAVIDARUM

Deidra Gradishar, RNC, BS

Hyperemesis gravidarum is a condition marked by severe, persistent nausea and vomiting and occasionally by excessive salivation. Prolonged extreme nausea and vomiting may require hospitalization and total parenteral nutrition to support fetal growth and maternal health.

ETIOLOGIES

The causes of this disorder are not precisely known. Hyperemesis is known to be influenced by a combination of emotional and hormonal factors.

CLINICAL MANIFESTATIONS

- The patient may experience dehydration, weight loss, decreased urine output and electrolyte disturbances.
- If the illness is not resolved, damage to the central nervous system, liver, and renal system may result.

CLINICAL/DIAGNOSTIC FINDINGS

- Ketosis
- More severe electrolyte derangements can be noted when nausea and vomiting persist beyond a short period of time.

▼

NURSING DIAGNOSIS: KNOWLEDGE DEFICIT

Related To new condition

Defining Characteristics
Apparent confusion about events
Multiple questions/lack of questions
Need for more information expressed
Inability to concentrate
Inability to retain information given

Patient Outcome
Patient will verbalize understanding of causes and treatment of hyperemesis gravidarum.

Nursing Interventions	Rationales
Assess knowledge of hyperemesis.	Many misconceptions exist among lay persons.
Provide information on the etiology of hyperemesis. Emphasize that while some factors (e.g., hormonal) are out of her control, other factors such as emotional are in her control.	
Describe available treatments and supportive measures	
1. antiemetics	Antiemetics may be prescribed in injection or suppository form. While hyperemesis traditionally occurs in the most sensitive period of gestational development—when all drugs are discouraged—the electrolyte imbalances and the nutritional deficiencies that occur from vomiting may become life-threatening if not adequately treated.
2. cold towels	
3. fluids and electrolytes	Fluid and electrolyte therapy is used to replace those lost through vomiting.
4. small/high carbohydrate meals	These meals prevent overload of stomach.

Nursing Interventions	Rationales
5. emotional support	Anxiety, fear, and ambivalence play a role in maternal adjustment. Hyperemesis is seen as a symptom that suggests the need to evaluate the meaning of the pregnancy and parenthood. Interaction with a therapist may be beneficial.
6. relaxation techniques	These techniques have been used to reduce the anxiety that accompanies this problem. Distraction techniques such as patterned breathing may shift focus away from nausea and vomiting. Guided imagery may promote positive feelings and acceptance in a patient feeling ambivalent. Progressive relaxation can promote a feeling of well-being which may reduce anxiety.
7. hospitalization	Is required when fluid and electrolyte derangements result in a maternal and subsequent fetal health risk.

▼

NURSING DIAGNOSIS: FLUID VOLUME DEFICIT
Related To hyperemesis

Defining Characteristics
Oliguria
Concentrated urine
Hypotension
Dry mucous membranes
General malaise

Patient Outcomes
Patient will maintain normal fluid volume, as evidenced by
- absence of vomiting
- normal blood pressure
- adequate urine output

Nursing Interventions	Rationales
Assess for signs of dehydration; monitor intake and output, specific gravity, daily weights, status of mucous membranes.	
Monitor serum electrolyte values.	
Administer antiemetics (parenteral or rectal) as needed.	Antiemetics may be required to prevent electrolyte imbalances and promote optimal nutrition. They may be the only effective tool to break the cycle of eating, nausea, followed by vomiting.
Administer fluid replacement as indicated. Consider total parenteral nutrition (TPN).	TPN may be indicated to prevent starvation in patients unresponsive to other measures.
Assess for subjective signs of hypoglycemia.	Symptoms may include dizziness, fatigue, fainting.
Advance diet from liquids to solids as tolerated.	Treatment goals include nutritional support during starvation, reduced complications, and resumption of normal diet.

▼

NURSING DIAGNOSIS: PAIN AND DISCOMFORT

Related To persistent nausea and vomiting

Defining Characteristics
Sore throat
Sour taste in mouth
Soreness of abdominal muscles
Generalized weakness
Ptyalism

Patient Outcomes
Patient will
- verbalize relief of emesis.
- appear relaxed and comfortable.

Nursing Interventions	Rationales
Assess for onset/frequency of emesis/vomiting.	
Instruct in need for/provide the following nonpharmacological measures to reduce discomfort: 1. positioning 2. muscular relaxation techniques 3. breathing techniques 4. distraction techniques 5. application of cold towel to forehead, neck 6. carbonated beverage, crackers, toast 7. mouth care 8. supportive contact	Because of vulnerability of the developing fetus to some ingested pharmaceutical, these measures are recommended.
Consult dietitian. Promote frequent small meals high in complicated carbohydrates. Recommend fluids between meals or 1 hour after rather than with meals.	This prevents the dumping of large amounts of fluid into stomach.
Remove trays immediately after meals.	Aromas may precipitate nausea.
Provide oral hygiene.	Sour taste in mouth may precipitate nausea/vomiting.
Provide emotional support during vomiting.	

▼

NURSING DIAGNOSIS: HIGH RISK FOR INEFFECTIVE INDIVIDUAL COPING

Risk Factors
- Situational and maturational crisis of pregnancy
- Personal vulnerability
- Multiple life changes
- Inadequate support systems

Patient Outcomes
Patient will
- verbalize ability to cope with pregnancy and its complications.

- identify one support person.
- identify methods/resources available to her in managing stress.

Nursing Interventions	Rationales
Assess patient's acceptance of pregnancy and her concerns about her ability to parent.	These issues may be central to resolving the psychological aspects of hyperemesis gravidarum.
Allow patient to verbalize positive/negative feelings.	Patient may be reluctant to disclose negative feelings (anger, dependence, etc.) unacceptable to her and presumably to others. Nurse who can adopt a nonjudgmental approach to patient's expressions will foster environment in which healing/adjustment can occur.
Assess support systems available now, and after birth of baby.	
Examine critical/stressful issues that may coincide with pregnancy (i.e., change in residence, interpersonal relationships).	
Encourage patient to reduce major life changes during emotionally tumultuous period of pregnancy. Assist in simplifying unavoidable major changes.	Tremendous physical, emotional, and biological changes occur in pregnancy. Changes may evoke severe anxiety in normally strong, less vulnerable people. Women who experience some vulnerability/ emotional lability in normal circumstances may find feelings exaggerated in pregnancy.
Assist in setting priorities and using energy only for critical tasks if patient is unable to meet personal obligations. Assist in evaluating personal, financial, etc., resources that might help her meet obligations.	
Assess effectiveness of stress-relief measures. If ineffective, determine whether patient can/will consider new/alternate methods to deal with stress.	

Nursing Interventions	Rationales
Support patient in application/use of coping measures used in past to deal with stress.	In time of unusual stress, patient may be overwhelmed by fears/concerns; fails to use long-standing coping measures. However, new circumstances may require new mechanisms.
Instruct patient in use of alternate coping measures: 1. guided imagery 2. breathing modifications 3. progressive relaxation	Advanced techniques may be required by specialized staff.
Assess patient's willingness to participate in counseling sessions.	

▼

DISCHARGE PLANNING/CONTINUITY OF CARE

Once patient has been stabilized, normal prenatal care is advised.

REFERENCES

Boyce, R. A. (1992). Enteral nutrition in hyperemesis gravidarum: A new development. *Journal of the American Dietetic Association, 92*(6), 733–736.

Devitt, N. F. (1991). Hyperemesis gravidarum: A case report suggesting new concepts and research needs. *Family Practice Research Journal, 11*(3), 279–282.

Hillard, P. A. (1990). Coping with morning sickness. *Parents, 65*(8), 143–144.

Vitamin B6 for nausea/vomiting of pregnancy. (1991). *Nurses Drug Alert, 15*(9), 70.

Zibell-Frisk, D., Jen, K. L., & Rick, J. (1990). Use of parenteral nutrition to maintain adequate nutritional status in hyperemesis gravidarum. *Journal of Perinatology, 10*(4), 390–395.

▼

$\mathcal{H}$YPERTENSION, PREGNANCY-INDUCED/ HELLP SYNDROME

Sarah Cohen RN
Valerie Wolf, RN, BSN

Pregnancy-induced hypertension (PIH) is marked by a significant increase in blood pressure in a pregnant woman who is otherwise normotensive. This increase generally occurs after the 20th week of gestation. Hypertension occurring before the 20th week of gestation is generally considered to be a function of chronic (perhaps undiagnosed/ asymptomatic) hypertension. PIH complicates about 5% to 7% of all healthy pregnancies and affects 20% to 40% of women found to have preexisting renal or vascular disease. Eclampsia represents the phase of PIH during which convulsions occur.

HELLP syndrome is a laboratory marker which reflects organ damage and a progression of the disease. The acronym HELLP represents the following: H stands for hemolysis, EL stands for elevated liver enzymes; LP stands for low platelets (thrombocytopenia).

ETIOLOGIES

Pregnancy-induced hypertension
The precise etiology of PIH has not been clearly established. Theories include:
- nutritional deficiency, most particularly
  - zinc
  - calcium
  - protein
  - total caloric intake
- immunological deficiency
  - an immune response to the pregnancy, placenta and fetus

- genetic
  - may be related to a single recessive gene (daughters and mothers often share the illness)
- uterine ischemia
  - results in the release of a vasoconstrictor into general circulation

HELLP syndrome

- Arterial spasms cause lesions in the vessel walls.
- Platelets collect on the lesion and a fibrin network is formed.
- Red blood cells are damaged as they are forced through the narrow lumen of the vessels (hemolysis).
- The liver is damaged by small circulating emboli.
- Hepatic distention may lead to rupture of the liver and maternal death.
- The volume of platelets circulating decreases as platelets adhere to damaged sites resulting in low platelets.

CLINICAL MANIFESTATIONS

Increased blood pressure

- Mild preeclampsia:
  - B/P >140/90 mmHg
  - systolic increase 30–60 mmHg
  - diastolic 15–30 mmHg above normal
- Severe preeclampsia:
  - B/P ≥ 160/110
  - systolic increase ≥ 60mmHg
  - diastolic increase ≥ 30 mmHg
- May also be associated with
  - headaches
  - nondependent edema (3 to 4+)
  - hyperreflexia
  - visual disturbances
  - proteinuria
  - epigastric pain
  - characteristic seizures called eclamptic seizures

With HELLP syndrome

- Thrombocytopenia
  - petechiae
  - ecchymosis, large bleed in joint, soft tissue
  - bleeding from any mucosal membrane
  - oozing from injection, IV puncture, wound, episiotomy
  - malaise, fatigue, weakness
  - tachycardia, shortness of breath
  - hypotension
  - restlessness, diaphoresis
  - shock

- Hemolysis: microangiopathic hemolytic anemia
  - fatigue, lassitude, weakness
  - apnea
  - edema
  - pallor
- Right upper quadrant pain or epigastric pain
- Hepatic rupture:
  - shock
  - oliguria, fever
  - leukocytosis, increase in white blood count
  - intraperitoneal hemorrhage
  - increased pain
- Nausea, vomiting
- Fluid retention, edema in ankles, sacral, ascites
- Oliguria: urine output less than 10 ml/hr, dark yellow urine
- Hypoglycemia
- Jaundice

CLINICAL/DIAGNOSTIC FINDINGS

- Proteinuria
- Increased plasma uric acid
- Increased AST (aspartate aminotransferase), SGPT (serum glutamic-pyruvic transaminase), LDH (lactic dehydrogenase)
- Hematocrit may be elevated
- May see increased clotting time and decreased platelet count

With HELLP
Laboratory data
- Hemolysis–abnormal, fragmented red blood cells
- Platelet count <100,000
- Normal partial thromboplastin
- Normal fibrinogen

Associated laboratory findings
- Haptoglobin < 60
- Hemoglobin and hematocrit decreased out of proportion to blood loss
- AST (aspartate aminotransferase) ≥60 u/liter
- Increased SGPT (serum glutamic-pyruvic transaminase)
- LDH (lactic dehydrogenase) ≥600 u/liter
- Alkaline phosphatase >100 mg/dl
- Hyperbilirubinemia ≥ 1.2 mg/dl

NURSING DIAGNOSIS: KNOWLEDGE DEFICIT

Related To unfamiliarity with condition

Defining Characteristics
Multiple questions
Lack of questions

Patient Outcome

Patient will describe pathophysiology, symptoms, and treatment of pregnancy-induced hypertension and its complications.

Nursing Interventions	Rationales
Assess knowledge of PIH and its effects on mother and fetus.	
Assess for family history.	There seems to be a familial tendency, with mothers and daughters often sharing the disease.
Instruct patient of subjective danger signs for developing PIH: 1. headache 2. blurred vision 3. dizziness 4. epigastric pain 5. sudden weight gain	
Teach patient regarding pathophysiology of disease: 1. precise etiology not understood 2. three major effects: • decreased blood perfusion to all organs • fluid shifts • changes in blood clotting 3. effects on mother: • damage to kidneys and liver, visual changes • edema, nausea/vomiting, headaches, convulsions • changes in clotting	These are related to decreased perfusion to target organs. These are related to fluid shifts from intravascular to intracellular space. This is associated with development of disseminated intravascular coagulation, or HELLP syndrome. A decrease in platelets is caused by intense vasospasm of PIH; this causes loss of vascular endothelial integrity with platelet adherence and fibrin deposition. Hemolysis of red blood cells in HELLP syndrome is marked by abnormal, fragmented red blood cells on peripheral blood smear.

Nursing Interventions

4. effects on fetus:

   - small for gestational age babies

   - fetal stress/distress

5. prognosis:
   - fetal outcomes dependent on blood pressure control
   - PIH not always responsive to patient or medical interventions

6. Treatment:
   - meticulous surveillances of both subjective and objective symptoms
   - weekly office visits for blood pressure/proteinuria/weight and monitoring growth of fetus
   - antepartum fetal assessment (nonstress test, oxytocin contraction test, biophysical profiles)
   - biochemical testing AST (aspartate aminotransferase), SGPT (serum glutamic-pyruvic transaminase), LDH (lactic dehydrogenase), urine proteins, uric acid
   - bed rest
   - home monitoring—sometimes is an alternative to prolonged hospitalization
   - hospitalization
   - delivery if/when the intrauterine environment becomes hostile to the growth of the developing fetus

Rationales

This is related to decreased perfusion to intervillous space and reduced placental performance, as well as decreased oxygen reserves.

This will indicate depletion of placental O_2 reserves resulting from maternal hypertension episodes/seizures.

NURSING DIAGNOSIS: HIGH RISK FOR INJURY TO MOTHER

Risk Factors
- Decreased blood perfusion to all organs
- Fluid shifts from intravascular to intracellular space
- Development of coagulopathies

Patient Outcome
Risk for injury is reduced due to early assessment and intervention.

Nursing Interventions	Rationales
Renal Failure Assess for signs of decreased renal function/failure: 1. proteinuria 2. increased uric acid 3. oliguria 4. edema	Renal changes related to decreased blood flow and reduced glomerular filtration rate.
Administer fluids/challenges as ordered. Titrate fluids closely.	
Monitor 1. intake and output 2. specific gravity	
Hepatic Damage Assess for epigastric pain and liver tenderness.	Pain may result from liver distention caused by obstruction in hepatic sinus blood flow. Obstruction produced by fibrin deposits in hepatic sinuses.
Assess for impaired liver function: 1. elevated AST (aspartate aminotransferase) 2. elevated SGPT (serum glutamic-pyruvic transaminase) 3. LDH (lactic dehydrogenase) >600 u/liter 4. high indirect bilirubin 5. hyperbilirubinemia 6 nausea/vomiting 7. jaundice 8. oliguria/dark-yellow urine 9. fluid retention	SGPT is a very good indicator of acute liver damage. SGPT values are higher than AST if liver has necrosed.

Nursing Interventions	Rationales
Observe for changes in bowel functions.	Clay-colored stool may indicate liver destruction.
Assess for signs of hepatic rupture.	Epigastric pain reflects possible impending rupture.
Visual Changes Assess for visual disturbances: 1. scotoma 2. blurred vision	This is caused by retinal arteriolar spasms.
Assist with funduscopic examination.	
Fluid Shifts Assess for weight gain of > 2 lb/week or > 6 lb/month.	This may represent significant fluid shifts.
Assess for circumorbital as well as generalized edema of face, hands, and abdomen.	
Assess for pitting edema following 12 hours of bed rest.	
Assess hematocrit.	An elevation may reflect hemoconcentration secondary to decreased intravascular volume.
Assess for signs and symptoms of impending eclampsia: 1. scotomata or blurred vision 2. epigastric pain 3. persistent or severe headache 4. vomiting 5. neurological hyperactivity 6. pulmonary edema or cyanosis	
Place patient in quiet, nonstimulating environment with subdued lighting. Limit visitors.	Seizure activity may be prevented by limiting central nervous system stimulation.
Maintain seizure precautions: 1. Pad side rails on bed; keep side rails pulled up; keep bed in low position.	
2. Maintain bed rest.	This serves to protect patient from injury.

Nursing Interventions	Rationales
3. Have emergency equipment available: • suction and oxygen • medications for treatment for eclamptic seizure 4. Keep call light within reach.	
Administer magnesium sulfate as ordered. (Usual loading dose of 4–6 g over 15–20 minutes). Monitor deep tendon reflexes and respirations closely. Initiate continuous drip of 1–3 g/hr. The magnesium sulfate infusion may be maintained 12–24 hours after delivery.	Magnesium sulfate decreases central nervous system irritability and lowers the seizure threshold. Therapeutic levels: >4–7.5 mEq/L.
Observe for signs and symptoms of hypermagnesia: 1. flushing 2. feeling of extreme warmth 3. diminished reflexes 4. respirations <12 breaths per minute 5. magnesium level > 10–12 mEq/L.	
Keep calcium gluconate 10% solution at bedside.	Calcium gluconate is an antidote for magnesium overdose.
If diastolic pressure increases to >110 mmHg, anticipate the administration of an antihypertensive medication for control: 1. hydralazine	 Hydralazine is a potent antihypertensive that acts directly on vascular smooth muscle. Its vasodilator action increases systemic and uterine blood flow. Note: Observe the patient closely for sudden precipitous drops in blood pressure, headache, and palpitations. Uteroplacental insufficiency has been associated with diastolic pressures that fall below 90 mmHg.

Nursing Interventions	Rationales
2. labetalol hydrochloride.	This beta-blocker causes vasodilation without significantly increasing heart rate or cardiac output; it may be used in preference to or in addition to hydralazine.
3. sodium nitroprusside (Nipride).	Women with severe, labile hypertension may require this agent, especially if they have been unresponsive to other medications. Its use in pregnancy is controversial, since it breaks down into cyanide; its use is normally reserved for the postpartum period.
Titrate intravenous fluids. Maintain accurate intake and output.	Titration is important to reduce risk of pulmonary edema.
If seizure occurs, provide prompt efficient care:	This minimizes risk to mother and infant.
1. Administer magnesium sulfate or Dilantin.	
2. Wedge hip.	This position displaces gravid uterus off vena cava and optimizes perfusion.
3. Maintain airway.	
4. Administer O$_2$.	
5. Suction as needed.	
6. Notify physician/ anesthesiologist.	
7. Prepare for emergency delivery.	
Coagulapathies Assess for changes in coagulation studies (increased clotting time, decreased platelet count).	This may indicate the development of HELLP syndrome or DIC.
Assess for signs of thrombocytopenia: 1. hematuria 2. petechiae 3. ecchymosis 4. hematemesis 5. oozing from intravenous/incision site and mucous membranes	This will indicate the possibility of a derangement in the coagulation profile.

Nursing Interventions	Rationales
Assess for vaginal bleeding, uterine tenderness.	This may indicate placental abruption or hemorrhage.
Have patient's blood typed and cross-matched.	Blood must be kept available for emergency transfusion.
Instruct patient to notify nurse of dizziness or bleeding from intravenous insertion sites, mucosa, hematemesis, etc.	
Prepare patient for emergency cesarean birth on physician order.	
Prepare for delivery of compromised fetus.	
See also treatment of disseminated intravascular coagulation in Chapter 46: Intrauterine Fetal Demise.	

▼

NURSING DIAGNOSIS: HIGH RISK FOR INJURY TO FETUS

Risk Factors
- Decreased placental perfusion caused by hypertensive events
- Cessation of blood flow to intervillous space during eclamptic seizures
- Uterine contractions

Patient Outcome
Injury risks to fetus are reduced through early assessment and initiation of necessary interventions.

Nursing Interventions	Rationales
Continuously monitor fetal heart rate electronically; assess and record every 30 minutes.	

Nursing Interventions	Rationales
Notify physician if signs of fetal stress occur: 1. fetal bradycardia or tachycardia 2. loss of fetal heart tones 3. meconium-stained fluid 4. decreased baseline variability (<5 beats per minute) 5. presence of ominous periodic patterns, including late decelerations.	Prompt identification and interventions for potentially compromised fetus may prevent fetal mortality/morbidity.
Maintain patient in left lateral position.	Placental/fetal perfusion is maximized by alleviating compression of aorta and inferior vena cava.
Administer O_2 to mother via re-breather mask at 10 L/min.	This increases O_2 saturation of circulating blood and may increase O_2 saturation in intervillous space.

▼

NURSING DIAGNOSIS: HIGH RISK FOR INEFFECTIVE INDIVIDUAL COPING

Risk Factors
- Concern for self/baby
- High-risk status of pregnancy
- Long-term hospitalization/bed rest

Patient Outcomes
Patient will
- verbalize feelings regarding high-risk pregnancy.
- demonstrate positive coping mechanisms.
- identify available resources as indicated by physical status.

Nursing Interventions	Rationales
Assess patient's response to: 1. high-risk diagnosis 2. loss of control over course of pregnancy 3. long-term hospitalization/bed rest	The nurse may need to help the patient to process these feelings. If these feelings are unresolved and the patient remains conflicted, compliance with the plan of care may be poor.

Nursing Interventions	**Rationales**
Encourage patient to verbalize fears, frustrations, anger, and other feelings regarding pregnancy.	Expressing feelings can help diffuse emotions.
Assess support systems and patient's ability to use them at this time. Determine their understanding of the diagnosis and treatment regimen.	Mothers may look healthy, yet require bed rest, intensive home management, even long-term hospitalization.
Emphasize the positive aspects of the pregnancy and the positive effects compliance with the treatment regimen is having on the pregnancy.	The closer to term the pregnancy can be brought while still controlling blood pressure, the less likely will be the risk to fetus from premature delivery.
Assess for: 1. changes in behavior/communication patterns 2. inappropriate use of defense mechanisms 3. depression 4. expressions of inability to cope 5. sleep/eating disturbances	
Integrate social services, occupational therapy, home nursing/homemaker services, and counseling into the treatment plan as needed.	
Provide diversional activities, stimulating environment, contact with friends and family if patient is to be confined to bed in the hospital or at home.	Maintaining a normal sensory environment will enhance patient's emotional adaptation.
Involve patient in decision-making in all aspects of care.	

▼

DISCHARGE PLANNING/CONTINUITY OF CARE

- Arrange routine early postpartum checkup with special focus on blood pressure status. (If blood pressure is still elevated, a workup for chronic hypertension should be initiated.)

- Refer to social services, home nursing, homemaker services as indicated.

REFERENCES

Doan-Wiggens, L. (1990). Pregnancy induced hypertension: Combating the dangers. *Emergency Medicine, 22*(6), 29–31, 34–35.

Heaman, M. (1992). Stressful life events, social support, and mood disturbances in hospitalized and nonhospitalized women with pregnancy-induced hypertension. *Canadian Journal of Nursing Research, 21*(1), 23–37.

Krening, C. (1992). Perinatal hypertensive crisis. *NAACOG's Clinical Issues in Perinatal and Women's Health Nursing, 3*(3), 413–419.

The National History of HELLP Syndrome. (1991). Patterns of disease prognosis and regression. *American Journal of Obstetrics and Gynecology,* June: 1500–1513.

Newman, V. & Fullerton, J. (1990). Role of nutrition in the prevention of preeclampsia: Review of the literature. *Journal of Nurse-Midwifery, 35*(5), 282–291.

Sweet, Arvon A. Y. & Brown, Edwin E. G. (1991). *Fetal and Neonatal Effects of Maternal Disease.* St. Louis, MO: C. V. Mosby.

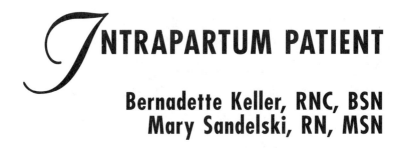

$\mathscr{I}$NTRAPARTUM PATIENT

Bernadette Keller, RNC, BSN
Mary Sandelski, RN, MSN

The intrapartum period begins with the onset of labor or rupture of membranes and ends with the delivery of the baby and placenta. The intrapartum period is a time of increased risk to the mother and fetus requiring close observation. Appropriate emotional and psychosocial support is provided to create the kind of environment in which the family will begin to embrace their new child.

ETIOLOGIES

N/A

CLINICAL MANIFESTATIONS

Regular uterine contractions, which, when timed, become closer together, stronger in intensity and accomplish progressive cervical dilation and effacement with or without rupture of the bag of water.

▼

NURSING DIAGNOSIS: HIGH RISK FOR INJURY TO FETUS

Risk Factors
- Physiological stress of labor
- Effects of medications (e.g., oxytoxics, analgesics, anesthetics)
- Result of maternal complications: infection, hypertension, hemorrhage, diabetes, etc
- Cord compression
- Head compression
- Placental insufficiency
- Decreased uterine blood flow

397

Patient Outcome

Risk of injury will be reduced through frequent assessment and early intervention in response to fetal stress.

Nursing Interventions	Rationales
Assess and document fetal heart rate (FHR) and contractions every 30 minutes in the first stage of labor, and every 15 minutes in the second stage. During delivery the FHR is auscultated after each contraction. Report: 1. baseline changes/abnormal baseline 2. late decelerations, moderate to severe variable decelerations 3. baseline variability <5 beats per minute	FHR variability is an important indication of fetal well-being.
Monitor and alert physician to changes in fetal heart rate parameters. If fetal heart rate pattern indicates fetal stress: 1. Institute position changes. 2. Increase intravenous drip rate. 3. Initiate O_2 per rebreather mask.	Changes in any parameter could signal acutely deteriorating condition requiring intervention.
Observe for changes in amniotic fluid from clear to meconium-stained.	
Monitor results of scalp sample.	A scalp pH <7.20 requires immediate intervention/delivery.
Prepare for possibility that operative delivery may be performed.	Prompt intervention will reduce complications.
Prepare for possible compromised infant.	

▼

NURSING DIAGNOSIS: PAIN

Related To

- Uterine contraction
- Discomfort from examination and medical procedure
- Patient expectation of degree of pain during labor

- Displacement of intraabdominal organs
- Distention and stretching of vagina and perineum
- Tissue trauma

Defining Characteristics
Discomfort
Moaning/crying/writhing
Restlessness/trembling
Request for pain medication
Withdrawn behavior/abrupt mood change

Patient Outcome
Patient verbalizes ability to cope with pain.

Nursing Interventions	Rationales
Determine level of discomfort related to labor.	Pain perception and experience varies among individuals.
Allow ambulation and position changes.	Ambulation/upright position during labor results in stronger, more efficient contractions. Labor may be shortened; patient may be less likely to adopt a "sick role."
Encourage use of relaxation measures:	
1. Perform massage if patient desires.	Backrubs ease muscular tension, promote circulation. Sacral counterpressure during contraction may relieve back labor.
2. Teach effleurage.	Effleurage acts as distractor, enhances muscular relaxation.
3. Encourage muscle relaxation through gentle touching.	Such activity reduces tension and anxiety by diminishing feeling of abandonment; provides stimulation other than that associated with contraction.

Nursing Interventions

Teach breathing modifications:
1. In early phase of labor
   - Slow, deep chest breathing. Instruct patient to take deep breaths through nose; exhale through pursed lips, 10–15 per minute. Entire body should be relaxed with this breathing pattern.

2. In active phase of labor
   - Accelerated/decelerated breathing. Instruct patient to take rapid shallow breaths, beginning slowly, then increasing in rate along with the intensity of the contraction, then decreasing respectively. Ensure that the rate is not too fast, resulting in hyperventilation.

3. In transitional phase of labor (especially to counteract urge to push)
   - Modified panting. Instruct patient to start with accelerated-decelerated breathing. When the urge to push begins, instruct patient to blow.

Rationales

Breathing modifications may promote abdominal/genital muscle relaxation and act as a distraction during contractions.

Blowing through contraction should alternate with accelerated-decelerated breathing to prevent hyperventilation. As a general rule, any breathing modifications devised as alternatives to the pattern breathing techniques described above can be equally effective, when one breathing modification is found to be useless, another should be tried.

Nursing Interventions	Rationales
Provide pharmacological interventions as ordered.	Analgesics have central nervous system depressant effect, diminishing pain perception. Intravenous medications are given over 5–10 minutes during contractions. When contractions occur, blood flow to intervillous space is decreased; therefore, less medication crosses placental barrier.
Time the administration of narcotic analgesics so that infant is not born with respiratory depression.	
Observe and document 15 and 30 minutes after administration of medication:	
1. fetal heart rate patterns	Patterns establish fetal response to depressant effects of analgesia. Intervene as indicated.
2. contraction pattern	Analgesia administered in latent phases may prolong labor by decreasing effectiveness, regularity of contractions.
3. blood pressure and pulse	Medications that relax smooth muscle may decrease maternal blood pressure through vasodilation.
4. patient's perception of pain and effectiveness of pain relief measures	
Assist significant other in supporting patient.	Degree of significant other's participation in labor process varies according to individual beliefs, culture, and expectations. Participation is significant in establishing favorable family relationships, self-esteem, and parenting skills.

Nursing Interventions	Rationales
Minimize external factors that may contribute to discomfort: 1. Decrease excessive noises. 2. Provide soft lighting. 3. Promote privacy. 4. Minimize temperature extremes.	It is important to provide environment conducive to relaxation.
Keep patient and significant other informed of labor progress.	This will enhance their sense of participation and decreases anxiety.
See also Pain Management during Labor, p. 445.	

▼

NURSING DIAGNOSIS: HIGH RISK FOR INJURY TO MOTHER

Risk Factors
- Infection
- Hemorrhage
- Hypertension
- Effects of regional anesthesia

Patient Outcome
Injury to mother will be prevented/reduced through early assessment and intervention.

Nursing Interventions	Rationales
Maintain aseptic techniques during procedures.	
Infection Notify physician of: 1. temperature >37.5°C 2. fetal tachycardia (heart rate: >160 beats per minute) 3. maternal tachycardia 4. malodorous vaginal discharge	Increased maternal infection risk associated with prolonged rupture of membranes, frequent vaginal examinations, failure to use consistent aseptic technique, poor perineal care.
Administer antibiotics as ordered.	
Hemorrhage Observe for excessive vaginal bleeding. Institute perineal pad count if indicated.	Blood loss must be quantified to guide treatment.

Nursing Interventions	Rationales
Monitor blood pressure, pulse, respiration, and fetal heart rate every 15–30 minutes in presence of excessive vaginal bleeding.	
If hemorrhage is noted:	
1. Institute administration of intravenous fluids or increase in drip rate.	Fluids increase blood volume and systemic perfusion.
2. Place bed in Trendelenburg position.	This position increases blood return from lower extremities and increases cerebral blood flow.
3. Administer oxygen at 10 L/min.	Supplementary oxygen increases oxygen saturation which increases the blood's capacity to perfuse tissue.
4. Prepare for emergency delivery of potentially compromised fetus.	The potential for hemorrhage increases in the following clinical situations: prolonged labor, uterine atony or rupture, placental or fetal malposition, cervical/vaginal lacerations.
Hypertension Assess and document blood pressure every 15 minutes if pressure is >150/90 mmHg, or if there is a 30 mmHg systolic or 15 mmHg diastolic increase from baseline.	
Assess for complications indicative of pregnancy-induced hypertension: 1. elevated blood pressure 2. visual disturbances 3. proteinuria 4. hyperreflexive deep tendon reflexes 5. epigastric pain	Pregnancy-induced hypertension (PIH) may be a late presenting complication of pregnancy. Diagnosis is made when two or more of the symptoms listed are noted.
If PIH occurs, see p. 384.	

Nursing Interventions	**Rationales**
Anesthesia reaction Assess for signs of reaction: 1. altered sensorium 2. hypotension 3. bradycardia 4. nausea/vomiting 5. decreased fetal heart rate variability/bradycardia 6. decreased respiratory rate	Complications from epidural anesthesia may result from intravascular injection of the anesthetic agent, the level of the anesthesia agent migrates too high and anesthetizes respiratory muscles, hypotension results from the sympathetic blockade, and decreased perfusion to the fetal-placental unit secondary to maternal hypotension.
Administer rapid intravenous infusion (500–2000 ml) of Lactated Ringer's solution prior to administration of regional anesthesia.	Fluid-loading may diminish or prevent hypotension.
Position patient in left lateral position or displace uterus to left by wedging hip after epidural administration.	Left lateral position reduces risk of supine hypotension associated with vena cava compression. In vena cava compression, blood return to left atrium is diminished resulting in decreased cardiac output and maternal hypotension, and decreased placental perfusion and fetal bradycardia.
Provide for safety; change position, support extremities, and keep side rails up.	Patient may have little or no movement/sensation in extremities following regional blockade.
Increase intravenous drip rate, apply O$_2$, turn patient to left lateral position for maternal hypotension and/or fetal bradycardia.	

▼

NURSING DIAGNOSIS: SELF CARE DEFICIT

Related To
- Pain
- Preoccupation with labor

Defining Characteristic
Inability to care for self

Patient Outcome

Patient maintains hydration/hygiene activities with assistance

Nursing Interventions	Rationales
Maintain hydration: 1. Provide ice chips and clear liquids if ordered. 2. Administer parenteral fluids as ordered.	Solid food intake and fluids by mouth may be restricted. IV fluids may be necessary to maintain hydration, particularly if patient experiences vomiting or is NPO.
Assist with bladder elimination: 1. Encourage voiding every 1–3 hours. 2. Assist with bedpan. 3. Observe for bladder distention.	Descent of fetus can be impended by full bladder. Increased risk of bladder trauma, urinary tract infection, and uterine atony may occur after delivery if bladder not evacuated regularly.
Provide frequent hygiene measures: 1. Assist with oral hygiene every 2 hours as needed. Moisturize lips if needed. 2. Assist with body hygiene: • Assist patient to shower/bathe every 8 hours. • Provide frequent perineal care every 1–2 hours as needed. • Maintain dry, wrinkle-free linen.	Hygienic measures promote comfort and relaxation. Oral hygiene moisturizes dry mucous membranes. Perineal care and bathing remove uncomfortable secretions, diminish odors, and reduce potential for infection.

▼

NURSING DIAGNOSIS: FAMILY COPING: POTENTIAL FOR GROWTH

Related To birth of a new family member

Defining Characteristics

Ability to see addition of new family member as challenge and opportunity for growth
Expressions of caring/concern
Demonstration of interactions, which suggest growth

Patient Outcome

Family will verbalize positive feelings about baby's presence in family unit.

Nursing Interventions	Rationales
Assess the changes family members anticipate in response to the birth of their child.	
Assess the perception of siblings and extended family members.	If problems with siblings are anticipated, nurse may be able to make helpful recommendations.
Reinforce the positive aspects of the growing/changing family consultation.	

▼

DISCHARGE PLANNING/CONTINUITY OF CARE

Routine postpartum check-up

REFERENCES

Bernat, S. H., Wooldridge, P. J., Marecki, M., & Snell, L. (1992). Biofeedback-assisted relaxation to reduce stress in labor. *Journal of Obstetrical, Gynecologic, and Neonatal Nursing, 21*(4), 295–303.

Biancuzzo, M. (1993). Six myths of maternal posture during labor MCN. *American Journal of National/Child Nursing, 18*(5), 264–269.

Chapman, L. (1992). Expectant father's roles during labor and birth. *Journal of Obstetrical, Gynecologic, and Neonatal Nursing, 21*(2), 114–120.

McKay, S. & Barrows, T. (1991). Holding back: Maternal readiness to give birth. *American Journal of Maternal-Child Nursing, 16*(5), 250–254.

Wheeler, D. (1991). Intrapartum bleeding. *NAACOG's Clinical Issues in Perinatal and Women's Health Nursing, 2*(3), 381–384.

▼

$\mathcal{I}$NTRAUTERINE FETAL DEMISE (STILLBIRTH)

Maripat Tomaszkiewicz, RN, MSN
Linda Escobar, RN, BSN

Intrauterine fetal demise (stillbirth) is the death of a baby in utero after the 20th week of gestation and before the time of birth. (A fetal demise before 20 weeks is termed a spontaneous abortion).

ETIOLOGIES

Stillbirth has been associated with
- Genetic diseases
- Congenital malformations incompatible with life
- Medical conditions that become exacerbated during pregnancy
  - diabetes
  - hypertension
  - heart disease
  - lupus
- Isoimmunization
- Cord accidents
- Placental abnormalities

CLINICAL MANIFESTATIONS

The mother may note decreased or absent fetal movement, or the death of the fetus may go unobserved. No fetal heart rate will be detected upon auscultation and no cardiac activity will be observed upon ultrasound. Spontaneous labor may begin or labor may be induced.

CLINICAL/DIAGNOSTIC FINDINGS

- Absence of fetal heart tones
- No cardiac activity noted on ultrasound
- Absence of fetal movement

▼

NURSING DIAGNOSIS: GRIEVING

Related To loss of fetus

Defining Characteristics
Anger
Bargaining
Crying
Denial
Disbelief
Shock

Patient Outcomes
Patient will demonstrate some positive aspects of grieving, as evidenced by
- expression of sadness or anger
- use of available support systems

Nursing Interventions	Rationales
Assess parent's response to the birth of their baby.	When a child dies in utero, grief is felt whether the child was wanted or unwanted. If the work of grief is not completed, grief can become dysfunctional, causing behaviors damaging to personal safety, and to the family's future and relationships.
Determine the influence, if any, of culture/religion on grieving process.	Individual's coping methods are affected by many factors.
Provide physical care; meet dependency needs thoughtfully, unhurriedly.	
Allow significant other to remain with patient throughout labor, delivery, recovery.	Significant other's participation acknowledges his loss.
Provide private room for labor, delivery, recovery. Minimize number of staff in room with patient.	Sensory overload can make coping more difficult.

Nursing Interventions	Rationales
Assist parents to identify and verbalize their feelings about: 1. loss of their baby 2. anger 3. helplessness, powerlessness 4. strangeness of own feelings 5. seeing other infants and parents	Expressing feelings can help diffuse emotions.
Encourage mother and significant other to view fetus.	Viewing fetus can promote acceptance of the death, reduce unreal mental images of fetus now or later, and promote reality.
Be accepting of all manifestations of grief provided they are not destructive.	
Accept mother's decision not to view fetus.	Patients have right to beliefs/behaviors that may conflict with those of nurses.
Arrange for baptismal rites/last rites if desired.	
Proceed with postmortem care with respect, dignity.	
Offer footprints, hat, lock of hair, or picture to patient if she wants them at time of birth; otherwise keep on file in labor rooms for social worker access.	Viewing pictures, and touching or holding baby's personal belonging may be helpful and may initiate acceptance of loss.

▼

NURSING DIAGNOSIS: SITUATIONAL LOW SELF-ESTEEM

Related To
- Perception of role in intrauterine fetal demise
- Feeling of inadequacy, inferiority, powerlessness
- Inability to bear living child

Defining Characteristics

Self-maligning statements
Overt expression of guilt and blame
Refusal to make eye contact

Patient Outcomes

The mother/parents will begin to verbalize positive expressions of continued self-worth.

Nursing Interventions	Rationales
Assess patient's/couple's self-perceptions as individuals and parents.	As the perinatal mortality rate continues to fall, perinatal death becomes an increasingly uncommon event. When it does occur, it is a shock to both the mother and family.
Assess degree to which patient assumes responsibility for fetal loss. Assist patient to express feelings about self and to verbalize any feelings of guilt and blame.	Stillbirth cannot be anticipated in most cases; an autopsy may not always provide the answers about cause of death.
Evaluate family's response to loss; note blame placed by members.	
Provide as much realistic and truthful information about what is known about the cause of fetal loss as possible.	
Respect and support patient's choice to be introspective at various times.	
Ensure that patient/family has the resources they may need to successfully grieve their child (e.g., support groups, social services, church and support of families and friends).	Grief is a process that will only begin in the hospital setting. The family will need resources to assist them over the months ahead.
Explain to parent that the majority of women who have a stillbirth become pregnant again and give birth to live children.	Such information may provide hope for future.

▼

NURSING DIAGNOSIS: PAIN

Related To uterine contractions

Defining Characteristics

Verbalized pain
Thrashing in bed

Grimacing
Hyperventilation/hypoventilation
Muscle tension

Patient Outcome
Patient will verbalize ability to cope with uterine contraction pain.

Nursing Interventions	Rationales
Elicit perception of uterine contraction discomfort.	Each patient demonstrates/experiences a unique response to pain.
Apply external contraction monitor as ordered.	
Assess patient's understanding of the need to accomplish/induce labor.	
Explain the cyclic nature of uterine contraction pattern.	Preparing patient for normal labor progression and assisting through the various stages help her cope with discomfort more effectively.
Evaluate current mechanisms being used to manage discomfort, and whether they are effective.	Unsuccessful mechanisms may need change.
Use nonpharmacological comfort measures when appropriate.	Physical and behavioral interventions can be useful in altering the perception of pain.
Administer analgesic medications as ordered; give patient choice of medications.	Providing choices allows patient to assume some control over situation.
Administer antiemetics, antidiarrheals, and analgesics per order if patient having a Prostin induction.	

▼

NURSING DIAGNOSIS: HIGH RISK FOR INJURY TO MOTHER

Risk Factors
- Prolonged retention of products of conception leading to sepsis
- Uterine rupture or abruption related to labor induction
- Disseminated intravascular coagulation (DIC)

Patient Outcome

Risk for injury is reduced through early assessment and intervention.

Nursing Interventions	Rationales
Infection Assess for signs of infection/sepsis: 1. elevated temperature 2. elevated white blood count left shift 3. malodorous vaginal discharge 4. maternal tachycardia 5. chills/flushing	Prolonged retention of the products of conception can lead to infection. Treatment is dependent on two key components: quick evacuation of the uterus and aggressive IV antibiotics.
Administer antibiotics as ordered if infection present.	
DIC Assess and document bleeding/clotting abnormalities: 1. hemoglobin and hematocrit 2. clotting studies: prothrombin time (PT), partial thromboplastin time (PTT), fibrinogen 3. inappropriate bleeding from vagina, venipuncture, parenteral sites, mucous membranes	Signs of DIC include hypofibrinogenemia, decreased platelets, prolonged prothrombin and partial thromboplastin time, increased fibrin, and fibrin split products.
Observe for signs of shock.	
Transfuse blood/blood products per order when necessary.	
Rupture of uterus Assess for signs/symptoms of rupture of uterus/abruption: 1. rising uterine resting tone 2. sudden hemorrhage 3. signs/symptoms of shock (see above) 4. increasing abdominal girth, increasing fundal heights 5. patient reports extreme pain "tearing in nature" which suddenly ceases	Hypertonic uterine contractions resulting from oxytocin use have been associated with abruptio placentae and in extreme cases, uterine rupture.
Notify physician of sudden changes in baseline parameters and implement care plan for the emergency delivery of the fetus.	Quick action will reduce life-threatening blood loss for the mother.

▼

DISCHARGE PLANNING/CONTINUITY OF CARE

- Refer family to social services for grief counseling.
- Encourage family to consider participation in a support group for fetal/neonatal loss.
- Instruct regarding mother's postpartum checkup.

REFERENCES

Cubberly, D. A. (1987). Fetal death: Diagnosis of fetal death. *Clinical OB/GYN, 30,* 259–267.

Page-Lieberman, J. & Hughes, C. B. (1990). How fathers perceive perinatal death. *American Journal of Maternal-Child Nursing, 15,* 320–323.

Parkman, S. (1992). Helping families say good-bye. *American Journal of Maternal-Child Nursing. 17*(1), 14–17.

Pitkin, R. M. (1987). Fetal death: Diagnosis and management. *American Journal of Obstetrics and Gynecology, 57,* 583–589.

Ryan, P. F., Cote-Arsenault, D. & Sugarman, L. L. (1991). Facilitating care after perinatal loss: a comprehensive checklist. *Journal of Obstetrical, Gynecologic, and Neonatal Nursing, 20,* 385–389.

▼

NEWBORN ASSESSMENT FROM BIRTH TO TWO HOURS OF LIFE

Bernadette Keller, RNC, BSN
Mary Sandelski, RN, MSN

The immediate period following birth is the most critical period for the newborn. During this time the infant's bodily functions change/adjust to operation in an extrauterine environment. Careful assessment identifies those infants who will require more intensive stabilization measures and continued close observation. The infant also initiates the first interactions with family members.

ETIOLOGIES

N/A

CLINICAL MANIFESTATIONS

N/A

▼

NURSING DIAGNOSIS: HIGH-RISK FOR ALTERED RESPIRATORY FUNCTION

Risk Factors
- Transition to extrauterine life
- Traumatic delivery
- Intrauterine fetal stress
- Meconium aspiration
- Congenital anomalies
- Prematurity

Patient Outcomes

Infant will maintain adequate respiratory functions, as evidenced by
- patent airway
- respirations of 40–60 per minute

Nursing Interventions	Rationales
Assemble resuscitation equipment before delivery.	
Assess for visible anomalies affecting normal respiratory function.	
Maintain patency of airway	
1. Suction nose and oropharynx with bulb syringe or secretions trap.	Suctioning reduces possible obstruction from aspiration of secretions.
2. Position infant in modified Trendelenburg's position.	This facilitates secretion drainage by gravity and reduces aspiration risk.
Stimulate crying by gently tapping feet or rubbing sternum.	Crying increases air movement.
Assess factors affecting respiratory status: 1. prematurity 2. meconium-stained amniotic fluid 3. type of delivery 4. maternal medication 5. fetal stress during labor	
Evaluate need for ventilatory assistance. Administer free O_2 per Ambu bag tail at 10 L/min with tube at an angle and 1–2 in. from nose for cyanosis, nasal flaring, or mild retractions. Provide warmed humidified oxygen.	Sudden gusts of air may startle infant into holding breath. O_2 delivered via Ambu bag tail more diffuse, less likely to startle infant.

▼

NURSING DIAGNOSIS: HIGH-RISK FOR HYPOTHERMIA

Risk Factors
- Altered environment
- Poor infant temperature regulation
- Unstable environmental temperature

Patient Outcome

Infant will maintain normal temperature of 37°C.

Nursing Interventions	Rationales
Dry infant (especially head) with warm blankets immediately after delivery.	Such action reduces heat loss from evaporation.
Place infant in heated radiant warmer: 1. Preset temperature at 37°C (98.6°F).	
2. Expose unwrapped body to radiant heat.	Warmer will heat only exposed surfaces (e.g., blanket on wrapped infant will be exposed to heat instead of skin).
3. Tape temperature probe to abdomen.	
4. Place cap on infant's head.	Infant's head is large in proportion to its surface area; can account for large amount of heat loss.
Assess newborn for signs of hypothermia: 1. Determine axillary temperature after birth.	To obtain baseline and to assure that infant did not suffer cold stress at birth. Thermoregulation is dependent upon a balance between heat being produced and lost by the infant.
2. Observe skin and mucous membrane changes from pink to cyanotic (other than acrocyanosis).	
3. Auscultate and observe for respiratory pattern change: • respiratory rate <40 or >60 breaths per minute • marked fluctuation in depth/rate of respiratory pattern • periods of apnea with subsequent decreased heart rate • nasal flaring, retractions	

Nursing Interventions	Rationales
Provide temperature maintenance during bonding:	
1. Dry infant during/before bonding.	Drying decreases heat loss caused by evaporation.
2. Allow maternal/infant skin-to-skin contact.	Maternal warmth can help stabilize infant temperature during bonding.
3. Cover both with warm, dry blankets.	
Maintain temperature during transport: 1. Use prewarmed transporter on stand-by. 2. Keep portholes closed.	Infant has poor thermoregulation and quickly responds to even small environmental temperature changes.
Observe for weakness/absence of reflexes.	This reflects cold stress in the infant.
If hypothermia is present, assess for hypoglycemia with Chemstrip.	Infants generate heat by burning brown fat where glucose is stored. Insulin secretion is increased in response to the greater circulating amounts of glucose, resulting in a relative state of hypoglycemia.

▼

NURSING DIAGNOSIS: HIGH-RISK FOR INJURY TO INFANT

Risk Factors
- Difficult adaptation to extrauterine life
- Birth trauma or anomalies

Patient Outcome
Potential for injury to infant is reduced by early assessment and intervention.

Nursing Interventions	Rationales
Evaluate physical status immediately after birth:	This will identify anomalies/trauma and ensure newborn well-being.

Nursing Interventions	**Rationales**

Apgar Score
1. Assign and document Apgar score at 1-, 5-, and 10-minute intervals:
 	
   • 7–10: no special interventions required.
   • 4–6: ensure infant's airway; provide ventilatory support per Ambu bag; call for pediatric assistance.
   • 0–3: institute resuscitative measures immediately (consult hospital cardiopulmonary resuscitation (CPR) policy).
	Score aids in identifying the infant who will require more aggressive resuscitation measures and observation following birth.

Cardiovascular system 1. Palpitate umbilical cord to assess heart rate. 2. Note infant's color. 3. Note number of vessels in umbilical cord, (normal = 3).	Heart rate should be >100 beats per minute. Approximately 1% of all umbilical cords have two vessels. This variation has been associated with congenital anomalies, including Sirenometia (fused legs), Vaters syndrome, and Trisomy 13 and 18, and renal anomalies.

Neurologic system
 	
1. Observe for presence and symmetry of reflexes:
   • motor activity
   • sucking
   • grasp
   • cry
 	
2. Elicit reflexes and notify pediatrician of weakness or asymmetry.
 	
3. Handle infant in a calm gentle manner.
	Abnormalities may indicate central nervous system depression or defects. Early detection allows for early intervention.
	
	Infants are calmed by gentle touch. A hyperstimulated infant's nervous system is difficult to evaluate.

Apgar Score

	2	1	0
Heart Rate	>100	<100	Not palpable
Respiratory Rate	Lusty cry	Slow irregular respiration only	Absent
Reflex	Cry	Grimace	Absent response
Muscle Tone	Flexed	Some flexion	Limp
Color	All pink	Body pink; extremities blue	Pale

Nursing Interventions	Rationales
4. Document • unusual size and shape of head • paralysis of face or extremities • poor reflex response • shrill cry • poor temperature control	
Musculoskeletal system 1. Inspect all limbs and digits. 2. Check for alignment of trunk and extremities. 3. Observe for normal range, motion, and flexion of extremities.	Polydactyly, syrodactaly, absent or malformed extremities, hip dysplasia, and presence of fractures are common birth anomalies/trauma. Specialized tests may be required to confirm presence of congenital abnormalities such as hip dysplasia.
Integumentary system 1. Inspect skin for deviations from normal appearance. 2. Report: • rash • blisters • lacerations • forceps marks • petechiae • scalp wounds (scalp electrode site).	Povodine iodine ointment to site protects against bacteria entering break in integumentary system.

Nursing Interventions	**Rationales**
Genitourinary system 1. Observe for urination. Document amount. 2. Assess penis for hypospadias or epispadias. 3. Observe for abnormal external genitalia.	
Gastrointestinal system 1. Observe for passage of meconium stool. 2. Note color of amniotic fluid. 3. Check for presence of cleft palate. 4. Document abdominal distention. 5. For omphalocele, apply sterile dressing moistened with warm saline to exposed abdominal/ contents.	Passage of stool is reassuring as it indicates a patent, functional gastrointestinal system.

▼

NURSING DIAGNOSIS: DEVELOPMENT OF PARENT/INFANT ATTACHMENT

Related To
- Delivery of newborn
- Existence of other offspring

Defining Characteristics

Initial face-to-face (visual) contact between parents and infant, including smiling with infant

Initial tactile contact between parent and infant, including hugging and kissing

Initial auditory contact between parents and infant, including calling infant by name if one has been selected or by affectionate term and speaking in a higher pitched voice to infant

Attempting to identify family characteristics in infant

Reaching for infant when infant is given to parents rather than passively receiving infant

Accepts sex of infant

Realistically appraises physical appearance of infant

Comments on beauty of infant

Patient Outcome

Positive bonding behaviors will be initiated, as evidenced by holding and talking to baby.

Nursing Interventions	Rationales
Place mirror or position patient/ significant other for viewing delivery when requested/possible; assist if necessary.	Encourage significant other's participation (e.g., cutting cord, footprinting infant.)
Increased involvement with infant promotes attraction to infant; enhances total birth experience.	Allow patient to hold infant immediately after delivery or as soon as possible.
This facilitates attachment and allows mother to get acquainted through touch.	
Identify visible anomalies before giving infant to parents.	Parents envision a perfect child and may have difficulty integrating a child with variations. Preparation may reduce the shock.
Encourage parent 1. to examine infant head to toe, visually. 2. to touch infant. 3. to talk to infant.	
Allow breast feeding when requested. Aid patient when necessary.	Immediately after birth the baby is in a quiet, alert state and apt to suckle with minimal assistance.
Reinforce patient's/significant other's positive bonding behavior. Allow family time alone with infant.	Fosters a sense of connectedness.
Point out infant's positive responses to parent's actions (e.g., quieting when parents stroke or talk to infant).	Such actions increase parents' pleasure with infant and increases feelings of mutual relationship with the infant.
Allow patient and infant to remain together as long as patient desires, and if the infant is not compromised.	Increased parent/infant contact promotes parent's attachment to infant.

Nursing Interventions	Rationales
Inform mother of a baby in the special care nursery that, when her own condition permits, she can see infant in special care nursery at any time.	
Bring pictures/infant from nursery to patient if she must remain in birth rooms because of complications of pregnancy/delivery.	

▼

DISCHARGE PLANNING/CONTINUITY OF CARE

First visit with pediatrician usually scheduled within a month after birth.

REFERENCES

Graves, B. W. (1992). Differential diagnosis of respiratory distress. *Journal of Nurse-Midwifery, 37*(2) (Suppl.), 27S-35S.

Graves, B. W. (1992). Newborn resuscitation revisited. *Journal of Nurse-Midwifery, 37*(2) (Suppl.), 36S-42S.

Lang, M. H. & Hsia, L. S. Y. (1992). The role of the CNM in newborn management. *Journal of Nurse-Midwifery, 37*(2) (Suppl.), 8S-17S.

Swartz, M. K. (1992). Primary care and differential diagnosis of the newborn. General considerations for the CNM. *Journal of Nurse-Midwifery, 37*(2) (Suppl.) 18S-26S.

NEWBORN ASSESSMENT FROM FIRST TWO HOURS OF LIFE TO THREE DAYS

Catherine Folker-Maglaya, RN, MSN, IBCLC
Charlotte Razvi, RN, MSN, Ph.D.

Continued assessment throughout the first three days enables the nurse to identify variations in the newborn and assurance that the transition to extrauterine life occurs without complications. Risks to the neonate will be reduced by early recognition of deviations and early intervention.

INDICATION

Newborn birth

▼

NURSING DIAGNOSIS: HIGH RISK FOR INEFFECTIVE BREATHING PATTERN

Risk Factors
- Inadequate surfactant levels
- Cold stress
- Hyperthermia
- Low hemoglobin
- Prenatal/intrapartum stressors resulting in Type II respiratory distress syndrome
- Maternal analgesia/anesthesia

Patient Outcomes
Infant will maintain patent airway, as evidenced by respiratory rate within normal limits.

Nursing Interventions	Rationales
Assess respiratory status immediately after admission to nursery. Report: 1. respirations <30 or >80 breaths per minute 2. generalized cyanosis 3. retraction of respiratory muscles 4. marked nasal flaring 5. auscultated or audible expiratory grunting 6. absence of lusty cry 7. choking 8. excessive secretions 9. apnea other than transient or occasional	
Clear airway; suction oropharynx by bulb syringe or DeLee mucous trap.	This helps remove accumulated fluid, enhances respiratory effort, and prevents aspiration.
Monitor apical pulse while suctioning.	Suctioning of oropharynx may cause vagal stimulation leading to bradycardia.
Place infant on side or in modified Tendelenburg's position.	Proper positioning facilitates drainage.
Administer appropriate tactile stimulation if infant is manifesting problems with respiration.	Stimulates respiratory effort and may increase inspired oxygen.
Evaluate need for ventilatory assistance. Administer supplemental O_2 as indicated by infant's condition.	
Assess blood glucose level.	Respiratory distress can result from hypoglycemia.
Perform Dubowitz assessment to determine infant's gestational age and predisposition to respiratory distress syndrome in relation to gestation age.	Dubowitz is a guide for the rating of external and neurological criteria elicited in the newborn; it is a tool that enables the examiner to make a gestational age assessment.
Note symmetry of chest movement.	Asymmetry may indicate pneumothorax (may have resulted from previous resuscitative measures).

Nursing Interventions	Rationales
Note Rh factor and blood group of infant and mother; note results of Coombs test.	
Assess hemoglobin and hematocrit levels and arterial blood gases.	

▼

NURSING DIAGNOSIS: HIGH RISK FOR DECREASED CARDIAC OUTPUT

Risk Factors
- Pneumomediastinum
- Emphysema
- Hypotension (hypovolemia, shock)
- Hypertension (coarctation of aorta)

Patient Outcomes
Infant will maintain optimal cardiac output, as evidenced by
- heart rate within normal limits
- adequate blood pressure
- absence of cyanosis

Nursing Interventions	Rationales
Evaluate heart rate on admission: 1. Average 130 beats per minute; may be irregular, especially when infant is crying. 2. Variation for brief periods; 100–180 beats per minute is normal.	Having a baseline makes it easier to assess or interpret the significance of changes in the infant.
Evaluate blood pressure.	
Assess infant's color over head and trunk. Check mucous membranes.	Feet and hands may remain cyanotic for 48 hours, especially if cold.
Refer to physician for further evaluation when cardiovascular dysfunction signs/symptoms are present.	

▼

NURSING DIAGNOSIS: HIGH RISK FOR INEFFECTIVE THERMOREGULATION

Risk Factors
- Unstable or low temperature
  - sepsis
  - respiratory distress syndrome
  - prematurity
  - cold
- High temperature
  - infection
  - dehydration
- Maternal analgesia

Patient Outcomes
Infant will maintain normal temperature of 37°C, and remain free of signs of hypo-/hyperthermia.

Nursing Interventions	Rationales
Prevent exposure and chilling: 1. Keep neonate snugly wrapped in a lightweight blanket. 2. Accomplish care and treatments quickly in a draft-free, warm environment.	This prevents heat loss.
Maintain nursery/mother's room temperature within recommended range of 72°–76°F (22.2°–23.3°C) with 40–60% humidity.	An environmental temperature decrease of 2°C. (3.6°F) is sufficient to double oxygen consumption of term neonate.
Measure axillary temperatures at least every 2–4 hours.	Temperature stabilization may not occur for 12 hours after birth.
Postpone bathing for 2–3 hours after birth until axillary temperature stabilizes 97.7°–98.6°F (36.5°–37.0°C).	
Provide extra warmth until body temperatures stabilizes but prevent overheating.	Neonates cannot perspire to prevent overheating.

▼

NURSING DIAGNOSIS: HIGH RISK FOR INFECTION

Risk Factors
- Deficiency of neutrophils
- Deficiency of specific immunoglobulin (IgA, IgM)
- Potential portals of entry for infectious organisms:
  - umbilical vessels
  - circumcision site
  - skin breaks
  - infant's delicate epidermal layer

Patient Outcome
Infection risk is reduced per early assessment and treatment.

Nursing Interventions	Rationales
Assess for signs and symptoms of infection: 1. elevated or lowered temperature 2. lethargy 3. poor weight gain 4. restlessness 5. jaundice 6. respiratory changes 7. visible lesions 8. positive culture results	
Assess maternal risk factors: 1. fever during week prior to birth 2. prolonged rupture >24 hours 3. foul-smelling amniotic fluid 4. presence of infectious disease	
Scrub hands with iodophor preparation prior to entering nursery, after contact with contaminated material and after handling each infant. Teach parents and siblings proper handwashing technique.	
Maintain individual equipment and supplies for each infant.	This helps prevent cross-contamination between infants.
Avoid excessive rubbing and use of soap. Gently pat infant's skin dry after bathing.	Rubbing may traumatize delicate skin; chemicals and perfume in soap may predispose infant's skin to rashes or breakdown.

Nursing Interventions	Rationales
Assess infant's skin daily while providing care. Distinguish between possible infectious rashes and erythematoxicum.	Vesicles or lesions caused by erythematoxicum contain eosinophils and are of no clinical significance.
Assess umbilical cord daily for: 1. redness 2. odor 3. discharge	
Expose cord stump to air by folding diaper below cord.	This promotes drying and healing, enhances normal sloughing, and eliminates moist medium for bacterial growth.
If infection is present, administer topical, oral, or parenteral antibiotics as ordered.	

▼

NURSING DIAGNOSIS: HIGH RISK FOR FLUID VOLUME DEFICIT

Risk Factors
- Dehydration as a result of
  - delayed feedings
  - reduced oral intake
  - excessive regurgitation
  - increased insensible water losses
- Hypotension
- Severe asphyxia
- Renal anomalies
- Poor suckling reflex

Patient Outcomes
The neonate will demonstrate
- rooting behavior
- effective grasp of nipple
- satisfactory sucking/swallowing behavior for adequate nourishment

Nursing Interventions	Rationales
Record initial and subsequent voidings: (scanty urine output: <2 voids in 24 hours, <30 ml in 24 hours).	Normal functioning may not be established until 24 hours following delivery.

Nursing Interventions	Rationales
Palpate bladder for distention if infant fails to void within 24 hours after birth.	This helps in determining presence of urine; may suggest a problem related to bladder or anomalies of urethra that may prevent voiding.
Assess for signs of dehydration.	
Initiate oral feedings.	The neonate requires approximately 24 oz of fluid/day for adequate weight gain (120 kcal/kg/day). Commercial formulas and breast milk contain approximately 20 cal/oz. Adequate fluid ingestion helps promote hydration and offset kidney's inability to concentrate urine and to conserve fluid during periods of high insensible losses and fluid and electrolyte stress.

▼

NURSING DIAGNOSIS: HIGH RISK FOR ALTERED NUTRITION—LESS THAN BODY REQUIREMENTS

Risk Factors
- Poor sucking reflex
- Inability to swallow or lack of gag reflex
- Rapid regurgitation
- Extreme fatigue
- High caloric requirement

Patient Outcomes
The neonate will
- demonstrate rooting behavior.
- effectively grasp nipple.
- effectively suck/swallow for adequate nourishment.
- gain weight steadily.
- feed comfortably on a regular schedule.
- sleep well between feedings.

Nursing Interventions	Rationales
Observe and record neonate's feeding behavior (e.g., reflex, level of arousal, ease of burping).	Extrauterine adjustment necessitates the independent acquisition of food, which may be complicated by an uncoordinated suck/swallow reflex, excessive secretions, anomalies, or maternal medications. Rapid metabolic rate predisposes neonate to fluid and electrolyte imbalance and hypoglycemia. The stomach empties in 2–4 hours, necessitating frequent feedings around the clock.
Demonstrate how to hold, feed, and burp neonate.	Provides role-modeling for new behavior.
Ask for return demonstration from parents. Provide support and positive feedback.	
Assess maternal-neonate interaction during feeding.	Parents may not know what to expect regarding feeding behaviors/needs of neonates and may provide inadequate nutrition. The neonate requires approximately 24 oz fluid/day (120 kcal/kg/day); commercial formulas and breast milk contain approximately 20 cal/oz.
Support parent's decision to breast- or bottle-feed.	
Encourage to hold neonate for feedings and let neonate set the pace.	
Stress importance of maintaining one feeding method in the early weeks of feeding.	The neonate uses different skills for breast feeding and bottle feeding.
Explain importance of placing neonate on side/abdomen after feeding.	Prevents aspiration of mild regurgitation of infant from air swallowed and temporary incompetence of cardiac sphincter. Any vomiting should be reported to physician.

▼

NURSING DIAGNOSIS: HIGH RISK FOR ALTERED BOWEL ELIMINATION

Risk Factors
- Infection
- Obstruction
- Congenital anomaly

Patient Outcome
Infant will pass stool within 48 hours.

Nursing Interventions	Rationales
Take rectal temperature.	Easy passage of thermometer indicates patency of anus and rules out imperforate anus.
Monitor passage of first meconium.	After first feeding is initiated, passage of meconium usually follows. If infant does not defecate in 48 hours, this may indicate intestinal obstruction.
Note frequency, color, consistency, and odor of stools.	This will vary whether human milk or formula is ingested. Usually meconium stools are present for 3–4 days followed by transitional stools, which are greenish-brown, and may last for 3–6 days. These stools are followed by formed or loose yellow stools. In breast-fed infants, the stool color is golden to mustard. In formula-fed infants, the stool is pale-yellow.

Nursing Interventions	Rationales
Assess abdomen for constant or intermittent distention. Note persistent vomiting.	Abdominal distention and persistent vomiting suggest obstruction. Obstruction that is high or complete is associated with vomiting soon after birth; more distal lesions are associated with later vomiting. Bile-stained gastric contents suggest duodenal obstruction. Paralytic ileus or partial obstruction is characterized by intermittent obstruction. Intestinal obstruction is the most frequent gastrointestinal emergency requiring surgery in the neonatal period.
Note cluster of gastrointestinal signs such as abdominal distention and tenderness, poor feeding, vomiting, presence of blood in stool, or presence of reducing substances in blood.	These signs indicate necrotizing enterocolitis (NEC), the onset of which ranges from the first day to the first month of life. NEC is associated with ischemic attack to intestines precipitated by systemic shock and hypoxia.

▼

NURSING DIAGNOSIS: HIGH RISK FOR INJURY

Risk Factors
- Birth trauma
- Congenital anomalies
- Hyperbilirubinemia and kernicterus
- Elevated levels of phenylalanine

Patient Outcome
Injuries/problems associated with birth or environment will be identified.

Nursing Interventions	Rationales
Assess for signs of birth trauma: 1. bruising 2. bleeding 3. obvious physical asymmetry	

Nursing Interventions	Rationales
Assess infant for evidence of jaundice. Note levels of direct and indirect bilirubin and behavior changes and central nervous system signs associated with kernicterus: 1. lethargy 2. listlessness 3. poor feeding 4. loss of Moro reflex	Increasing jaundice may indicate Rh or ABO incompatibility or breast milk-induced jaundice, with possible outcome of kernicterus if condition is left untreated.
Assess for congenital anomalies: 1. cleft lip 2. cleft palate 3. spina bifida 4. club foot 5. hip dislocation Monitor x-ray studies and assist with diagnostic testing as indicated.	Specialized tests may be required to confirm presence of congenital abnormalities, such as hip dysplasia.
Administer vitamin K (Aqua-Mephyton) intramuscularly as ordered.	Because newborn's intestinal tract is sterile at birth, and because feedings are delayed, infant does not have the intestinal flora needed to promote coagulation.
Perform heel-stick for PKU (phenylketonuria) test, preferably within 72 hours after initiating intake of protein.	This test identifies elevated serum levels of phenylpyruvic acid, which occur when phenylalanine is not converted to tryosine because of absence of the liver enzyme phenylalanine hydroxylase. Excessive levels of the acid can result in central nervous system involvement, mental retardation, seizures, growth retardation, and absence of melanin.

▼

NURSING DIAGNOSIS: EFFECTIVE PARENTING

Related To
- New experience with the childbearing process
- Infant care and nurturing
- Parenting role

Defining Characteristics

Parent holds baby closely to body
Parent establishes eye contact with baby
Parent calls baby by name and talks in soothing voice
Parent shows pleasure during nurturing activities (sings, smiles, rocks)
Parent readily receives baby
Parent asks questions about baby's behavior/care
Baby is content/soothed in parent's arms

Patient Outcomes

Positive parent-infant interaction

Nursing Interventions	Rationales
Provide mother extended contact with the baby. Encourage father to visit as much as possible.	Fosters a sense of connectedness.
Observe/assist with mother-infant interactions, initially exploring infant's face using fingertips, progressing to the entire body.	
Provide positive reinforcement, acknowledging positive maternal behaviors. Compliment mother.	Compliments enhance feelings of self-esteem.
When father is present, assess for his participation in care. Assist with caretaking activities.	It is important to assess both parental anxiety levels regarding infant care. Lack of confidence and anxiety may be misinterpreted as disinterest or unaffectionate behavior.
Appraise the level of understanding of infant's physiological needs: 1. maintenance of body temperature 2. nutrition 3. respiratory needs 4. bowel and bladder function	Accurate assessment provides baseline for intervention.
Provide opportunities for/assist mother (parents) with infant care (e.g., diaper changing, bathing, etc.). Praise efforts.	This promotes confidence in their ability to care for the baby.

Nursing Interventions	**Rationales**
Discuss newborn behaviors after the first and during the second periods of reactivity.	This helps parents to understand infant behaviors. After the first period of reactivity (30 minutes after birth), the infant usually falls into a deep sleep, followed by the second period of reactivity, which involves wakefulness, mucous regurgitation, gagging, and passage of first meconium stool.
Instruct the mother (parents) regarding normal infant behaviors that are in response to inner drives and not a rejection of caretaking capabilities: 1. frequently regurgitates feedings 2. grimaces and gurgles 3. maintains periods of sleeplessness 4. cries during changing, dressing, or bathing	Preparatory information reduces uncertainty.

Discuss different types of cries that the infant may use in communication and ways of assessing the infant's needs.
1. Crying does not always indicate hunger.
2. Other causes of cries include the need:
  • to be held
  • to be burped
  • for diaper to be changed
  • to express irritability or frustration (all babies tend to cry at a particular time of the day, often in early evening)
	Ability to console the infant impacts on parents' feeling of competence.

Perform newborn physical assessment in presence of parents. Provide information regarding variations in the newborn: 1. pseudomenstruation 2. breast enlargement 3. physiological jaundice 4. caput succedaneum 5. cephalohematoma 6. milia	This helps reduce anxiety and helps new parents recognize normal variations.

Nursing Interventions	Rationales
Discuss and demonstrate the normal newborn reflexes and describe when they disappear.	This provides parents with tools to help them recognize normal infant reactivity.
Demonstrate and instruct in care activities related to: 1. feeding 2. bathing 3. diapering 4. clothing 5. care of the circumcision 6. care of the umbilical cord stump	This promotes understanding of principles of newborn care and fosters parents' skill as caregivers.
Discuss newborn nail care and importance of trimming them while infant is asleep.	This prevents injury associated with movement during the cutting process.
Provide information about normal sleep patterns and ways of promoting sleep.	The infant usually requires at least 17 hours of sleep per day.
Discuss infant's nutritional needs, variability in infant appetite from one feeding to the next, as well as means of assessing adequate nutrition and hydration.	This helps to ensure adequate nutrition and hydration.
Discuss breast feeding: 1. importance of nursing infant every 2–3 hr/day until 3–4 weeks of age 2. no supplements for normal neonate 3. to ensure adequate intake, count 6 to 8 wet diapers per day after 4–5 days of life and at least one bowel movement every other day	
Discuss types of formula preparation, economics of each method, and necessary preparation and storage tips on selected formula.	This ensures proper preparation and administration of formula.
Discourage "bottle propping."	This prevents possible aspiration of formula as well as otitis media associated with drainage of nasal mucus or occlusion of duct when eustachian tube oriface opens during swallowing.

Nursing Interventions	Rationales
Instruct patient regarding positioning of newborn after feedings and the use of bulb syringe. 1. Position infant on the side after eating. 2. When infant is on the back in carrier seat or stroller, head should be elevated 30–45°.	Weak gag reflex predisposes infant to aspiration. Syringe removes secretions from nasopharynx, clearing air passages.
For premature infants, or a baby with congenital malformation: 1. Show acceptance of the baby and emphasize the positive features. 2. Allow the parents to see and touch the baby as soon as possible.	If long periods of time elapse from the time the parent(s) are informed of the complication and the moment they actually see the baby, fantasies worse than the actual situation may develop. There is then the burden of eliminating the fantasies before they can begin relating to the reality of the baby.
3. Invite parents to perform care-taking activities.	

▼

DISCHARGE PLANNING/CONTINUITY OF CARE

Emphasize importance of follow-up by pediatrician to monitor ongoing growth and development and to initiate program of immunizations.

REFERENCES

Graves, B. (1992a). Differential diagnosis of respiratory distress. *Journal of Nurse-Midwifery, 37*(Suppl.2):27S–35S.

Graves, B. W. (1992b). Newborn resuscitation revisited. *Journal of Nurse-Midwifery, 37*(Suppl.2), 365–425.

Swartz, M. K. (1992). Primary care and differential diagnosis of the newborn: General considerations for the CNM. *Journal of Nurse-Midwifery, 37*(Suppl.2):18S–26S.

▼

*O*XYTOCIN INDUCTION/ AUGMENTATION OF LABOR

Mary Christine McCarthy, RN, BSN
Mary Mullee, RN, BSN

Oxytocin induction is the artificial stimulation of uterine contractions through the use of synthetic oxytocic agents titrated carefully and administered via a fluid administration pump. If uterine contractions are present, but not frequent or strong enough, the same agents may be used to augment labor.

INDICATIONS

- Premature rupture of membranes
- Rh sensitization
- Pregnancy-induced hypertension
- Amnionitis
- Fetal growth retardation
- Postterm pregnancy
- Severe gestational diabetes
- Intrauterine fetal death
- Any clinical situation in which the benefits of delivery outweigh the benefits of continuing the pregnancy

▼

NURSING DIAGNOSIS: KNOWLEDGE DEFICIT

Related To unfamiliarity with labor induction/augmentation

Defining Characteristics
Apparent confusion about events
Multiple questions
Lack of questions
Expressed need for information
Expressed fear of chemical stimulation of labor

Patient Outcomes

Patient will describe specifics of labor induction/augmentation.

Nursing Interventions	Rationales
Assess knowledge of oxytocin induction of labor.	
Provide information regarding indications for procedure (see Indications)	
Explain the difference between spontaneously occurring versus induced contractions.	Studies indicate that induced labor/augmentation will result in active phase contractions (stronger, more frequent) during the early latent phases of labor when contractions would normally be softer and further apart.
Explain that: 1. Synthetic oxytocin is infused intravenously via a pump. 2. The dose is increased every 30–60 minutes until contractions occur 2–3 minutes apart and last 45–60 seconds; contractions are 50–80 mmHg in intensity. 3. When these endpoints are reached, the oxytocin drip rate is maintained.	

▼

NURSING DIAGNOSIS: PAIN

Related To uterine contractions

Defining Characteristics

Severe pain
Thrashing in bed
Facial grimacing
Hyperventilation

Patient Outcome

Patient will verbalize ability to cope with discomfort of labor.

Nursing Interventions	Rationales
Elicit patient's perception of uterine contraction discomfort.	Each patient demonstrates a unique response to pain.
Keep patient informed of labor progress and fetal status.	Cyclic nature of uterine contractions causes patient to lose sense of time and purpose. Reminding patient that pain "has a purpose" and induction promotes cervical changes is reassuring.
Determine mechanisms patient usually employs to manage discomfort.	
Provide nonpharmacological comfort measures when appropriate.	
Administer analgesic medications as ordered.	Patients with spontaneously occurring latent phase contractions rarely require medications for pain. In contrast, augmented/induced contractions are stronger and may require early medication.

▼

NURSING DIAGNOSIS: HIGH RISK FOR INJURY TO MOTHER

Risk Factors
- Hyperstimulation
  - failure to establish uterine resting tone between contractions
  - contraction frequency 5 in 10 minutes
  - contraction duration ≥90 seconds
- Abruptio placentae
  - increasing abdominal girth
  - rising fundus
  - boardlike uterus
  - severe restlessness
  - vaginal bleeding
  - fundal pain
  - apparent hemorrhage or signs and symptoms of occult bleeding
- Uterine rupture
  - vaginal bleeding
  - patient complaint of tearing/pain in uterus, then cessation of pain
  - apparent hemorrhage/shock

- Water intoxication
  - decreased urine output
  - hypotension
  - increased heart rate
  - headache and other central nervous system signs including confusion, nausea, vomiting

Patient Outcome

Potential for injury will be contained, or recognized and treated early.

Nursing Interventions	Rationales
Monitor contractions electronically: 1. contraction length, frequency, intensity	
2. uterine relaxation periods	Normal uterine resting tone in augumentive labor does not exceed 20 mmHg.
3. patient's description of contractions	This aids in early diagnosis of hyperstimulated contractions or early signs of impending abruption.
Discontinue infusion and notify physician if the uterus fails to relax between contractions or if there is an increase in abdominal girth or fundal height.	Oxytocin has a relatively short half-life. A decrease in uterine activity should be noted within minutes of discontinuing the infusion. There is an increased incidence of hyperstimulated contractions and abruptio placenta in induced labors.
Assess color and amount of vaginal bleeding. Implement pad count.	Excessive bleeding may indicate uterine rupture or abruptio placenta.
Monitor vital signs and level of consciousness.	Hypovolemic shock may result from abruptio placentae or uterine rupture.
Implement the following if shock occurs. 1. Maintain complete bed rest. 2. Administer parenteral fluids as ordered.	
3. Place patient in Trendelenburg position with hip wedged.	This displaces uterus off vena cava.

Nursing Interventions	Rationales
4. Prepare for delivery of a potentially compromised fetus.	
In the presence of water intoxication, decrease IV fluids to a keep-vein-open rate.	Water intoxication can be prevented by administration of balanced IV saline solution, maintaining balanced intake and output, and observing for symptoms.

▼

NURSING DIAGNOSIS: HIGH RISK FOR INJURY TO FETUS

Risk Factor
Uteroplacental insufficiency

Patient Outcome
Risk for injury will be contained, or injury will be recognized early and treated.

Nursing Interventions	Rationales
Assess fetal heart rate electronically for 15 minutes before initiating oxytocin infusion. Document fetal heart tones with each increase or decrease of infusion pump.	
Notify physician: 1. if fetal heart rate is <110 or >160 beats per minute	These changes may be associated with fetal stress in response to contraction.
2. of changes in fetal heart rate variability or reactivity.	Early recognition of signs of fetal stress allows for prompt intervention to reduce risk of fetal damage.
3. of presence of moderate or severe variable decelerations 4. of presence of late decelerations	

Nursing Interventions	Rationales
Decrease or discontinue oxytocin if signs of hypertonicity are noted: 1. five of more contractions within 10 minutes 2. failure of uterus to return to resting tone between contractions 3. <45 seconds relaxation between contractions.	Hypertonicity of uterus may cause decreased blood flow to intervillous space, resulting in fetal hypoxia.
If tracing denotes presence of fetal stress:	
1. Turn patient to lateral position.	Side position improves circulation to utero-fetal-placental unit.
2. Increase intravenous drip rate.	Fluids increase circulating blood volume, thereby increasing blood flow to intervillous space.
3. Apply O$_2$ at 10 L per rebreather.	Supplemental oxygen increases maternal PO$_2$, which increases oxygen concentration presented to intervillous space.
If fetal indicators do not improve, prepare for emergency delivery of a compromised neonate (one who will require resuscitation after delivery): 1. Notify pediatrician. 2. Check pediatric emergency equipment. 3. Check transporter.	

DISCHARGE PLANNING/CONTINUITY OF CARE

Make appointment with primary health care provider for 6-week postpartum visit.

REFERENCES

Blumenthal, P. & Ramanauskas, R. (1990). Trial of Dilapan and Laminaria as cervical ripening agents before induction of labor. *Obstetrics-Gynecology, 75*(3 Pt. 1), 365–368.

Brodsky, P. L. & Pelzar, E. M. (1991). Rationale for the revision of oxytocin administration protocols. *Journal of Obstetrical, Gynecologic, and Neonatal Nursing. 20*(6), 440–444.

Mandiville, L. K. & Toriano, N. H. (1992). *High-Risk Intrapartum Nursing*. Philadelphia, PA: J. B. Lippincott.

▼

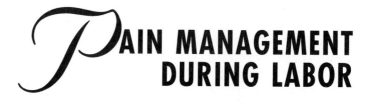

PAIN MANAGEMENT DURING LABOR

Joy C. Grohar, RNC, MS

The pain of childbirth is a very personal experience. A woman's perception of and responses to pain are influenced by culture, social status, personality, life experience, general health, quality of health care, and the amount of support she receives. For specific information on epidural anesthesia, see Chapter 38.

ETIOLOGIES

Etiology of pain in labor is not well understood. Hypotheses include
- Uterine ischemia
- Stretching of the cervix
- Traction upon the peritoneum and ligaments adnexa
- Distention of the vagina
- Pressure upon the bladder

CLINICAL MANIFESTATIONS

N/A

CLINICAL/DIAGNOSTIC FINDINGS

N/A

▼

NURSING DIAGNOSIS: PAIN

Related To
- Physiological processes of labor and delivery
  – uterine contractions

445

  – pelvic pressure
  – headache
  – leg cramps
  – bearing down
- Invasive procedures
  – vaginal examinations
  – intravenous catheter insertion
  – maternal/fetal monitoring
  – epidural placement

Defining Characteristics
Increase in respiratory rate
Increase in blood pressure
Increase in pulse
Diaphoresis
Crying/moaning
Grimaces
Writhing or thrashing movements

Patient Outcomes
- Patient will verbalize ability to manage pain.
- Partner will support patient through encouragement and the use of comfort measures.

Nursing Interventions	Rationales
Assess patient's pain source and intensity.	Pain during childbirth includes both physical and psychological components. Uterine contractions, pelvic pressure, backache, leg cramps, nausea, vomiting and other physical discomforts abound.
Assess other factors contributing to discomfort, e.g., fear, anxiety.	Sources of subjective distress include concern for self and baby, helplessness and fear.
Acknowledge patient's discomfort.	The mother's ability to cope with the discomforts of childbirth will depend, in part, on her sense of control over the event. The nurse's challenge is to assist the mother in facing childbirth with a sense of capability, "I can do it," and a feeling of support, "I will have help."

Nursing Interventions	**Rationales**
Assess support systems in place. Reassure patient/significant other that emotional support/care and pain management measures will be provided.	
Reinforce use of positive coping strategies.	The pain experience during childbirth can impact on the woman's/ couple's parenting experience. Her perceptions can positively or negatively color her feelings about herself, her behavior, and her future childbearing choices and experiences.
Provide comfort measures to reduce/eliminate painful stimuli: 1. touch (backrub, effleurage, accupressure) 2. oral hygiene, perineal care, fresh linen	
3. walking or position change.	The upright position has been shown to increase the effectiveness of contractions and to shorten labor with no increase in discomfort.
4. warm shower/ice or hot packs/ blankets 5. cool cloth 6. ice chips	
7. distraction • guided imagery • headphones with relaxation tapes, music • humor as appropriate • videotapes, television 8. medical therapeutics, as prescribed and desired by patient • analgesia • conduction anesthesia	Distraction can serve to build self-esteem and confidence as well as decrease the amount of pain medication needed.

▼

NURSING DIAGNOSIS: KNOWLEDGE DEFICIT

Related To
- Lack of experience with childbearing
- Lack of prenatal care
- Misinformation or misunderstanding of information
- Language barrier
- Cognitive deficit
- Fear contributing to avoidance or denial of information
- Immaturity

Defining Characteristics
Need for information
Lack of interest
Repeated questions on previously covered material
Lack of follow-through on information

Patient Outcomes
- Patient will verbalize potential sources of discomfort.
- Patient will demonstrate use of pain management measures at appropriate time.
- Partner will reinforce teaching to complement patient's understanding and use of pain management measures.

Nursing Interventions	Rationales
Assess need for teaching. Assess patient's desire for involvement of significant other.	
Encourage participation in prenatal classes.	

Nursing Interventions	**Rationales**

Provide information about:
1. labor process
2. options for delivery
  • labor-delivery-recovery setting (LDR)
  • single room maternity care (LDRP)
  • traditional hospital setting
  • nontraditional experiences, such as outpatient birth centers, home birth
3. pain management techniques to include, but not limited to
  • relaxation measures
  • breathing methods
  • positioning
  • (TENS) transcutaneous electric nerve stimulation
  • distraction
  • guided imagery
  • biofeedback
  • therapeutic touch
  • accupressure
  • doula/monitrice or labor coach
  • analgesia
  • anesthesia
	Approaches should be selected based on individual patient needs, e.g., stage of labor, anxiety level, acceptability to patient and availability. A variety of approaches may be necessary.

Validate level of understanding at frequent intervals throughout prenatal and intrapartum course.	

▼

NURSING DIAGNOSIS: POWERLESSNESS

Related To
- Inexperience with childbirth pain
- Lack of knowledge
- Loss of control
- Fear
- Hospital/institutional constraints
- Lack of involvement in decision-making
- Lack of privacy
- Unexpected complications

Defining Characteristics

Feelings of helplessness, uncertainty, and loss of control
Refuses to participate in decision-making
Demonstrates anxiety, depression, or hostility

Patient Outcomes

Patient will
- verbalize feeling a sense of control over her response to the pain experience.
- make informed choices.

Nursing Interventions	Rationales
Assess prenatally, patient's level of experience and knowledge with discomforts of labor.	This provides baseline for care planning.
Identify patient's perception of event(s) creating sense of power-lessness. Acknowledge patient's feelings and perceptions.	This respects patient's concerns and implies the nurse cares about her and will support her needs in an individualized way.
Assess for behaviors demonstrating loss of control: 1. acting out 2. aggressiveness 3. hostility 4. anxiety 5. apathy 6. demanding attitude 7. uncertainty	Setting limits in a caring manner assist patient in regaining control.
Acknowledge behavior and encourage verbalization of feelings and concerns.	This validates/clarifies patient's concerns and acknowledges she is doing the best she can. Acceptance is the greatest form of respect; it allows patient to share control with the nurse.
Discuss labor experiences in the context of decisions she may be faced with (e.g., type of analgesia/anesthesia). Provide scenarios and have patient/significant other practice decision-making skills.	

Nursing Interventions	**Rationales**
Discuss potential problem areas such as transition.	Patients may come to birth center with the preconceived notion that transition is the time in labor when they are likely to feel the most challenged to remain in control. Having strategies to deal with transition labor may be seen as helpful.
Assess support systems.	An effective support network can facilitate coping and improve problem-solving skills.
Assist patient/significant other in arranging tour of delivery suite and introduction to managers and staff.	
Employ pain management measures. Keep patient informed of labor progress.	Cyclic nature of uterine contractions causes patient to lose sense of time and purpose. Reminding woman that pain has a purpose may provide reassurance.

▼

DISCHARGE PLANNING/CONTINUITY OF CARE

- If patient had a very difficult labor and delivery, make arrangements for a home nursing visit.
- Consult with postpartum health care provider regarding need for discussion, support, and reassurance regarding her labor and delivery.
- Assist the family in processing the events surrounding this birth.
  - Review events
  - Clarify misconceptions.
  - Provide positive feedback when possible.

REFERENCES

Aderhold, K. (1991). Jet hydrotherapy for labor and postpartum pain relief. *Maternal Child Nursing, 16*(2), 97–99.

Andrews, S. & Chrzanowski, M. (1990). Maternal position, labor and comfort. *Applied Nursing Research, 3*(1), 7–13.

Duchene, P. (1989). Effects of biofeedback on childbirth pain. *Journal of Pain Symptom Management, 4*(3), 17–23.

Faure, E. (1991). The pain of parturition. *Seminars in Perinatology, 15*(5), 342–347.

Faut-Callahan, M. (1990). Postoperative pain control for the parturient. *Journal of Perinatal Neonatal Nursing, 4*(1), 27–40.

Hornett, E., & Osborn, R. A (1989). Randomized trial of the effects of Monitrice support during labor: Mothers' views two to four weeks postpartum. *Birth, 16*(4), 177–183.

Nicholson, C. (1990). Nursing considerations for the parturient who has received epidural narcotics during labor or delivery. *Journal of Perinatal Neonatal Nursing, 4*(1), 14–26.

Wuitchik, M., Hesson, K., & Bakal, D. (1990). Perinatal predictors of pain and distress during labor. *Birth, 17*(4), 186–191.

▼

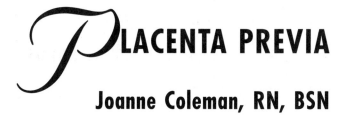

$\mathcal{P}$LACENTA PREVIA

Joanne Coleman, RN, BSN

$\mathbf{P}$lacenta previa is implantation of the placenta near or over the cervical os. Episodic, painless bleeding may occur from 24 to 40 weeks gestation as a result of cervical changes that dilate the cervix and disrupt the placenta. Previa may be classified as total, if the internal os is completely covered by the placenta; partial, if the os is not entirely covered; or marginal, if the placental edge lies close to the internal os. Partial and marginal previas may not bleed until the cervix begins to dilate or may never bleed.

ETIOLOGIES

- Multiparity
- Advanced age
- Previous cesarean sections or uterine surgery
- Defective vascularization of the decidua as a result of infection
- Atrophic changes
- Large placentas resulting from fetal erythroblastosis

CLINICAL MANIFESTATION

One or more episodes of bright red, painless vaginal bleeding

DIAGNOSTIC FINDINGS

- Decreasing hemoglobin and hematocrit levels
- Derangements in clotting factors

▼

NURSING DIAGNOSIS: HIGH RISK FOR INJURY TO MOTHER

Risk Factors
- Decreased circulating blood volume
- Hemorrhage
- Hypotension
- Hypovolemic shock

Patient Outcomes
Risk to patient from hemorrhage will be reduced through early identification and intervention.

Nursing Interventions	Rationales
Determine: 1. amount of blood loss 2. time bleeding began 3. whether pain accompanied bleeding 4. color of blood (pink or red) 5. activity before bleeding episode. Institute pad count.	Nurse needs to monitor patient closely because the patient is not always aware of actual bleeding episodes.
Place patient on bed rest.	Restricted activity is necessary to reduce chance of dislodging clot at cervical os; it may also shorten bleeding episode.
Monitor pulse, respirations, and blood pressure frequently until bleeding and vital signs stabilize.	Falling blood pressure and increasing maternal heart rate may indicate impending hypovolemic shock.
Assess labor status: 1. Only use external monitor to continuously assess status of uterine activity and fetal well-being.	Application of internal monitors may cause placental perforation and increased bleeding.
2. Report changes in fetal heart rate variability or presence of periodic patterns.	This may signal decreased placental perfusion caused by the hypovolemic state.
Avoid rectal and vaginal examinations.	Clot at os may be dislodged, causing bleeding. Placenta may be perforated during vaginal examination.

Nursing Interventions	Rationales
Record intake and output and specific gravity.	In hypovolemic states, urine output decreases/ceases.
Review serial hemoglobin/hematocrit results.	This will determine amount of blood loss.
Verify blood type and have cross-matched blood available.	Blood replacement may be indicated if blood loss becomes life-threatening.

▼

NURSING DIAGNOSIS: HIGH RISK FOR INJURY TO FETUS

Risk Factors
- Decrease in circulating blood volume
- Maternal hemorrhage
- Maternal hypovolemic shock
- Placental insufficiency

Patient Outcomes
Risk for injury to fetus is reduced due to early identification of threat and quick intervention.

Nursing Interventions	Rationales
Monitor fetal heart tones electronically. Notify physician of changes.	Change may indicate fetal compromise.
In event of fetal stress: 1. Have mother assume left lateral recumbent position.	This position removes pressure from vena cava, enhances tissue perfusion and fetal gas exchange.
2. Increase intravenous infusion flow rate.	Fluids increase circulating blood volume and blood flow to placenta.
Administer O_2 by rebreather at 10 L/min.	Supplemental oxygen increases maternal O_2 saturation; it may also increase O_2 saturation in fetal compartment.
If fetal stress is unresolved by interventions, prepare patient for emergency cesarean section.	

▼

DISCHARGE PLANNING/CONTINUITY OF CARE

- Routine postoperative delivery checkup
- Postpartum monitoring of hemoglobin and hematocrit
- Instructions in iron-rich diet and iron supplements as needed

REFERENCES

Lavery, J. (1990). Placenta previa. *Clinics in Obstetrics and Gynecology*, *33*(3), 414–421.

Lockwood, C. (1990). Placenta previa and related disorders. *Contemporary OB/GYN*, *35*(1), 47–68.

Oppenheimer, L. W., Farine, D., Ritchie, J. W., Lewinsky, R. M., Telford, J., & Fairbanks, L. A. (1991). What is a low-lying placenta? *American Journal of Obstetrics and Gynecology*, *165*(4), 1036–1038.

Saller, D. N., Nagey, D. A., Pupkin, M. J., & Crenshaw, M. C. (1990). Tocolysis in the management of third trimester bleeding. *Journal of Perinatology*, *10*(2), 125–128.

▼

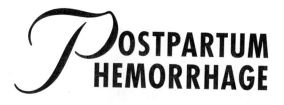

POSTPARTUM HEMORRHAGE

Theresa Vanderhei, RN
Mary Mullee, RN, BSN

A loss of more than 500 ml of blood during and after delivery is called postpartum hemorrhage. While approximately 4 percent of all deliveries are complicated by hemorrhage, only about 0.5 percent lead to hypovolemic shock.

ETIOLOGIES

A number of events may influence homeostasis following delivery, including:
- Uterine atony
- Retained placental fragments
- Cervical and/or vaginal lacerations
- Perforated uterus
- Hematomas

CLINICAL MANIFESTATIONS

- Uterine atony:
  - uterus fails to contract after delivery
  - boggy uterus Credé will result in the expulsion of clots and steady flow of blood
- Lacerations:
  - persistent bleeding with a firm uterus
- Hematoma:
  - bluish bulge on the perineum
  - extremely painful
  - occult bleeding
  - symptoms of shock

- Retained placenta:
  - persistent bleeding
  - placenta not intact

CLINICAL/DIAGNOSTIC FINDINGS

- Hemoglobin and hematocrit levels are decreased.
- Derangements in the clotting factors might be apparent if bleeding is extreme or persists over a protracted period of time.

▼

NURSING DIAGNOSIS: FLUID VOLUME DEFICIT

Related To excessive bleeding

Defining Characteristics
Decreased urine output
Concentrated urine
Decreased venous filling
Hypotension
Decreased pulse volume
Weakness

Patient Outcomes
Patient will maintain normal fluid balance, as evidenced by
- stable blood pressure.
- urine output >30 ml/hr.

Nursing Interventions	Rationales
Determine amount of uterine bleeding. Assess for signs of uterine atony.	Uterine atony is responsible for 90% of all postpartum hemorrhages.
If atony is present: 1. Massage fundus until firm. 2. Initiate breast feeding.	Breast feeding may stimulate uterine contractions.
Assess for retained placenta or bleeding from another site if bleeding persists despite a firm uterus.	Bleeding from the cervix and vagina, perineal tears, hematoma, or separation of episiotomy are additional causes of hemorrhage.

Nursing Interventions	**Rationales**
Review delivery history for: 1. use of forceps or excessive vaginal manipulation 2. precipitous or prolonged first or second stage 3. large baby, multiple gestation, or polyhydramnios 4. placental abnormalities 5. drugs that relax the uterus, including magnesium sulfate or general anesthesia 6. use of oxytocic agents that fatigue uterine muscle 7. infection	These events predispose to postpartum hemorrhage.
Review delivery record for documentation of sponge count. Inspect vagina for retained sponges.	This alone may be responsible for persistent bleeding.
Monitor vaginal bleeding.	
Institute pad count. Weigh bedpads and linen to estimate blood loss.	One ounce equals approximately 30 ml of blood.
Monitor vital signs at frequent intervals. Observe for signs and symptoms of impending shock.	
Start one or more intravenous infusions with large-bore needles, and infuse crystalloids or blood as needed.	Blood/fluids should be infused at rate needed to replace blood lost and support blood pressure.
Administer oxytocic agents and prostaglandins as ordered.	These medications are commonly used to promote uterine contractions/involution.
Palpate urinary bladder for distention.	A full bladder may displace the uterus, resulting in relaxation and increased bleeding.
Encourage patient to void or catheterize as needed.	
Monitor serial hemoglobin & hematocrit values. Perform clotting studies regularly. Type and cross-match as needed.	

Nursing Interventions	Rationales
Prepare patient for manual exploration of the uterus, dilatation and curettage (D&C), and surgical repair of lacerations.	Manual exploration and D&C are indicated for retained products of conception; abdominal surgery is necessary to explore source of bleeding or repair occult hematoma, laceration or perforated uterus.

▼

NURSING DIAGNOSIS: ACTIVITY INTOLERANCE

Related To
- Low hemoglobin
- Low hematocrit
- Reduced oxygen-carrying capacity

Defining Characteristics
Report of fatigue or weakness
Exertional dyspnea or discomfort
Increased heart rate response to activity

Patient Outcomes
Patient will
- maintain adequate periods of rest.
- perform required activities within limitations.

Nursing Interventions	Rationales
Assess to what degree acute bleed has depleted patient's ability to perform: 1. activities of daily living 2. child care routines	
Encourage mother to ingest iron-rich food and a balanced diet in other nutritional areas.	
Encourage patient to rest at frequent intervals throughout the day, and to rest when baby is resting.	Rest is necessary to conserve energy and ensure proper balance between activity and rest.
Administer iron replacements and vitamins as ordered.	These nutrients will increase the oxygen-carrying capacity of blood.

DISCHARGE PLANNING/CONTINUITY OF CARE

- Instruct patient in signs and symptoms of ongoing bleeding.
- Encourage proper nutrition; prescribe vitamins and iron supplements as needed for 4 to 6 weeks.
- Reinforce need for rest. Encourage patient to secure assistance in home maintenance during recovery period.
- Follow-up with routine postpartum checkups with evaluation of hemoglobin and hematocrit.

REFERENCES

American College of Obstetricians and Gynecologists. (1990). Diagnosis and management of postpartum hemmorrhage. *ACOG Technical Bulletin* 143. Washington, D.C.

Long, P. (1991). Bleeding in the third stage of labor. *NAACOG's Clinical Issues in Perinatal and Women's Health Nursing, 2*(3), 385–395.

Luegenbiehl, D. L. (1991). Postpartum bleeding. *NAACOG's Clinical Issues in Perinatal and Women's Health Nursing, 2*(3), 402–409.

$\mathscr{P}$REGNANT PATIENT IN FIRST TRIMESTER

Jill Kollmann, RN, BSN
Deidra Gradishar, RNC, BS

Pregnancy during the first trimester (weeks 1 through 12) is a period of immense change. It affects all dimensions—physical, mental, emotional, psychosocial, and spiritual. Health care workers can be a valuable asset to the patient by providing education, support, and referral to services not directly provided by the caregiver.

ETIOLOGIES

N/A

CLINICAL MANIFESTATIONS

N/A

▼

NURSING DIAGNOSIS: KNOWLEDGE DEFICIT REGARDING PRENATAL CARE, BODY CHANGES/DISCOMFORTS ASSOCIATED WITH FIRST TRIMESTER, AND POTENTIAL COMPLICATIONS

Related To first experience with pregnancy

Defining Characteristics
Desire for confirmation of pregnancy and estimated date of delivery
Many questions about pregnancy
Lack of questions
Verbalized misconceptions

Patient Outcomes
Patient will verbalize understanding of
• estimated date of delivery and how it was calculated

- importance of prenatal care and keeping appointments
- fetal development
- normal discomforts of early pregnancy and possible strategies to relieve them
- assessments of maternal well-being

Nursing Interventions	Rationales
Assess age and maturational level of patient.	Pregnancy and parenthood represent a developmental milestone in the maturational process. Individuals may require assistance to negotiate this rite of passage. This is even more critical if the mother is a teenager or lacks the family or financial support to master the skills necessary to parent effectively.
Explain need for assessment of health/pregnancy history.	Contributing factors such as family medical history, menstrual and pregnancy history, and sexual history provide valuable information.
Explain what information is derived from the physical examination/internal pelvic examination:	
1. pelvic diameter	This will determine adequacy of pelvis for vaginal delivery.
2. size of uterus as compared to weeks gestation from last menstrual period	
3. vaginal secretions	This examination is done to rule out infection.
4. pelvic structures	This will determine integrity, placement, changes associated with pregnancy.
Explain tests to confirm pregnancy: 1. serum/urine human chorionic gonadotropin levels 2. pelvic ultrasound	

Nursing Interventions	**Rationales**
Explain how the estimated date of delivery (EDD) is determined and reinforce that it is an *estimated* date.	EDD is based on findings of health history, Naegle's rule, and/or ultrasound examination.

Explain common risk factors:
1. history of
   • previous pregnancy losses
   • preterm births
   • immunization
   • elective abortions
2. age
   • <17 years
   • >35 years
3. family history
   • birth defects
   • pregnancy-induced hypertension
   • diabetes
4. alcohol or drug abuse
   • suspicious use of prescribed/over-the-counter drugs
   • use of tobacco products
5. uterine surgery, reproductive anomalies
6. malignancy
7. pregnant more than 5 times	

Assess patient's knowledge level regarding importance of prenatal care. Inform of schedule of care during pregnancy: 1. monthly through 7th month 2. every 2 weeks until last month 3. weekly during last month	
Inform patient of maternal well-being procedures/tests to be expected during course of prenatal care: 1. height and weight 2. urine testing for protein 3. blood pressure assessment 4. glucose screening 5. alpha-fetoprotein 6. ultrasound examination 7. *Rubella* titer	Increased understanding promotes compliance.

Nursing Interventions	**Rationales**
Inform patient of importance of keeping prenatal appointments.	Ongoing assessment of maternal and fetal well-being will help identify any problems that may arise.
Assess patient's knowledge of fetal growth and development. Explain that the first 12 weeks are the most rapid period of growth for the fetus.	All organs are formed by the end of the first trimester. The fetus begins to look like a human and weighs approximately ½ oz. and is approximately 3 in. long.
Inform patient of fetal well-being tests as needed:	
1. ultrasound examination	This test determines adequate growth for dates, is used to rule out fetal/placental anomalies, aids in assessment of well-being.
2. alpha-fetoprotein between 14 and 18 weeks gestation.	This test screens for neural tube defects/Down syndrome.
3. nonstress test, oxytocin contraction test, and biophysical profile.	These tests indirectly assess placental function in an attempt to predict fetal well-being.
4. fundal heights	This test ensures that size equals date.
Assess whether patient is experiencing any of the common discomforts of pregnancy: 1. breast changes (fullness, tenderness) 2. urinary frequency due to compression of bladder 3. nausea and vomiting related to hormonal changes 4. fatigue 5. mood swings 6. fetal movement	
Explain strategies for relieving some of these discomforts: 1. breast tenderness/enlargement: • supportive bra one or two sizes larger than usual	Large size bra needed to accommodate growth.

Nursing Interventions	Rationales
2. nausea and vomiting: • frequent small meals throughout day	Always having some food present in the stomach aids in absorbing hydrochloric acid.
• food high in carbohydrates, low in fats • minimum spices • dry carbohydrates eaten before getting out of bed if nausea is worse in morning	
• fluids between meals	Prevent stomach from getting overloaded during meals.
3. fatigue • rest for short intervals throughout day.	Energy usually returns in second trimester.
4. urinary frequency.	Due to pressure of the growing uterus on the bladder, urination is more frequent.
Inform patient of danger signs of pregnancy and need to notify physician if the following symptoms manifest:	
1. bleeding with or without cramping	Bleeding may indicate threatened abortion.
2. sudden gush or a persistent trickling of fluid from the vagina	This may indicate premature rupture of the membranes
3. pain on urination or urinary frequency	These may indicate urinary tract infection or pylonephritis.
4. sudden weight gain of more than 5 lb in a week, or swelling that persists even after 12 hours of bed rest	These conditions may indicate pregnancy-induced hypertension.
5. relentless vomiting/inability to keep food or fluids in stomach	This may indicate hyperemesis gravidarum.
6. headache, visual disturbances, epigastric pain	These are often associated with pregnancy-induced hypertension.
7. severe relentless abdominal pain	This pain may indicate preterm labor, placental abruptio.

Nursing Interventions	Rationales
8. fever	Fever indicates infection.
9. weight loss	Loss of weight may indicate development of gestational diabetes.
Explain the importance of avoiding drugs, alcohol, or tobacco during pregnancy.	Ingestion of substances during critical periods of growth and development may be harmful to the fetus.
Assess patient's usual pattern of exercise before pregnancy. Instruct her to continue with/initiate a regular exercise regimen such as walking 20–30 minutes three times per week.	Exercise helps maintain a healthy state during pregnancy. It provides an optimum environment for fetal development and a physically fit mother strong enough to do the work involved in labor and delivery.
Inform patient of need to allow for adequate rest periods, especially if urinary frequency or other discomforts interrupt her normal sleeping pattern.	

▼

NURSING DIAGNOSIS: HIGH RISK FOR ALTERED NUTRITION—LESS/MORE THAN BODY REQUIREMENTS

Risk Factors
- Nausea/vomiting
- Increased appetite

Patient Outcomes
Patient will verbalize understanding of what a balanced diet is and how it relates to a healthy pregnancy.

Nursing Interventions	Rationales
Assess current eating patterns and understanding of nutrition during pregnancy.	This provides basis for learning.

Nursing Interventions	Rationales
Provide patient with a plan for a balanced diet with sample menus: 1. protein sources: 2 servings a day (each group) • meat, fish, cheese or eggs • beans/legumes or nuts/seeds 2. dairy products: 4 servings a day • milk, yogurt, tofu, or cheese 3. grain products: 3+ servings a day • bread, cereal, pasta, rice, or wheat germ 4. vitamin C sources: 2+ servings a day • fruits and vegetables 5. leafy green vegetables: 1+ servings a day	
Provide information about maintenance of good hydration and nutrition during episodes of nausea and vomiting.	Nausea and vomiting is usually limited to the first trimester. Severe nausea and vomiting marked by the inability to maintain adequate food and fluid intake is termed Hyperemesis gravidarum. See, p. 377.

▼

NURSING DIAGNOSIS: HIGH RISK FOR ALTERED SEXUALITY PATTERNS

Risk Factors
• Discomfort of early pregnancy
• Impaired relationship with significant other

Patient Outcomes
Patient will
• engage in satisfying level of sexual activity.
• verbalize understanding of how her feelings about herself affect her sexuality.

Nursing Interventions	Rationales
Assess patient's comfort/anxiety level related to sexuality.	

Nursing Interventions	Rationales
Encourage patient and partner to verbalize feelings regarding their sexual relationship and how it is affected by pregnancy.	
Inform couple that intercourse is safe as long as it is not uncomfortable and membranes are not ruptured. If patient has a history of bleeding or preterm labor, discuss limitations on sexual activity with physician.	In the presence of preterm labor the patient may be cautioned against orgasm, which might precipitate contractions.
Inform couple that during the first trimester, libido is decreased.	This frequently occurs due to fatigue and the normal discomforts of pregnancy. During the second and third trimesters, libido will increase.
Provide information on other ways of sexual expression (e.g., alternate positions for intercourse, mutual masturbation, cuddling).	

DISCHARGE PLANNING/CONTINUITY OF CARE

- Provide sample meal plans for balanced nutrition.
- Provide written information on danger signs and potential complications.
- Provide listing of/refer to community services, which may include
  - childbirth education
  - parenting classes
  - breast-feeding classes
  - social service
  - Medicaid office
  - support groups
  - family planning clinics
  - county health department

REFERENCES

Alfonso, D. & Sheptak, S. (1990). Maternal themes during pregnancy. *American Journal of Maternal-Child Nursing, 18*, 147–166.

Hansell, M. (1991). Sociodemographic factors and the quality of prenatal care. *American Journal of Public Health*, *81*(8), 1023–1028.

Patterson, E. T., Freese, M. P., & Goldenberg, R. L. (1990). Seeking safe passage: Utilizing health care during pregnancy. *Image*, *22*, 27–31.

▼

$\mathscr{P}$REGNANT PATIENT IN SECOND TRIMESTER

Christine Potaczek McFadden, RN, BSN

The second trimester of pregnancy encompasses weeks 13 to 24. The mother begins to appear pregnant and to feel fetal movement. These changes allow the mother to begin to differentiate herself from her developing fetus. Nesting behaviors are noted, and the discomforts of early pregnancy are absent. She may now have concern about body image.

CLINICAL MANIFESTATIONS

The uterus rises out of the pelvis. Early discomforts of pregnancy are reduced as the uterus no longer presses on the bladder causing urinary frequency. The debilitating fatigue experienced in the first months is replaced by increased energy. Nausea and vomiting are absent.

▼

NURSING DIAGNOSIS: PAIN (LOW ABDOMINAL PAIN; LEG CRAMPS; BACKACHE; VARICOSE VEINS)

Related To
- Poor venous return from compression of vessels by the gravid uterus
- Dislodgement of internal organs
- Softening of connective tissue with resultant skeletal shifts
- Weight gain

Defining Characteristics

Aching, cramping, or stabbing pain in low abdomen—especially on sides and frequently related to changing position

Severe stabbing pains usually in calves of legs but sometimes in thighs or buttocks

Pressure and dull pain down back of legs and hips

Pressure in lumbosacral area upon standing or walking

Dilated or swollen veins on legs or vulva

Patient Outcomes

Patient will

- verbalize the knowledge of self-help measures to prevent/relief of pain/discomfort.
- express tolerance of pain/discomfort associated with pregnancy.

Nursing Interventions	Rationales
Assess patient's complaints of pain, especially in regard to location, degree, precipitating factors, and recurrence.	Accurate assessment facilitates detection of complications.
Visually check areas of patient's concern when possible, e.g., pain in legs or vulva.	Redness suggests phlebitis.
Abdominal pain • Teach patient signs of impending labor so she can differentiate rhythmic contractions—or "baby balling up"—from sudden episodes of pain due to stretching ligaments.	Information serves to reduce unnecessary anxiety related to pain.
• Instruct patient to get off her feet and rest in comfortable position when pain occurs. • If pain is due to stretching ligaments, suggest heating pad to lower abdomen for short periods of time (while patient is awake only). • Notify physician if pain is persistent.	
Leg pain • Instruct patient to stand up and attempt ambulation; point foot toward face, stretching the calf muscle; rub calf and apply heat.	These measures are aimed at "working out" the cramp.

Nursing Interventions	Rationales
• Recommend to patients that they shake their legs for 30 seconds before bedtime.	This improves circulation to the legs.
• If nighttime leg cramps are a recurrent problem, instruct patient to raise the foot of the bed 6 inches and sleep on side, not back.	This improves circulation, especially venous return, and relieves compression of pelvic nerves.
• Teach patients to avoid high phosphorous, low calcium foods such as processed snacks, colas, and soda pop.	Cramps may be due to disturbed calcium/phosphorous ratio.

Back pain
- Instruct patient to sit instead of standing when possible.
- Teach of importance of sleeping on firm mattress and sitting on straight back chair.

• Demonstrate proper body mechanics: bending from knees, not from waist; standing with erect posture; pelvic-rock exercises.	Back muscle strain is due to changed center of gravity.
• Recommend use of heating pad at 10-minute intervals.	
• Recommend wearing flat or low-heeled shoes and maternity girdle.	

Varicose veins
- Avoid prolonged standing, especially in one position.
- Instruct patient to sit with feet elevated when possible.
- Recommend maternity support pantyhose and a maternity girdle, especially for vulvar varicosities.

• Instruct patient to avoid knee-high stockings or round garters.	These constrict circulation.

▼

NURSING DIAGNOSIS: PAIN/DISCOMFORT (HEARTBURN; HEMORRHOIDS; CONSTIPATION)

Related To
- Physical changes of pregnancy
- Reflux resulting from smooth muscle relaxation
- Poor venous return
- Crowding of abdominal contents
- Reduced motility

Defining Characteristics
Heartburn
Burning pain or discomfort under sternum or upper abdomen, especially after eating spicy or fatty foods

Hemorrhoids
Dilated veins around anus and rectum
Pressure and pain when passing stool
Rectal bleeding

Constipation
Difficulty in/discomfort when passing stool

Patient Outcomes
Patient will
- verbalize knowledge of self-help measures to reduce occurrence of heartburn, hemorrhoids, and constipation.
- verbalize relief from discomfort.

Nursing Interventions	Rationales
Assess patient's complaints of discomfort.	Treatment is aimed at the cause.
Assess measures used to relieve problem and its effectiveness.	Previously unsuccessful methods require additional intervention.
Instruct in methods to treat heartburn: 1. Avoid spicy, fatty foods. 2. Eat small frequent meals during day rather than 3 large meals.	
3. Avoid lying flat after eating.	Heartburn is due to reflux of acidic secretions from stomach into lower esophagus.

Nursing Interventions	Rationales
4. Avoid straining to pass stool.	Straining may aggravate heartburn.
Instruct patient in methods to reduce/treat hemorrhoids: 1. Avoid constipation. 2. Use side-lying position with hips on pillow 20 minutes tid. 3. Use hemorrhoidal suppositories or cream after each bowel movement. 4. Apply witch hazel compresses to anal area. 5. Take frequent sitz baths in 3 inches warm water 20 minutes.	This relieves pressure of uterus on pelvic abdominal veins.
Instruct patient in methods to prevent/treat constipation: 1. Increase fiber in diet. Increase intake of grains, fruits, and vegetables. 2. Increase fluid intake, especially water (6–8 glasses daily). 3. Increase exercise. 4. Emphasize importance of never ignoring urge to defecate. 5. Recommend bowl of raisin bran or cup of hot water at bedtime.	Increased fiber promotes motility of gastrointestinal (GI) tract. Regular physical activity promotes GI motility.

NURSING DIAGNOSIS: HIGH RISK FOR ALTERED NUTRITION—MORE THAN BODY REQUIREMENTS

Risk Factor

Nutritional requirements are increased due to growing fetus and products of conception.

Patient Outcomes

Patient will

- verbalize good food choices to provide adequate energy for the growing fetus.
- gain sufficient weight during pregnancy.
- maintain hematocrit and hemoglobin levels to prevent anemia.

Nursing Interventions	Rationales
Assess patient's knowledge of nutrition and its importance in pregnancy outcome.	This provides baseline for subsequent diet instruction.
Evaluate current eating habits with patient.	
Plot patient's weight gain as pregnancy progresses.	Weight gain provides information on growth of fetus.
Assess fundal height as related to gestational age.	
Review laboratory work, especially hematocrit and hemoglobin levels.	Anemia is common during pregnancy.
Teach importance of four food groups in daily diet:	
1. breads and cereals	Carbohydrates provide quick, short-term energy and stored energy.
2. milk and milk products	Calcium is important for maternal and fetal musculoskeletal systems.
3. meat, poultry, fish, and beans	Protein is needed to build new tissues and restore cells.
4. fruits and vegetables	These provide fiber and vitamins.
Stress the importance of taking vitamins and supplemental iron. Instruct patient to take iron with a source of vitamin C to increase iron absorption.	

▼

NURSING DIAGNOSIS: KNOWLEDGE DEFICIT REGARDING BODY CHANGES, SELF-HELP MEASURES

Related To new experience with pregnancy

Defining Characteristics
Need for more information
Lack of questions

Patient Outcomes

Patient will verbalize
- knowledge of possible body changes associated with pregnancy
- self-help measures to treat problems experienced

Nursing Interventions	Rationales
Assess knowledge of body changes commonly associated with second trimester of pregnancy.	
Provide self-help information.	Giving patient some control over/ responsibility in treatment increases the probability of success.

1. Flatulence/bloating
  • Instruct patient to keep food log.
  • Teach patient to be aware of foods causing discomfort and flatulence. Foods to avoid: onions, dried beans, collard greens, cauliflower, cabbage, brussel sprouts and turnips.	

2. Edema
  • Instruct patient to monitor weight gain, and to observe for dependent edema of ankles and feet late in day, tight shoes and rings and indentation left on legs and feet from socks.
 	
  • Instruct that edema is normal in pregnancy, but a weight gain of 2 lb/week or more along with facial or hand swelling may signal a pregnancy-induced hypertensive disorder.
  • Instruct to avoid prolonged standing or sitting with legs dangling.
 	
  • Instruct to avoid constrictive clothing.
	Normal edema is due to increased pressure by gravid uterus on venous return, which causes stasis of fluid in lower extremities.

Nursing Interventions

- Instruct to lie on left side.

- Instruct to avoid added salt intake.
3. Tachycardia
   - Instruct patient that increased blood volume is normal in pregnancy, and results in increased heart rate.
   - Teach patient to monitor for feelings of breathlessness and palpitations, and to slow down physical activities to compensate.
4. Dizziness/fainting
   - Instruct patient to monitor for precipitating factors, e.g., position change, activity, timing of meals.

   - Instruct to avoid sudden position changes.

   - Instruct to avoid excessively hot showers or baths.

   - Instruct to avoid hypoglycemia.
   - Instruct to lie down or sit during episode of lightheadedness to avoid injury.
5. Diaphoresis/increased vaginal secretions/breast changes
   - Instruct patient that increased hormonal secretions are normal, but require frequent self-care and hygiene measures: showers, tub, baths, shampoos.

   - Remind patient that skin condition may change.

Rationales

This increases blood flow to kidneys and relieves pressure on abdominal veins, thereby increasing elimination.

Orthostatic hypotension is a significant cause.

Hot bathing causes vasodilation.

Oily skin may require astringent; oily hair may require change in shampoo selection.

Nursing Interventions	**Rationales**
• Instruct patient to report foul-smelling vaginal discharge or excessive vaginal itching.	May be sign of vaginal infection.
• Encourage patient to wear good support bra so heavier breasts will not sag. Pads may need to be worn to cover leaking nipples so clothes will not be stained.	
• Instruct patient to prepare nipples for nursing by exposing to air for a few hours once or twice per day. Wash nipples with water, not soap, as it may dry the skin.	
6. Skin pigmentation changes	
• Determine whether patient is experiencing chloasma, linea negri or alba, angiomas or vascular spiders.	These are hormonal effects that regress after pregnancy.
• Suggest use of sunblock with SPF (sun protection factor) of 15 or more.	Sun intensifies skin pigmentation changes.
7. Fatigue	
• Teach importance of 8 hours sleep each night; nap in afternoon (if home); rest at work with legs elevated.	Pregnancy makes increased demands on mother's body. She needs more rest, a good diet, and vitamins to meet these needs and stay healthy.
• Instruct patient on adequate diet, need for vitamin and iron supplements.	

▼

NURSING DIAGNOSIS: KNOWLEDGE DEFICIT REGARDING SAFE EXERCISE HABITS

Related To
• Previously inactive lifestyle
• Change in body size and shape

Defining Characteristics
Need for more information
Lack of questions

Patient Outcomes
Patient describes participation in safe exercise regimen.

Nursing Interventions	Rationales
Assess patient's past and current activity/exercise level.	
Teach patient importance of keeping active throughout pregnancy.	Strengthening and toning muscles stimulates circulation and increases oxygen intake. It produces a feeling of exhilaration, providing relaxation and a better night's sleep.
Recommend walking, swimming, dancing and prenatal exercise classes as good forms of exercise. Emphasize this is not a time to start an aggressive exercise regime but to increase healthy activities such as walking.	

▼

NURSING DIAGNOSIS: HIGH RISK FOR INJURY TO FETUS

Risk Factors
- Smoking
- Illicit drug use

Patient Outcomes
Patient will
- verbalizes dangers to fetus secondary to smoking and drug use.
- remain free of drug and cigarette use.

Nursing Interventions	Rationales
Assess smoking habits in initial interview; follow up throughout pregnancy.	

Nursing Interventions	**Rationales**
Instruct patient about dangers of smoking while pregnant.	Understanding of risks to fetus may facilitate reduction/cessation of such behaviors.
1. Carbon monoxide competes with oxygen for space on red blood cells so less oxygen is available to growing fetus.	
2. Nicotine constricts blood vessels so less nutrients pass to fetus and waste products are eliminated more slowly.	
3. Smoking mothers are at increased risk for placenta previa, placental abruption, premature labor and premature rupture of membranes, increased incidence of sudden infant death syndrome (SIDS) and lower birth weights due to decreased circulation and oxygenation.	Accurate information may promote healthy behavior.
Assess patient's use of alcohol.	No safe level of alcohol consumption has been demonstrated.
Teach dangers to fetus if drugs are used during pregnancy:	
1. Marijuana: same risks as cigarettes, but also increases the risk of prematurity, precipitous labor and antepartal meconium passage. Babies may have problems responding to environmental stimuli and have tremors. Usually these problems resolve by 1 month of age.	
2. Cocaine: increases risk of placental abruption and produces babies with neurological deficits, interactive behavior problems, depressed response to environmental stimuli, and lower birth weight.	

▼

DISCHARGE PLANNING/CONTINUITY OF CARE

- Routine prenatal visits
- Referral to social service, support group, drug treatment program as indicated

REFERENCES

Artal, R. (1992). Exercise and pregnancy. *Clinical Sports Medicine, 11*(2), 363–377.

Lowe, T. (1990). Normal pregnancy. *Current Opinions in Obstetrics and Gynecology, 2*(6), 768–772.

McElroy, D. (1992). Pica: Nutritional and medical concerns . . . bizarre food cravings and aversions. *International Journal of Childbirth Education, 7*(1), 7.

Richardson, P. (1990). Women's experiences of body change during normal pregnancy. *American Journal of Maternal-Child Nursing, 19*(2), 93–111.

Zeanah, M. & Schlosser, S. (1993). Adherance to ACOG guidelines on exercise during pregnancy: Affect on pregnancy outcome. *Journal of Obstetric Gynecologic and Neonatal Nursing, 22*(4), 329–335.

$\mathcal{P}$REGNANT PATIENT IN THIRD TRIMESTER

Deidra Gradishar, RNC, BS

During the third trimester the woman accommodates to enormous physical changes as the pregnancy advances. Emotionally she deals with issues about impending labor and delivery, parenthood, and integrating the new child into her life and family. This period of time is marked by preparation for feeding, clothing, sheltering, and nurturing her child.

ETIOLOGIES

N/A

CLINICAL MANIFESTATIONS

N/A

▼

NURSING DIAGNOSIS: KNOWLEDGE DEFICIT REGARDING PROCESS OF LABOR AND BIRTH, PARENTING

Related To
- New experience
- Lack of resources
- Unfamiliar with information resources

Defining Characteristics
Articulates concerns about being capable of tolerating childbirth
Expresses concerns about her ability to competently provide care for her newborn child
Asks questions relative to her concerns
Seeks advice from friends and family members
Seeks out classes in childbirth preparation/parenting

Patient Outcomes

Patient will
- seek out required information.
- identify appropriate resources.
- enroll in prenatal class.

Nursing Interventions	Rationales
Assess patient's experience with/ knowledge about childbirth and child care practices.	This provides information about patient's current knowledge base.
Ask patient to describe special areas of interest/concern.	The adult learner responds best to information about her own interests.
Assess interest in participating in childbirth preparation programs, parenting, and breast-feeding classes.	Many patients still hold the misconception that childbirth preparation classes are only for those desiring an unmedicated birth. Patients often need support and encouragement to access these learning opportunities. Women from single-parent homes or those lacking family support may hesitate to enroll in classes due to their lack of a partner.
Encourage participation in preparation programs.	
Ask specific questions about her birth plans and intentions regarding infant feeding/child care issues.	Gives health care provider a sense of patient's learning needs. Stimulates client to begin to think about and seek out information in areas she is uncertain about. Many clients presume that they will instinctively understand what is happening to their bodies during birth and how to care for a newborn.

Nursing Interventions	Rationales
Assess family and other resources available to patient during birth and early days as a new parent. Encourage her to identify people who can be available to help and teach her when she first brings her infant home.	Historically families provided support to the new mother during her pregnancy and her early days as a parent. However, family members may be located at a distance the new mother might be estranged from or reluctant to ask friends and family for support and help, expecting that the transition will be easy.
Provide the patient with written materials, a book list, and video resources.	The woman in the third trimester often experiences an exquisite readiness to learn about childbirth and child care as birth becomes imminent.
Encourage patient to utilize expert resources to answer her most important questions.	Friends and family are eager to aid the new parent by sharing information, but there is always a risk that misinformation will accompany the valuable information.
Review danger signs of pregnancy and reinforce the necessity of notifying physician. (See "Care of Patient in First Trimester", p. 462, for complete listing of symptoms.)	
Instruct patient on the phases and stages of labor and provide information on measures which may be helpful in coping with the discomforts. Refer to care plan, "Care of the Intrapartum Patient", see p. 397, for description of coping measures.	

Nursing Interventions	**Rationales**
Prodromal phase: Symptoms include	This phase precedes the actual initiation of labor, but physical changes are occurring which prepare the body for labor.
1. lightening	The baby settles down into the pelvis. Clothes fit differently. The patient experiences relief of the symptoms of breathlessness as the diaphragm is better able to expand; however, she now feels increased urinary frequency as the baby compresses the bladder.
2. rupture of membranes	May be apparent as a slow leak or a sudden gush of fluid from the vagina. Labor can begin before or not at all after the membranes rupture. Patients need to notify care providers once the membranes begin to leak or break.
3. increased Braxton-Hicks contractions	Contractions have been present throughout pregnancy, but the strength, frequency, and regularity increase and mimic labor.

• To determine whether patient is in true or false labor, instruct patient to
  – attempt to sleep if contractions begin at night.
  – "challenge" the contractions to abate by walking around.
  – come to the hospital when the membranes rupture, if contractions are 10 minutes apart for the multipara or 5 minutes apart for the primipara
	Braxton-Hicks contractions will space out and become softer with activity. True labor contractions will increase in frequency and intensity with activity and over time.

Nursing Interventions	Rationales
4. bloody show	As the cervix softens and begins to dilate through the action of more coordinated Braxton-Hicks contractions, the mucous plug, which has been sealing the cervical os, might be expelled. The blood tinge may be the result of tiny capillaries in the cervix breaking with the stretching action of the cervix.
5. burst of energy	Probably the result of hormonal surges, this burst of energy often manifests for several days before labor begins.
Stage 1 of labor	
1. early latent phase	During this time contractions are effacing the cervix and resulting in some dilation. Contractions may be inadequate, or regular but widely spaced. Patients are instructed to continue with normal activities of daily living until they become too uncomfortable. Contractions should be timed and care provider consulted.
2. active phase of labor	Contractions are closer together and increase in intensity. Effacement has been accomplished and the cervix continues to dilate to 10 cm. Patient will need distraction and relaxation techniques to negotiate the contractions. Anesthesia or analgesic may be used.
Stage 2 of labor	Patient actively pushes fetus down birth canal during contractions. Begins with the complete dilation of the cervix and ends with the birth of the baby.
Stage 3 of labor	The third stage ends with the delivery of the placenta.

Nursing Interventions	**Rationales**
Explain normal newborn behaviors and needs:	This teaches parents to note the signals that babies give to indicate needs.

1. crying
  • a mechanism to communicate specific needs (hunger, desire for physical and emotional comfort)
2. reflexes
  • an indication of an intact central nervous system
3. facial expressions that mirror and engage parent
4. quiet alert state
  • baby is subdued, eyes are open and infant is prepared to take in stimuli from environment/parent
5. yawning, turning away from or closing eyes
  • indicate a state of overload and is a clue that infant needs a decrease in stimulation	

Suggest that patient find infants and mothers to observe. Recommend that she volunteer to care for infants during last months of pregnancy.	This will promote confidence and provide opportunities for gaining new skills.

▼

NURSING DIAGNOSIS: ALTERED SEXUALITY PATTERNS

Related To
• Discomforts associated with late pregnancy
• Decreased libido
• Restrictions due to high-risk status

Defining Characteristic
Reported difficulties, limitations, or changes in sexual activities

Patient Outcomes
Patient will
• engage in satisfying level of sexual activity to personal comfort level.

- find a mechanism for expressing/experiencing love, comfort, and physical intimacy with partner.

Nursing Interventions	Rationales
Assess the degree to which patient is comfortable discussing sexual activities.	The patient may perceive these matters to be highly personal in nature and inappropriate to discuss. However, she may still require information about sexual changes associated with late pregnancy.
Encourage patient and partner to discuss: 1. effect altered sexual response has had on them personally 2. alternatives to intercourse that would be mutually acceptable	
If medical restrictions have been placed upon a couple's sexual activity, be certain that couple clearly understands the rationale for these recommendations.	Understanding promotes acceptance and compliance.
Acknowledge that couples may experience a decrease in libido during the third trimester despite need for affection and love.	Men may be fearful of hurting their partner or the baby while women may feel discomfort during intercourse from the gravid uterus, inability to tolerate certain familiar positions, and decrease in sexual drive.

▼

NURSING DIAGNOSIS: DISCOMFORT/PAIN

Related To advanced pregnancy

Defining Characteristics
Will vary from client-to-client. Can include:
Constipation
Fatigue
Swelling of feet and hands
Varicose veins
Frequent urination
Insomnia

Patient Outcomes

Patient will

- verbalize relief of discomfort, or ability to tolerate.
- appear relaxed and comfortable.

Nursing Interventions	Rationales
Instruct patient on preventive/self-directed remedies for last trimester discomforts:	
1. avoidance of constipation. Recommend: • increase in vegetable and fruit consumption in diet • ingest whole grain breads • drink plenty of fluids • maintain a regular program of exercise	Constipation is caused by gastric motility changes resulting from hormone changes and crowding of intestines.
2. fatigue. Recommend: • rest at intervals in response to fatigue • curtailing activities during late part of day when fatigue is greatest • rest periods while performing strenuous activities • modification of workload to respect reduced tolerance	Fatigue is often related to sleepless nights or interrupted sleep, weight gain, difficulty breathing related to inadequate pulmonary inflation.
3. swelling of hands or feet and varicose veins. Recommend: • elevating extremities at intervals throughout day, especially if extremities are in dependent position • wearing support hose.	Edema is related to poor venous return.
4. frequent urination. • stress importance of adequate fluid intake • recommend regular emptying of bladder • limit fluids at night.	Frequent urination may be related to decreased bladder capacity due to crowding or pressure from the fetus.

Nursing Interventions	Rationales
5. insomnia. Recommend: • sleep when the baby sleeps • develop strategies to relax prior to bedtime or upon wakening to maximize ability to get to or return to sleep • limit fluid before bedtime	May be related to fetal movement becoming apparent while mother is at rest; disturbance by dreams and anxiety; frequent trips to bathroom to void.

▼

DISCHARGE PLANNING/CONTINUITY OF CARE

- Provide information on educational programs related to childbirth/parenting.
- Provide written materials for patient to read at her leisure.
- Provide book and video lists.

REFERENCES

Bonovich, L. (1990). Recognizing the onset of labor. *Journal of Obstetrical, Gynecologic, and Neonatal Nursing, 19*(2), 141–145.

Imle, M. A. (1990). Third trimester concerns of expectant parents in transition to parenthood. *Holistic Nursing Practice, 4*(3), 25–36.

Mackey, M. C. (1990). Women's preparation for the childbirth experience. *American Journal of Maternal-Child Nursing, 19*(2), 143–173.

McClanahan, P. (1992). Improving access to and use of prenatal care. *Journal of Obstetrical, Gynecologic, and Neonatal Nursing, 21*(4), 280–284.

Sherwin, L. N. (1990). Stress factors related to antenatal teaching during high-risk pregnancy. *Journal of Perinatology, 10*(2), 195–197.

▼

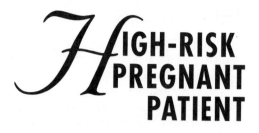

HIGH-RISK PREGNANT PATIENT

Deborah Schy RNC, MSN

A pregnancy is considered high-risk when either the mother or fetus is at increased risk of morbidity or mortality compared to the general population. Determination of risk status may occur at any time during the pregnancy—before conception or during the antepartum, intrapartum, or postpartum period.

ETIOLOGIES

- *Medical factors*
  - Hypertension
  - Autoimmune disease
  - Systemic lupus erythematosus
  - Neurological conditions
  - Cardiac problems
  - Diabetes mellitus
  - Renal disease
  - Pulmonary disease
  - Hemoglobinopathies
  - Endocrine disorders
  - Eating disorders
  - Metabolic disease
  - Gastrointestinal disease
  - Emotional disorders
  - Mental retardation
  - Malignancies
  - Infectious disease
  - Major congenital anomalies of the reproductive tract
- *Obstetrical factors*
  - late or no prenatal care
  - Rh sensitization

- inappropriate fetal size (small for gestational age or large for gestational age)
- premature labor
- pregnancy-induced hypertension
- multiple gestation
- polyhydramnios
- premature rupture of the membranes
- antepartum bleeding (previa or abruptio)
- abnormal presentation
- postmaturity
- abnormality in fetal well-being assessments
- maternal anemia
- ectopic or multiple spontaneous abortions
- grand multiparity
- stillborn or neonatal death
- uterine/cervical anomalies
- previous multiple gestation
- previous premature labor/delivery
- previous prolonged labor
- previous classical cesarean
- previous low birth weight
- previous macrosomia infant
- previous midforceps delivery
- previous baby with neurological deficit
- birth injury or malformation
- previous hydatidiform mole
- choriocarcinoma
- *Socioeconomic/demographic factors*
  - Inadequate finances
  - Poor housing
  - Severe social problems
  - Unwed or no social support
  - Minority
  - Nutrition deprivation
  - Parental occupation
  - Maternal age <16 or >35 years
  - Overweight or underweight prior to pregnancy
  - Height <5 feet
  - Maternal education <11 years
  - Smoking during pregnancy
  - Regular alcohol intake including binging
  - Drug use/abuse
- *Family History*
  - Severe inherited disorders
  - Medical complications

CLINICAL MANIFESTATIONS

Maternal findings related to Etiologies.

▼

NURSING DIAGNOSIS: KNOWLEDGE DEFICIT

Related To unfamiliarity with testing procedures

Defining Characteristics
Noncompliance
Many questions
Need for additional information
Inappropriate behavior related to information given

Patient Outcomes
Patient will
- verbalize an understanding of testing procedures and the results obtained.
- be compliant with recommendations regarding self-care as well as medical care.

Nursing Interventions	Rationales
Assess knowledge of possible testing to be performed: 1. fetal movement counting 2. nonstress testing 3. oxytocin challenge testing 4. ultrasound 5. Doppler flow studies 6. biophysical profile 7. amniocentesis 8. biochemical assessment	Depending on the condition, all or some of these tests will be used.
Explain subsequent interventions to be implemented when results indicate further actions.	
Clarify what information each test can and cannot provide.	Not all tests give the same information. Patients need to understand limitations and need for multiple tests.
Clarify that different tests are helpful at different points during pregnancy.	Testing at inappropriate times may lead to erroneous results.

Nursing Interventions	Rationales
Caution the patient not to make assumptions based on one piece of information (e.g., a normal amniocentesis means no genetic abnormalities are present, not that the baby is perfect).	
Clarify words like reactive, positive, negative, which can have multiple connotations to medical staff versus lay person (e.g., a nonstress test that is reactive is good; a negative oxytocin challenge test is also good).	
Provide information about special testing; include special points of interest: **Nonstress Test** 1. indications: <ul><li>chronic hypertension/pregnancy-induced hypertension</li><li>chronic renal disease</li><li>diabetes mellitus (insulin-requiring)</li><li>cyanotic congenital heart disease</li><li>Rh or other isommune disorders</li><li>homozygous twins</li><li>hemoglobinopathies</li><li>maternal use of alcohol/cigarettes/drugs</li><li>previous unexplained stillborn</li><li>fetal growth retardation</li><li>postdatism</li><li>hydramnios/oligohydramnios</li><li>decreased fetal movement</li><li>multiple gestation</li><li>premature rupture of membranes</li><li>third trimester bleeding</li><li>arrhythmia</li><li>maternal collagen vascular disease</li></ul>	

Nursing Interventions	Rationales

2. results:
  • fetal heart rate response to fetal activity
  • reactive: meets protocol of two fetal heart rate accelerations of 15 beats per minute × 15 seconds in a 20-minute window
  • nonreactive: less than two fetal heart rate accelerations meeting criteria within a 40-minute time period; no fetal heart rate accelerations in 40 minutes of testing
  • unsatisfactory: tracing of poor quality or noninterpretable
3. special points of interest:
  • may begin testing as early as 26 weeks, although many normal fetuses will not be reactive until later; most physicians begin testing between 28 and 32 weeks gestation
  • a nonreactive test may be followed up with another form of antepartum testing
  • the nonstress test is predictive for 3–4 days without any change in condition of mother or baby
  • protocols throughout the United States vary as to length of time and number of accelerations.
Oxytocin Challenge Test (OCT)
1. assesses uteroplacental function and requires the use of electronic-fetal monitor and intravenous pitocin or nipple stimulation
2. indications:
  • same as nonstress test
  • any condition indicating uteroplacental insufficiency
  • nonreactive nonstress test	

Nursing Interventions	**Rationales**
3. contraindications: • preterm labor • bleeding • preterm premature rupture of membranes (PPROM) 4. results: • three contractions in 10-minute period obtained either with pitocin or nipple stimulation • negative: no fetal heart rate decelerations noted. • equivocal: some fetal heart rate decelerations noted with uterine contractions but not consistent; retest within 24 hours • positive: late fetal heart rate decelerations noted with uterine contractions • hyperstimulation: too many uterine contractions; discontinue test; give oxygen; wait at least 30 minutes and repeat test • unsatisfactory: – fetal heart rate cannot be traced – no uterine contractions 5. special points of interest: • test is thought to be predictive for a 7-day period • late decelerations tend to be earlier warning sign of fetal compromise than loss of reactivity	

Nursing Interventions	Rationales

Biophysical Profile (BPP)
1. Indications:
  • suspect uteroplacental insufficiency
  • multiple gestation
  • contraindication of oxytocin challenge test
2. results:
  • test is based on 5 areas: non-stress test, fetal movements, fetal breathing movements, fetal tone, amniotic fluid volume
  • maximum of 10 points achievable
  • ultrasound must be used
  • test takes ~60 minutes to complete
  • scores of <6 are suspect for chronic hypoxia	

Nursing Interventions

Discuss pregnancy's effect on medical problems and the effect of medical problems on pregnancy. Instruct patient of warning signs in pregnancy:

1. bleeding from the vagina
2. severe nausea or vomiting
3. pain or burning when urinating
4. fever and chills
5. gush or trickle of water from the vagina
6. no activity of the baby for 12 hours
7. severe pain in the abdomen
8. signs of pregnancy-induced hypertension:
   - severe persistent headache
   - sudden swelling of face, hands, feet or ankles
   - sudden, unexplained weight gain
   - blurred vision or spots before the eyes
9. signs of premature labor:
   - contractions that occur every 10 minutes or more frequently
   - menstrual like cramps in the lower abdomen, which may come and go or be constant
   - dull backache felt below the waistline; may come and go or be constant
   - pressure in the pelvis
   - abdominal cramping with or without diarrhea
   - spotting or bleeding from the vagina
   - watery discharge from the vagina

Encourage the use of fetal movement counting by the patient.

Rationales

Problems may signal danger, will vary depending on the patient's medical condition. For example, uterine contractions may be dangerous for the client with a previous classical cesarean delivery; difficulty in breathing may be normal in the third trimester for the normal pregnant women, but for the client with a cardiac condition this may signal heart failure.

This is an ongoing assessment that indicates how the fetus is doing.

Nursing Interventions	Rationales
Instruct patient to: 1. Lie quietly on her left side approximately half an hour after eating. 2. Record each time she feels the baby kick during 1 hour. 3. Notify her physician if less than 3 movements are felt during 1 hour. 4. Stop counting if more than 10 movements are felt during 1 hour. 5. Count 3 times per day.	
Encourage the patient and support person to take a high-risk pregnancy class.	Many women experiencing high-risk pregnancies feel isolated and different. These classes can help patients to feel as though they are not alone.
Encourage the patient to keep all test appointments.	

▼

NURSING DIAGNOSIS: ANXIETY

Related To
- High-risk pregnancy
- Threat of death to self or fetus

Defining Characteristics
Fear of unspecific consequences
Worried
Anxious
Symptoms related to catecholamine release, including fetal arrhythmia, increased heart rate, insomnia, nervous habits

Patient Outcomes
Patient will
- express fears about pregnancy.
- demonstrate appropriate coping strategies for the situation.

Nursing Interventions	Rationales
Assess for physiological characteristics of anxiety/stress.	
Question patient concerning stress and the pregnancy.	
Provide access to health care that will help to alleviate anxiety.	Knowing that health care professionals are available 24 hours per day may help to alleviate stress/anxiety as questions or problems can be addressed as they arise.
Encourage the patient to verbalize fears, frustrations, anger, or other feelings regarding the pregnancy. Assist the patient in assessing the situation realistically.	
Reinforce positive aspects of pregnancy.	This helps to increase confidence and focus on some of the "good" aspects of the pregnancy.
Instruct in methods to reduce anxious feelings: 1. relaxation techniques. 2. reducing sensory stimuli. 3. distraction/visualization.	

▼

NURSING DIAGNOSIS: ALTERED ROLE PERFORMANCE

Related To high-risk pregnancy and possible physical limitations

Defining Characteristics
Changes in self-perception of role
Expresses feelings of abnormalcy, low self-worth
Changes in physical capacity to continue/resume role
Change in usual patterns of responsibility
Investment in pregnancy appears limited
Fails to demonstrate appropriate psychological adaptation to pregnancy

Patient Outcomes
The patient will progress through the physical and emotional stages of pregnancy while undergoing a high-risk pregnancy.

Nursing Interventions	Rationales
Evaluate patient's perceptions of pregnancy.	This will help her integrate the fact that she is pregnant as well as having other medical problems.
Identify patient's fantasies about what the pregnant woman's role is and how she is or is not meeting it.	Some women need to be able to carry on regular roles as wife and mother; to have pregnancy noticed and acknowledged by others; to be seen in public in maternity clothes; to participate in baby showers and plans for baby. However, being in a high-risk pregnancy may mean bed rest and confinement that conflicts with this.
Discuss the normal changes of pregnancy as well as the high-risk changes the patient can expect.	
Observe interaction with other pregnant clients.	
Encourage the client and her support person to attend childbirth classes (either high-risk or traditional.)	These classes will help the client to focus on some of the roles and tasks of pregnancy. She will also come into contact with other pregnant women and can share information.
Assess feelings at various points in pregnancy.	

▼

NURSING DIAGNOSIS: DIVERSIONAL ACTIVITY DEFICIT

Related To
- Bed rest
- Activity restrictions

Defining Characteristics
Complaints of boredom
Feelings of apathy
Usual hobbies cannot be undertaken

Patient Outcomes

The patient will participate in diversional activities that will help her cope with bed rest and restricted activities.

Nursing Interventions	Rationales
Assess how the patient is coping with bed rest and/or restricted activity.	
Determine which activities previously/presently is participating in.	
Identify changes in activity tolerance.	
Provide positive feedback for complying with limited activity.	Patient may feel guilty about being inactive. This will help her to feel good about the role she is playing in supporting the pregnancy.
If bed rest is required, encourage active/passive range of motion exercises.	This will help to prevent muscle wasting and speed up the recuperation period.
When the patient must be active (e.g., clinic appointments), encourage her to pace activities and allow for sufficient rest periods.	
Suggest diversional activities that are appropriate for those on restricted activity. Some suggestions include: 1. recopying books 2. putting together photo albums 3. crafts 4. telephone research 5. letter writing 6. writing a diary to the baby about the pregnancy	This can be a time to do those activities patient never had time for. It is also a way to do special tasks for others who may be helping out, like family and neighbors.

▼

NURSING DIAGNOSIS: POWERLESSNESS

Related To

- Illness-related regimen
- Dependence on others; necessity to relinquish control to others
- Inability to control pregnancy outcome

Defining Characteristics
Verbal expressions of having little or no control over situation or outcome
Apathy
Depression

Patient Outcomes
The patient will become an integral part in participating with her own treatment regimen, as evidenced by compliance with prescribed treatments.

Nursing Interventions	Rationales
Assess patient's perceptions of/attitude toward pregnancy and required medical treatment.	
Evaluate patient's compliance with treatment regime. Assess ability to be active participant in self-care.	When individuals participate in their own care they tend to feel more in control and follow through with recommendations.
At each outpatient visit, ask patient specific questions about herself, the family and the pregnancy.	
Give the patient options that are safe for both herself and her baby, e.g., do you want your test in the morning or afternoon?	This will help the patient feel a part of the planning, even though her options may be limited.
Provide positive feedback for all the positive contributions she has made since last visit.	This will acknowledge compliance and the difficulties of a high-risk pregnancy.

▼

DISCHARGE PLANNING/CONTINUITY OF CARE

- Refer patient to services that may help the family during this stressful time. Services may include, but are not limited to
  - social workers
  - visiting nurses
  - religious support
  - financial assistance
  - child care support
  - dietitian
- Provide information about a support network. This might include telephone support or group support.
- Refer to support groups as appropriate. Groups such as High-Risk

Moms, Parent Care, American Diabetes Association, and Spina Bifida Association can provide support and accurate information about the specific problem the patient has.

REFERENCES

Dineen, K., Rossi, M., Lia-Hoagberg, B., & Keller, L. O. (1992). Antepartum home-care services for high-risk women. *Journal of Obstetrical, Gynecologic, and Neonatal Nursing, 21*(2), 121–125.

Harvey, M. (1992). Humanizing the intensive care unit experience. *NAACOG's Clinical Issues in Perinatal and Women's Health Nursing, 3*(3), 369–376.

Heaman, M. (1990). Psychological aspects of antepartum hospitalization. *NAACOG's Clinical Issues in Perinatal and Women's Health Nursing, 1*(3), 333–341.

▼

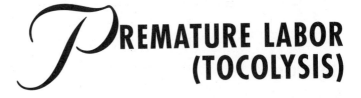

$\mathscr{P}$REMATURE LABOR (TOCOLYSIS)

Denise Talley-Lacy, RN, MSN
Mary Christine McCarthy, RN, BSN

Uterine contractions causing progressive cervical dilation and effacement that occur after the 20th week and before the 36th week of gestation. About 5 to 10 percent of all labors are premature and is referred to as premature labor, and cause 70% of all perinatal morbidity and mortality.

ETIOLOGIES

- Multiple gestations
- Polyhydramnios
- Premature rupture of membranes
- Third trimester bleeding
- Pregnancy-induced hypertension
- Premature dilation of cervical os
- Vaginal infections
- Recurrent urinary tract infections
- Poor nutritional state
- Renal disease
- Age younger than 18 years or older than 40 years

CLINICAL MANIFESTATIONS

- Regular uterine contractions with or without pain
- Dull, low backache, pressure, or pain
- Intermittent lower abdominal or thigh pain
- Intestinal cramping with or without diarrhea or indigestion
- Change in vaginal discharge

CLINICAL/DIAGNOSTIC FINDING

Vaginal secretions may be nitrizine- or fern-positive.

▼

NURSING DIAGNOSIS: KNOWLEDGE DEFICIT

Related To unfamiliarity with premature labor, hospital environment, nursing procedures

Defining Characteristics

Expressed need for information
Confusion about early hospitalization
Restlessness/agitation
Apprehension
Selective inattention

Patient Outcomes

Patient will verbalize understanding of the causes and treatment of premature labor.

Nursing Interventions	Rationales
Assess knowledge of premature labor.	
Provide information on conditions that predispose women to premature labor (see Etiologies).	
Explain need for hospitalization for each bout of preterm labor; give rationale for close observation. Explain that intensive observations and management can help conduct of remaining pregnancy and fetal outcome.	Some women believe that small/premature baby is easier to deliver. Better survival rates for premature infants have led women to believe that premature labor symptoms can be ignored, particularly if a woman is tired of pregnancy.
Instruct patient on how to recognize premature labor activity and to report symptoms immediately.	Mother may be more accurate than electronic monitor in detecting contractions. However, signs of preterm labor may be silent.

Nursing Interventions	Rationales
Symptoms may include: 1. painless uterine contractions, which sometimes feels like the baby is "balling up" 2. backache 3. menstrual cramps 4. pelvic pressure 5. diarrhea, stomach cramps 6. watery vaginal discharge 7. premature rupture of membranes	
Arrange a tour of the special care nursery when possible.	Parents gain reassurance from knowledge of technology and staff available to support premature infant, if necessary.
Provide information about fetal growth and development for gestational age of fetus.	Allows parents to begin to deal realistically with potential outcome for baby if it becomes impossible to stop labor.
Discuss common medications used to treat premature labor: 1. magnesium sulfate (in hospital only) 2. ritodrine (in hospital only) 3. terbutaline (hospital or home).	Selection of drug is dependent on progression of the preterm labor as well as physician preference. Whether the patient is managed/treated in the hospital or at home with monitoring is controversial at this time.
Advise patient to notify staff if experiencing difficulty breathing, palpitations, or chest pain.	Magnesium sulfate is usually well tolerated at therapeutic levels. Terbutaline and ritodrine at therapeutic levels cause jitteriness and tremors secondary to sympathomimetic effects and are to be expected. However, more severe side effects such as chest pain, shortness of breath, and palpitations must be reported.
Discuss other interventions used in the treatment of preterm labor: 1. bed rest 2. decreased strenuous activity	Restricted activity decreases stimulation of muscle activity.

Nursing Interventions	**Rationales**
3. decreased work hours or decreased activity on the job	
4. increase fluid intake.	Fluid loading increases perfusion to uterus.
Begin discharge teaching: 1. Reinforce patient's knowledge on how to recognize preterm contractions. 2. Instruct patient that if she experiences symptoms she should: • assume left lateral position until contractions subside.	
• drink 4–5 cups of water.	Fluids cause increased uterine blood flow and decreased myometrial activity.

• empty bladder.
  • continue to observe for contraction symptoms.
  • call physician if symptoms persist for >1 hour.	

• call physician immediately if membranes rupture or bleeding is noted.	As the cervix begins to open, small capillaries may break and result in a bloody show.
3. Remind patient to discontinue sexual activity that leads to orgasm.	Orgasm increases uterine contractions.
4. Instruct patient to refrain from breast stimulation (as in nipple massage), sometimes used to prepare breasts for breast feeding.	Stimulation can result in endogenous oxytoxin release, which can precipitate uterine contractions.
5. Encourage patient to reduce physical and employment activities which seem to precipitate bouts of premature labor.	

▼

NURSING DIAGNOSIS: HIGH RISK FOR INJURY TO FETUS

Risk Factor
Preterm labor

Patient Outcomes
Mother will participate in treatment regimen aimed at recognizing and halting preterm labor, as evidenced by
- maintaining restricted activity.
- taking prescribed medications.
- notifying staff of contraction activity.

Nursing Interventions

Assess for possible causes of preterm labor:
1. Dehydration
   - Assess fluid intake.
   - Administer intravenous fluid infusion as ordered (usually 1 liter of solution over 30 to 45 minutes).
   - Assess patient after first liter is infused. If contractions are spaced out, give second liter over a 2-hour period.
   - If contractions and cervical dilation stops, give a third liter over a 6-hour period.
   - If contractions persist or cervical dilation progresses, stop hydration therapy, and anticipate administration of tocolytic agents.

2. Urinary tract infection
   - Assess for urinary burning, frequency/urgency.
   - Obtain clean-catch urine specimen.

Rationales

Rapid fluid loading causes increased uterine blood flow and decreased myometrial activity. Use of fluid loading as a treatment for preterm labor has been recommended for:
- effectiveness
- risk of fluid over-load

Both symptomatic and asymptomatic bacteremia are associated with preterm labor.

Nursing Interventions	Rationales
3. Vaginal infection • Assess for infections, including chlamydia, gonorrhea, and beta-streptococcus. • Administer antibiotics as ordered.	These infections are associated with preterm labor.
Assess for contractions, which may be experienced as low back pain, flank pain, or "pressure in the vagina."	The risk to the fetus is not related to the contractions per se, but rather to the preterm labor.
If contracting, encourage patient to maintain left lateral recumbent position.	This allows optimal blood flow to the uterus.
Administer tocolytic agents per protocol:	Tocolytic protocols and medication preparations/concentrations may vary across institutions.
1. terbutaline • Administer subcutaneously (0.25 mg) every 20–30 minutes, up to 6 doses. If contractions fail to stop, begin intravenous administration. • Suggested intravenous solution: 10 mg per 100 ml fluid. Using infusion pump, begin dosing at 10 µg/min (or 6 ml/hr). Titrate flow rates per protocol until contractions cease, maximum dose is delivered, or if pulse rate exceeds 120 beats per minute or blood pressure is <90/60. • Wean dosage per protocol. Note: Terbutaline can be given by mouth to maintain tocolysis, but the doses are variable.	Terbutaline is a receptor agonist that exerts preferential effect on the β_2-adrenergic receptors of uterine smooth muscle; relaxes uterine muscle and vessel walls.

Nursing Interventions	**Rationales**
2. ritodrine hydrocholoride	Ritodrine is a β_2-adrenergic agonist that has a preferential affinity for β_2-receptors, which inhibit uterine contractions.

- Suggested solution: 150 mg/500 ml of fluids administered intravenously. Using infusion pump, begin dosing at 50 μg/min (or 10 ml/hr). Titrate flow rates per protocol until contractions cease, maximum dose is delivered (0.35 mg/min), or if pulse rate exceeds 120 beats per minute or blood pressure is <90/60.
- Wean dosage per protocol.
- After cessation of labor, administer 20 mg of oral ritodrine, and follow with 10 mg every 2 hours.
- Discontinue intravenously administered ritodrine 1/2 hour after first oral dose.

Note: For patients receiving ritodrine or terbutaline, obtain baseline blood glucose and electrolyte levels before initiating tocolytic treatment, and monitor regularly throughout treatment.

Nursing Interventions	Rationales

3. magnesium sulfate
  • Suggested solution: 4–6 g in 100 ml fluids. Administer intravenously as a loading dose over a 15 to 20 minute period.
  • Following the loading dose, prepare 40 g MgSO₄ in 1000-ml fluids. Using infusion pump, administer 2–3 g/hr.
  • Titrate dose against contractions, respiratory rate, magnesium levels, and deep tendon reflexes.
  • Draw baseline and serial magnesium levels.
  • Discontinue administration if respiratory rate falls below 12, deep-tendon reflexes become absent, and serum values exceed 10–12 g/hr.
	Magnesium sulfate suppresses the contractile response at the target organ, the myometrial cell, by antagonizing the flow of calcium. This decreases the frequency of muscle cell action potential, uncouples the excitation and contraction of smooth muscle, and relaxes the contractile elements.

• Keep calcium gluconate 10% at bedside.	Calcium gluconate is an antidote for magnesium sulfate overdose.
If contractions are not halted, prepare for the delivery of a premature infant. Take measures to prevent a precipitous delivery.	Prompt action may prevent birth trauma.

▼

NURSING DIAGNOSIS: PAIN

Related To uterine contractions

Defining Characteristics

Grimacing

Thrashing in bed
Verbalization of pain

Patient Outcomes
Patient will verbalize reduced or more manageable pain/discomfort.

Nursing Interventions	Rationales
Assess and document: 1. length/frequency of contractions 2. location/intensity of pain	
Use nonpharmacological measures when appropriate: 1. positioning 2. muscle relaxation techniques 3. breathing modification 4. distraction techniques	These techniques may help decrease anxiety, fatigue, and uterine tension.
Encourage patient to void frequently.	Voiding prevents bladder distention; may reduce lower abdominal pressure and pressure on uterus that causes uterine irritability.
Explain that analgesic agents may mask labor contractions, consequently they may not be ordered. Analgesics may also result in neonatal respiratory depression if labor is not suppressed and infant is born.	Some analgesic agents may cross the placenta. If a premature fetus is born when drug is still in the infant's system, it may cause respiratory depression.

▼

DISCHARGE PLANNING/CONTINUITY OF CARE

- Ensure that patient can list signs/symptoms of preterm labor.
- Consider referral to home monitoring service for continued monitoring/tocolysis at home.
- Stress importance of pregnancy maintenance/preterm labor preventive program in deterring premature labor:
  - bed rest/activity limitations
  - fluid intake
  - medications
  - follow-up appointment

REFERENCES

Egonhouse, D. J. & Burnside, S. M. (1992). Nursing assessment and responsibilities in monitoring the preterm pregnancy. *Journal of Obstetrical, Gynecologic, and Neonatal Nursing, 21*(5), 355–363.

Freda, M. C. (1991). Professionally speaking—Home care for preterm birth prevention: Is nursing monitoring these interventions? *American Journal of Maternal-Child Nursing, 16*(1), 9–14.

Freda, M., Damus, K., & Merkatz, I. (1991). What do pregnant women know about preventing preterm birth? *Journal of Obstetrical, Gynecologic, and Neonatal Nursing, 20*(2), 140–145.

Lynam, L. C. & Miller, M. A. (1992). Mothers and nurses' perceptions of the needs of women experiencing preterm labor. *Journal of Obstetrical, Gynecologic, and Neonatal Nursing, 21*(2), 126–136.

Reynolds, H. D. (1991). Bacterial vaginosis and its implications in preterm labor and premature rupture of membranes: A review of the literature. *Journal of Nurse-Midwifery, 36*(5), 289–296.

Roberts, W., Morrison, J., Hamer, C. & Wiser, W. (1990). The incidence of preterm labor and specific risk factors. *Obstetrics and Gynecology, 76*(1) (Suppl.), 855–895.

Stanton, R. (1991). Comanagement of the patient on subcutaneous terbutaline pump therapy. *Journal of Nurse Midwifery, 36*(3), 204–208.

▼

PRETERM PREMATURE RUPTURE OF MEMBRANES

Reneau A. Buckner, RNC, MS

"Preterm" premature rupture of membranes (PPRMO) is defined as the rupture of the amniotic sac prior to 37 completed weeks of gestation. "Premature" rupture of membranes alone implies the rupture of membranes before the onset of labor.

ETIOLOGIES

Largely unknown. May be seen in association with vaginal infections.

CLINICAL MANIFESTATIONS

- May occur as a sudden gush or continuous leak of amniotic fluid
- The patient may also experience mild uterine cramping, backache, or abdominal pressure prior to the rupture.

CLINICAL/DIAGNOSTIC FINDINGS

- Nitrazine: positive
- Ferning: positive
- C-reactive protein may be increased in presence of infection
- L/S (lecithin/sphigomyelin ratio) and P/G (phosphatidyglycerol ratio) for fetal lung maturity (will vary depending on fetal age)

▼

NURSING DIAGNOSIS: HIGH RISK FOR INJURY TO MOTHER AND FETUS

Risk Factor
Rupture of amniotic sac

Patient Outcome

Risk of injury is reduced through early assessment and intervention.

Nursing Interventions	Rationales
Assess for presence and characteristics of leaking amniotic fluid. Notify physician of suspected rupture of membranes.	
Instruct mother to wear perineal pad; change frequently.	Pads can help nurse assess characteristics of amniotic fluids. However, they may create environment for nurturing bacteria; they should be changed every 1–2 hours.
Assist with speculum examination. Observe for cervical dilation/effacement.	Examination allows direct visualization of vaginal canal, posterior vaginal pool and cervix which aids in the diagnosis of preterm premature rupture of membranes (PPROM). Cervical dilation resulting from labor may be apparent when the cervix is visualized.
Limit vaginal/speculum examinations.	Frequency increases risk of infection.
Assess last menstrual period, fundal height, obstetrical ultrasound.	This will pinpoint the gestational age of the fetus with as much precision as possible.
Assess fetus for accurate gestational age and estimated fetal weight.	It is important to have an accurate evaluation of gestational age and weight to clarify plans for management of PPROM and interventions should birth occur. Possible fetal injury may include deformities of the extremities from amniotic bands, craniofacial defects, and hypoplastic lungs if rupture occurs at <28 weeks gestation.

Nursing Interventions	Rationales
If membranes rupture on antepartum unit: 1. Note and record date and time of rupture. 2. Note characteristics of amniotic fluid. 3. Immediately take fetal heart tone.	
Observe mother for contractions, excessive abdominal pain, vaginal bleeding, prolapsed cord, or prolapse of presenting part of fetus.	Patient needs ongoing assessment to rule out labor, infection, or fetal compromise. If preterm fetus is delivered, the neonate is at risk for complications related to prematurity, such as respiratory distress syndrome (RDS).
Assist with transfer to labor rooms, if necessary.	Patient should be transferred to the Labor and Delivery room for intensive observation should signs and symptoms of labor or infection occur. Mother may need to be transferred to a tertiary care facility to optimize maternal-fetal outcome.

▼

NURSING DIAGNOSIS: HIGH RISK FOR PERINATAL INFECTION

Risk Factors
- Invasion by Group B beta-*Streptococcus*
- Chlamydia
- *Haemophilis influenzae*
- Chorioamnionitis

Patient Outcomes
- Mother will be afebrile.
- Fetus will not demonstrate signs of infection.
- If infection occurs, it will be treated early and effectively.

Nursing Interventions	Rationales
Observe mother for signs of infection: 1. fever/chills 2. tachycardia 3. uterine tenderness/irritation/ contractions 4. purulent cervical drainage 5. malodorous vaginal discharge	
Monitor results of complete blood count/differential, C-reactive protein, and endocervical cultures.	
Monitor fetal heart tones.	Mild tachycardia (161–180 beats per minute) to marked tachycardia (>180 beats per minute) have been associated with PPROM.
Instruct mother to observe decreases in fetal movement; notify staff of changes.	Ascending infections may result in chorioamnionitis and maternal/fetal sepsis. If intrauterine infection presents, fetus must be delivered regardless of gestational age.
Encourage increased oral fluid intake.	
Administer antibiotics, tocolytics, or steroids as ordered.	The use of tocolytics and antibiotics following PPROM remains controversial. The benefits of prophylactic antibiotics in the absence of proven infection have not been well documented. Tocolytics should not be used in the presence of chorioamnionitis, but they have been used to prolong delivery for up to 48 hours, during which time steroids may be given to accelerate fetal lung maturity.

▼

NURSING DIAGNOSIS: HIGH RISK FOR DIVERSIONAL ACTIVITY DEFICIT

Risk Factors

Medical restrictions on activity

Patient Outcomes
Patient will
- follow physical activity limitations.
- participate in diversional activities that help her cope with restricted activity.

Nursing Interventions	Rationales
Assess mother's ability to comply with activity limitations.	Patient may be placed on complete bed rest or bed rest with bathroom privileges according to diagnosis and condition. Activity can increase uterine activity and can cause active labor.
Provide positive feedback to patient for complying with limited activity.	This helps patient to feel good about the role she is playing in supporting the pregnancy.
Provide comfort measures for mother on bed rest: 1. egg crate mattress 2. back massage 3. pillows 4. change in position	Comfort may facilitate compliance with restrictions and interest in diversional activity.
Assist mother to identify meaningful activities.	This can be a time to do those activities she never had time for.
Assist patient/family to adapt environment to accommodate desired activity.	
Consult the occupational therapy department.	

▼

NURSING DIAGNOSIS: HIGH RISK FOR FEAR

Risk Factors
- Coping with "high-risk" pregnancy
- Potential for long-term hospitalization
- Potential for preterm infant with complications

Patient Outcomes
Patient will verbalize fears and concerns related to pregnancy outcome and infant's condition.

Nursing Interventions	Rationales
Assess mother's ability to cope with management and prognosis of pregnancy.	
Encourage mother/family to express fears about outcome.	Fear of unknown and misconceptions can increase anxiety.
Focus on positive aspects of pregnancy, but share all aspects of management as mother and family can handle information.	Realistic information provides the family with the opportunity to process their feelings about the status of the pregnancy and of the fetus.
Update mother/family with test results, changes in management strategies, etc.	Families appreciate the opportunity to actively participate in decision-making.
Encourage mother to visit special care nursery before delivery if preterm delivery anticipated.	Parents gain reassurance from knowledge about the technology available and introduction to the staff who will care for their premature infant.
Use strategies to reduce mother/father's fears.	Some fears may be unwarranted and can be reduced by providing information at the appropriate moment.

▼

NURSING DIAGNOSIS: KNOWLEDGE DEFICIT

Related To
- Unfamiliarity with PPROM, treatment and outcome
- Possible discharge if patient successfully reaches 36 weeks gestation

Defining Characteristics
Multiple questions
Expressed need for more information
Overt confusion about events

Patient Outcomes
Patient will verbalize knowledge of self-care management required in the hospital and outpatient setting.

Nursing Interventions	Rationales
Assess knowledge about self-care management during PPROM.	
Explain need to monitor for signs of infection:	
1. Take temperature four times a day.	Temperature elevation and odorous discharge may reflect infection.
2. Observe for malodorous vaginal discharge.	
3. Monitor complete blood count (CBC) and C-reactive protein as prescribed.	An elevation in white count or C-reactive protein may be noted in the presence of infection.
Instruct in techniques to reduce risk of infection:	
1. Change perineal pads frequently.	The dark, warm, moist environment is the ideal medium for bacterial growth.
2. Avoid tub baths.	Tub baths might result in ascending infections.
3. Wipe from front to back after toileting.	This precaution will prevent contamination from fecal material.
4. Avoid vaginal douching, tampons, and vaginal/rectal intercourse.	This will prevent introduction of bacteria higher into the vagina.
Instruct patient regarding activity limitations.	
Instruct patient in signs of labor.	

DISCHARGE PLANNING/CONTINUITY OF CARE

Instruct mother to notify primary health care provider/hospital of:
- Temperature elevations.
- Signs and symptoms reflecting labor.
- The presence of malodorous vaginal secretions.
- Changes in the color or character of amniotic fluid.

REFERENCES

Fortunato, S., Welt, S., Eggleston, M, Cole, J., Bryant, E., & Dodson, M. (1990). Prolongation of the latency period in preterm premature rupture of the membranes using prophylactic antibiotics and tocolysis. *Journal of Perinatology, 10*(3), 252–256.

Iams, J. D., Stilson, R., Johnson, F. F., Williams, R. A., & Rice, R. (1990). Symptoms that precede preterm labor and preterm premature rupture of the membranes. *American Journal of Obstetrics and Gynecology, 162*(2), 486–490.

Levine, C. D. (1991). Premature rupture of the membranes and sepsis in preterm neonates. *Nursing Research, 40*(1), 36–41.

▼

PROLAPSED CORD/ EMERGENCY CESAREAN SECTION

Elicita A. Chavez, RN
Cheryl A. King, RN, BSN

The umbilical cord descends past the presenting part through the dilated cervix after rupture of the membranes. The cord becomes impinged between the presenting part of the fetus and the maternal pelvis or soft parts. At no time does this place the mother at risk, but prolapsed cord constitutes a life-threatening emergency for the fetus. When complete impingement of the cord occurs, oxygen exchange and carbon dioxide disposal cannot take place between the fetal cord and maternal compartments. This plan of care also discusses the measures taken to prepare a patient for Cesarean birth. In true life-threatening emergencies, the measures to prepare the patient are accelerated to facilitate quick delivery.

ETIOLOGIES

- Artificial or spontaneous rupture of membranes with the fetus at a high station
- Polyhydramnios
- Breech presentation
- Prematurity
- Multiple gestation

CLINICAL MANIFESTATIONS

- Protrusion of cord from vagina
- Palpation of cord on vaginal examinations
- Sudden morbid and precipitous decrease in fetal heart rate with prolonged bradycardia
- Absence of fetal heart tones
- Rupture of membranes with unengaged presenting part

▼

NURSING DIAGNOSIS: HIGH RISK FOR INJURY TO FETUS

Risk Factors
- Cord compression
- Uteroplacental insufficiency

Patient Outcomes
Injury to the fetus will be reduced/prevented through early assessment and intervention.

Nursing Interventions	Rationales
Notify physician of evidence of sudden and prolonged bradycardia following suspected/certain rupture of membranes.	This may indicate cord prolapse and impingement.
Check vagina/introitus for cord. Note protrusion from vagina.	Sudden rupture of membranes may result in the rapid descent, prolapse, and impingement of the umbilical cord.
Place patient in knee-chest position with examiner's hand in vagina to elevate presenting part.	Maneuvers reduce cord compression and prevent occlusion until delivery is accomplished.
Call for assistance to prepare for emergency delivery.	
After decision on route of delivery is made: 1. Expedite delivery. 2. Prepare for immediate delivery of potentially compromised fetus.	

▼

NURSING DIAGNOSIS: KNOWLEDGE DEFICIT

Related To
- Life-threatening condition to fetus
- New/unexpected surgical procedure

Defining Characteristics
Expressed need for information
Multiple questions or lack of questions
Confusion

Patient Outcomes

Patient will verbalize
- understanding of cord prolpase.
- understanding of sequence of events in cesarean delivery.

Nursing Interventions	Rationales
Assess patient's understanding of fetal distress caused by cord prolapse.	
Provide patient/significant others with information about known/ possible causes of prolapsed cord.	Providing patient/significant other information facilitates supporting each other and focusing on baby's well-being.
Explain need for expeditious preparation for and probable delivery. Assess patient's knowledge of cesarean birth.	There may be little time to spend on explanations if fetal well-being is compromised.
Explain "normal" preoperative procedures as they are being carried out 1. obtaining informed consent for surgery and anesthesia 2. recording fetal heart rate 3. drawing blood for complete blood count (CBC), electrolytes, type and cross-match 4. obtaining urine for urinalysis 5. insertion of Foley catheter. 6. starting an intravenous infusion for emergency access 7. choosing type of anesthesia (general, spinal, or epidural) 8. maintaining NPO status 9. preparing preoperative site with an antimicrobial scrub and a shave 10. removing dentures, contact lenses, jewelry, fingernail polish. 11. administering preoperative medications, e.g., Maalox or sodium citrate.	Understanding can reduce anxiety and may increase cooperation. Patient will feel more involvement in her own care and less powerless. This will keep the bladder empty during surgery so it is not obstructing surgical field. Changes pH of stomach contents in the event regurgitation occurs, and contents are aspirated.

▼

NURSING DIAGNOSIS: ANXIETY

Related To
- Potential loss of fetus
- Increased activity by medical personnel and rapid sequence of events
- Unexpected operative procedures

Defining Characteristics
Multiple questions
Lack of cooperation
Crying
Inability to offer accurate health history
Impatience with procedures
Inability to maintain eye contact

Patient Outcomes
Patient will demonstrate reduced anxiety, as evidenced by
- calmer appearance
- cooperation with procedures

Nursing Interventions	Rationales
Assess patient's awareness and understanding of situation.	
Observe for nonverbal signs of fear/anxiety.	
Explain all actions taken.	
Repeat explanations when necessary.	Because of swiftness of events, patient may not be able to remember what was said during emergency.
Encourage patient to verbalize concerns.	Patient may be intimidated by procedures, equipment, and medical personnel
After delivery Allow patient to see and touch infant before transport to nursery.	This reassures parents of infant's well-being and promotes bonding.

Nursing Interventions	Rationales
Provide realistic information on probable neonatal outcome.	When a favorable outcome is expected, parent's concerns can be relieved; information may also help to prepare family if poor outcome is anticipated.
Provide patient/significant other with positive feedback.	Patient/significant other may adjust perceptions to include cesarean birth as acceptable alternative to vaginal birth.
Visit patient on postpartum unit to review labor/delivery events.	Sequence of events may be unclear to patient. Postpartum visit gives patient an opportunity to process the events and their feelings surrounding this birth experience.

▼

DISCHARGE PLANNING/CONTINUITY OF CARE

Instruct patient to make appointment for postoperative/postpartum checkup.

REFERENCES

Barrett, J. M. (1991). Funic reduction for the management of umbilical cord prolapse. *American Journal of Obstetrics & Gynecology, 165*(3), 654–657.

Green, M. & Pickett, S. (1993). Nursing management of umbilical cord prolapse. *Journal of Obstetric Gynecologic, and Neonatal Nursing, 22*(4), 311–315.

Miser, W. F. (1992). Outcome of infants born with nuchal cords. *Journal of Family Practice, 34*(4), 441–445.

Tighe, D. & Sweezy, S. R. (1990). The perioperative experience of Cesarean birth: Preoperative considerations and complications. *Journal of Perinatal and Neonatal Nursing, 3*(3), 14–30.

▼

$\mathcal{V}$AGINAL DELIVERY: POSTPARTUM CARE

Connie J. Campbell, RN, MSN, MJ

Nursing care in the postpartum period is wellness oriented, focusing on the physiological and psychological adaptation of the mother, infant, and family after delivery. Recognition of deviations from normal and initiation of appropriate interventions is essential in positively affecting the health of the postpartum patient and her family.

ETIOLOGIES

N/A

CLINICAL MANIFESTATIONS

N/A

▼

NURSING DIAGNOSIS: PAIN
Related To
- Involution of the uterus
- Perineal trauma
- Episiotomy
- Hemorrhoids
- Engorgement of the breasts

Defining Characteristics
Communication of the presence of pain
Guarding or protective behavior/positioning
Increase in pulse, blood pressure, and respiration
Evidence of inflammation (redness, heat, swelling)

Patient Outcomes

Patient will
- experience relief or control of pain.
- verbalize methods that provide relief of pain and effectiveness after implementation.

Nursing Interventions	Rationales
Assess location, intensity, quality, and duration of pain.	Medications will be available for cramping, episiotomy, and hemorrhoidal pain.
Assist patient to explore methods for alleviation/control of pain.	
Administer analgesics as ordered to relieve pain and document response to medication.	
Uterine involution Provide heat to abdomen.	Heat relaxes the smooth muscle of the uterus and may reduce cramping.
Perineal/rectal pain Provide ice packs (24 hours following delivery), or ice sitz bath.	This is done to decrease edema and discomfort in perineal orea.
Provide hot sitz bath after first 24 hours.	Complaints of *severe* vulvar pain (usually from her "stitches"), or severe rectal pressure, is often the first indication of the formation of hematoma. Hematomas occur as a result of injury to a blood vessel, often without noticeable trauma, and may accumulate up to 500 ml of blood rapidly.
Use anesthetic sprays, creams, or local anesthetics.	These are used to decrease episiotomy and hemorrhoidal pain or pain from perineal stretching.
Position to relieve discomfort.	

Nursing Interventions	Rationales
Breast engorgement Advise patient on how to care for lactating breasts: 1. Provide supportive bra. 2. Put infant to breast and empty breasts on a regular basis. 3. Massage breasts. Teach patient to express milk manually or with a breast pump.	These measures will encourage the establishment and enhancement of the milk supply.
Advise patient on how to care for nonlactating breasts: 1. Provide supportive bra or binder. 2. Apply ice packs to breasts. 3. Use minimal stimulation to breasts.	These measures will decrease milk supply for the mother who will not be breast feeding.

▼

NURSING DIAGNOSIS: HIGH RISK FOR FLUID VOLUME DEFICIT

Risk Factors
Blood loss

Patient Outcomes
Patient will
- progress through the stage of uterine involution without incident.
- maintain normal fluid volume as evidenced by stable vital signs and a hematocrit of >30%.

Nursing Interventions	**Rationales**
Assess and document fundal height, position, and tone every 15 minutes for 1 hour, once an hour for 2 hours, and then every 4 hours for 24 hours. Afterwards, assess every shift until discharge.	Immediately following the expulsion of the placenta, the uterus should contract firmly to the approximate size of a large grapefruit. During the first few hours after birth, the fundus of the uterus decreases to the level of the umbilicus. A fundus that is above the level of the umbilicus or boggy is associated with excessive uterine bleeding or the passing of clots. The uterus remains at the level of the umbilicus for a day following delivery. The rate of uterine involution then is 1 fingerbreadth per day beginning 24 hours after delivery.
Massage fundus and express clots if the uterus is not firm. Explain massage to patient and encourage her to assess and massage her own fundus.	Patient is better able to provide continuous massage to her own uterus.
Assess amount/type of vaginal bleeding.	Postdelivery uterine discharge is initially bright red, changing to a dark red or reddish brown (lochia rubia). After 3–4 days the flow pales, becoming pinkish or brownish (lochia serosa). At approximately 10 days after delivery, the drainage becomes yellowish to whitish (lochia alba). Persistence of lochia rubia early in the postpartum period suggests problems with uterine involution. If the bloody discharge spurts or continues to seep into the vagina, cervical or vaginal tears may be present in addition to the normal lochia.

Nursing Interventions	Rationales
Notify physician for any excessive vaginal bleeding (more than one saturated pad per hour). Weigh peripads if necessary to determine a more accurate estimate of blood loss.	Postpartum lochia is excessive if the patient saturates more than 6–8 pads in 24 hours.
Monitor vital signs.	Hypervolemia during pregnancy allows most women to tolerate a considerable blood loss at delivery; however, patient must be assessed for signs of hypovolemia.
Monitor hemoglobin and hematocrit.	
Administer medications to maintain uterine tone as ordered by physician.	Pitocin or ergots may be ordered to enhance uterine contraction and resultant involution.

▼

NURSING DIAGNOSIS: URINARY RETENTION

Related To
- Labor and delivery
- Anesthesia
- Apprehension

Defining Characteristics
Bladder distention
Large residual urine volumes
Urinary hesitancy

Patient Outcomes
Patient will resume normal pattern of urination, as evidenced by
- output >100 ml per void
- bladder not distended

Nursing Interventions	**Rationales**
Assess bladder elimination pattern.	
Observe bladder for distention during the first 8 hours after delivery or until patient voids. Palpate bladder after voiding.	Increased bladder capacity, swelling, and bruising of the tissues around the urethra, decreased sensation of bladder filling and inability to void in the recumbent position, put the puerperal woman at risk for over distention, incomplete emptying, and buildup of residual urine. In addition, women who have had conductive anesthesia have inhibited neural functioning of the bladder and are more susceptible to bladder complications.
Stimulate spontaneous voiding by such measures as: 1. assisting patient to bathroom 2. providing privacy 3. providing the auditory stimulus of running water	
4. pouring alternate warm/cold water over the perineum.	Tactile, thermal stimulus.
5. encouraging the patient to take a sitz bath	
6. assisting patient to assume normal position for voiding	Bladder distention presents an immediate problem. Stasis increases risk of urinary tract infection.
Catheterize as ordered per physician.	Distention of the bladder promotes uterine atony. Note drifting of the fundus to the right or left of the umbilicus, rising fundal height without loss of uterine tone, or excessive vaginal bleeding.
Encourage daily fluid intake of at least 2000 ml/day.	

▼

NURSING DIAGNOSIS: HIGH RISK FOR CONSTIPATION

Risk Factors
- Labor and delivery
- Anesthesia
- Apprehension

Patient Outcomes
Patient will
- resume normal pattern of bowel elimination.
- have a bowel movement within 48–72 hours of delivery.
- verbalize absence of gas pains.

Nursing Interventions	Rationales
Assess previous bowel elimination pattern.	
Assess food/fluid intake during labor.	The practice of limiting fluids and solid food during labor causes a delay in the first bowel movement.
Assess for complaints of abdominal distention/feeling of rectal fullness.	The bowel tends to be sluggish after birth due to the lingering effects of progesterone and decreased abdominal muscle tone. In addition, the pain from the episiotomy, any lacerations, and hemorrhoids may lead the woman to delay elimination for fear of increasing pain or "tearing" her stitches open.
Encourage fluid intake and early ambulation.	
Encourage roughage in diet.	Roughage provides bulk to stimulate bowel.
Give stool softener or laxative as ordered by the physician.	
Encourage immediate response to urge to defecate and provide privacy.	

▼

NURSING DIAGNOSIS: HIGH RISK FOR INFECTION

Risk Factors

- Prolonged labor
- Hemorrhage
- Premature and/or prolonged rupture of membranes
- Soft tissue trauma
- Invasive techniques (e.g., internal fetal monitoring, frequent vaginal examinations)
- Operative procedures (e.g., forceps, vacuum extraction)
- Maternal exhaustion, malnutrition, anemia, or a debilitated condition

Patient Outcomes

Patient will
- remain free of infection, as evidenced by
  - temperatures < 38°C
  - white blood count within 15,000–30,000/mm (normal puerperal limits)
  - negative cultures
  - no foul-smelling lochia
  - clean, healing episiotomy/perineum
- verbalize risk factors associated with infection and practice appropriate preventive measures.

Nursing Interventions	Rationales
Assess for fever or chills; check temperature every 4 hours × 24 hours, then every shift if below 100.4°F (38°C).	Postpartum infections will manifest with temperature elevations.
Observe perineum every shift. Assess perineal area and episiotomy incision for heat, discoloration, approximation, swelling, pain, and drainage.	These symptoms may reflect infection.
Evaluate degree of healing using the REEDA scale (redness, edema, ecchymosis, discharge, approximation).	

Nursing Interventions

Report signs and symptoms of infection immediately:
1. uterine subinvolution
2. foul-smelling lochia
3. uterine tenderness
4. severe lower abdominal pain
5. fever
6. elevated white blood cell count
7. chills
8. malaise
9. lethargy
10. tachycardia
11. nausea and vomiting
12. abdominal rigidity

Rationales

Nursing Interventions	Rationales
Note character and amount of lochia.	
Instruct patient to perform perineal care after each void and bowel movement. Instruct her on the proper method to remove and replace peripads.	Pericare promotes removal of feces and urine contaminates from perineum. Frequent pad changes decrease media for bacterial growth.
Promote normal wound healing by encouraging: 1. sitz bath 2–4 times daily for 10–15 minutes 2. diet high in protein, vitamin C and iron 3. fluid intake to 2000 ml/day 4. early ambulation	Warm water is soothing and cleansing and promotes healing through increased vascular flow to affected area. Essential nutrients are needed for wound healing. Ambulation promotes drainage of lochia.
Obtain cultures and administer antibiotics as ordered.	
Provide comfort measures: 1. ice packs 2. heat lamp 3. anesthetic sprays or creams 4. pads soaked in witch hazel (can be refrigerated)	

NURSING DIAGNOSIS: FAMILY COPING, POTENTIAL FOR GROWTH

Related To addition of new family member

Defining Characteristics

Family members attempt to describe impact of new infant on own values, priorities, goals, and relationships

Family members move in direction of promoting and enriching family life that supports integration of new family member and choose experiences that optimize wellness

Patient Outcomes

Patient will demonstrate appropriate bonding/attachment behaviors, as evidenced by

- eye-to-eye contact in en face position (holding, cuddling, calling infant by name, talking to infant)
- describing infant characteristics to visitors
- seeking out opportunities to carry out care giving of baby

Nursing Interventions	Rationales
Provide information about infant development and characteristics.	
Observe and document relevant information about progressive parental bonding/attachment.	The process of attachment is linear, beginning during pregnancy, intensifying during postdelivery, and being constant and consistent once it is established. Attachment is critical to mental and physical health across the lifespan.
Encourage father/support person to participate in infant caregiving activities.	
Encourage rooming-in and sibling visitation.	This provides opportunities for the family to have infant contact.
Review sibling rivalry and appropriate interventions to promote sibling acceptance of the new baby.	Introduction of a new baby may pose problems for parents as they are faced with the task of caring for the new child while not neglecting the others. Parents need a learn to distribute their attention fairly to all children.
Offer support and encouragement as parents/support person relate positively to infant and engage successfully in infant care activities.	Recognition and praise of success increases the mother's feeling of competence and control in her abilities. Feelings of self esteem are increased through positive feedback.

NURSING DIAGNOSIS: HIGH RISK FOR ALTERED FAMILY PROCESSES

Risk Factors

Addition of new family member

Patient Outcomes

Parents will demonstrate good coping skills and acceptance of roles and responsibility as parents, as evidenced by

- family members express feelings freely and appropriately
- family members involved in infant caregiving
- appropriate solutions determined for situation/crises as they arise
- realistic plans for self and infant care
- no persisting postpartum depression

Nursing Interventions	Rationales
Determine knowledge level and teaching/learning needs related to infant and self-care.	
Assess role expectations of mother and family member. Determine emotional and physical support systems available.	Adequate assessment of the mother's psychological adjustment to parenting this new child is an integral part of postpartal evaluation. The birth of a child along with the role changes and increased responsibilities it produces is a time of emotional stress. Assessment should focus on mother's general attitude, feelings of competence, available support systems, and care giving skills.
Encourage verbalization of feelings related to pregnancy, labor and delivery, present condition, and the baby.	
Provide self-care and infant care based on learning needs. Include father/support person in teaching and discharge planning.	Fathers may feel inadequate to provide care. Fostering confidence and permission to care for their child will facilitate their transition to parenthood.
Discuss the potential for postpartum blues related to emotional and hormonal changes.	During the early postpartum days, mood swings and tearfulness are common as the body adjusts to the nonpregnant state. Normally occurs 3–10 days postpartum but may occur anytime during the 6 weeks postpartum period.
Schedule nursing care to correspond with infant's periods of wakefulness and encourage resting intervals throughout the day.	Fatigue reduces coping ability.

Nursing Interventions	Rationales
Encourage expression of concerns, fears, or feelings related to changes in role (e.g., working, mothering, sexuality).	

▼

DISCHARGE PLANNING/CONTINUITY OF CARE

- Provide information on signs/symptoms of infection/hemorrhage.
- Provide information on family planning as needed.
- Routine postpartum checkup.
- Routine well-baby care visit at regular intervals.

REFERENCES

Jordan, P. J. (1990). Laboring for relvance: Expectant and new fatherhood. *Nursing Research, 39*(1), 11–16.

Lowe, N. K. (1991). Maternal confidence in coping with labor: a self-efficacy concept. *Journal of Obstetrical, Gynecology, and Neonatal Nursing, 20,* 457–463.

OGN Nursing Practice Resource. (1991). *Postpartum Nursing Care: Vaginal Delivery.* Nurses' Association of the American College of Obstetricians and Gynecologists (NAACOG).

▼

Health Teaching Guides

▼

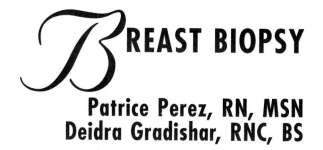

REAST BIOPSY

Patrice Perez, RN, MSN
Deidra Gradishar, RNC, BS

1. Assess patient's awareness and previous experience with breast biopsy.
2. Explain purpose: To determine whether a breast irregularity (cyst or lump) is cancerous.
3. Describe the needle biopsy procedure:
   a. Local anesthetic injected to numb skin over cyst.
   b. Tiny amounts of the abnormal lumps are aspirated through the needle for cytologic evaluation.
   c. Several samples are collected from different angles/areas of the lump.
4. Describe a surgical biopsy:
   a. Involves the removal of the complete, or portion of a lump for pathology evaluation.
   b. Local or general anesthesia may be used.
   c. The breast is scrubbed with antiseptic solution.
   d. The physician makes an incision and removes the lump.
   e. The incision is closed.
   f. Complete pathology evaluation takes 1 to 2 days, after which more aggressive surgery might be planned.
5. Explain that findings might reveal a number of conditions that are not cancerous, including mastitis, papilloma, fat necrosis or fibrocystic disease.
6. Instruct patient in care of biopsy site, including:
   a. Maintaining cleanliness.
   b. When sutures can be wet.
   c. Applying dressing.
   d. When to return for suture removal.
7. Instruct patient to self-medicate with analgesic prescribed by physician.
8. Advise patient how and when she will be made aware of pathology results.
9. Instruct on need for ongoing self-breast examination.

REFERENCES

Dow, K. H. (1991). Newer developments in the diagnosis and staging of breast cancer. *Seminars in Oncology Nursing. 7*(3), 166–174.

Haller, K. B. (1991). One out of every nine women . . . breast cancer. *Journal of Obstetric, Gynecologic, and Neonatal Nursing. 20*(6), 438.

MacFarlane, M. E. & Sony, S. D. (1992). Women, breast lump discovery, and associated stress. *Health Care for Women International. 13*(1), 23–32.

CIRCUMCISION CARE

Caroline Reich, RN, MS

---

1. Teach parents care of the circumcised penis:
   a. Keep the glans of the penis covered with a petroleum gauze dressing the first 24 hours after the procedure.
   b. Once the dressing has been removed, apply a small amount of petroleum jelly directly to the glans for several days postprocedure. (Petroleum jelly protects the fresh circumcision site from adhering to the diaper and from direct contact with urine or feces.)

   NOTE: Petroleum jelly is NOT needed in an infant who had a bell circumcision. No special dressing is required. The bell will fall off 7–10 days after the procedure.

   c. Cleanse the penis only with clear water during the first few days after the gauze is removed. (Soap may be irritating.)
   d. Wait until after the circumcision site has healed before manipulating the foreskin remnants in an attempt to prevent adhesions. Forcibly attempting to "loosen" the remnants of the foreskin can cause bleeding of the freshly circumcised penis and is unnecessarily traumatic.
2. Instruct parents to check with their health care provider to ascertain whether any additional measures are needed to prevent adhesions from developing. (This is dependent on the technique of the physician who performed the circumcision. Individual practice may vary as to how much foreskin remains postprocedure.)
3. Teach parents the characteristics of the healing process, signs and symptoms of infection, and other complications.
   a. Instruct parents that any bleeding, lack of or difficulty voiding, odor, or discharge should be reported to the physician.
   b. Instruct parents that a yellowish, adherent exudate (which is part of the granulation process) may appear on the penis and should not be removed. (This exudate is a normal part of the healing process.)
4. Teach parents comfort measures that can be employed for several days postprocedure such as:

a. Applying the diaper loosely and positioning the infant on his side. (This will prevent undue pressure against the penis and will make the infant more comfortable.)
b. Using cloth diapers instead of disposable diapers. (Some practitioners believe that cloth diapers are less irritating to the circumcision site than disposables.)

REFERENCES

Lund, M. M. (1990). Perspectives on newborn male circumcision. *Neonatal Network*. 9(3), 7–12.

Marchette, L., Main, R., Redick, E., Bagg, A., & Leatherland, J. (1991). Pain reduction interventions during neonatal circumcision. *Nursing Research*, 40(4), 241–244.

Roberts, J. A. (1990). Is routine circumcision indicated in the newborn? An affirmative view. *Journal of Family Practice*. 31(2), 185–188.

$\mathcal{C}$ONTRACEPTION METHODS

Margo Elizabeth Lewis-Brown, RN, MS

1. Determine the reason the patient is seeking information.
2. Assess patient's previous experience with contraception.
3. Obtain a complete reproductive history including:
   a. Onset of menses.
   b. Characteristic of personal menstrual cycle.
   c. Patterns of sexual activity.
4. Obtain a complete medical history; ask specifically about:
   a. High blood pressure.
   b. Clotting disorders.
   c. Allergies.
   d. Age.
5. Provide information on all available methods of contraception.

   NOTE: True informed consent mandates disclosure on all available alternatives.

FERTILITY AWARENESS METHODS

1. Fertility awareness methods may include one or more of the following techniques:
   a. Rhythm or calendar method.
   b. Basal body temperature method.
   c. Mucous/ovulation method.
   d. Symptothermal method.
2. Description: These techniques help the woman to determine probable periods of fertility. With this information she can:
   a. Plan pregnancy.
   b. Pinpoint days when pregnancy is likely and the use backup methods to ensure that pregnancy does not occur.
   c. Pinpoint days when pregnancy is not probable and unprotected sex is less likely to result in pregnancy.
3. Advantages:
   a. Accepted by religious groups that have prohibitions against other types of contraception.
   b. Teaches a woman about her own reproductive physiology.

549

    c. Safe, inexpensive, or free.

    d. Teaches couples to work together on family planning.

4. Disadvantages:

    a. Requires much information about physiological parameters.

    b. Monitored symptoms are sometimes vague or subtle.

    c. Women with irregular cycles may find the calendar and basal body temperature methods ineffective.

    d. Requires planning, partner cooperation.

    e. May diminish spontaneity.

5. Effectiveness: Since failure to implement abstinence during projected period of fertility results in potential failure, there is a broad range of effectiveness reported in the literature for each method or combination of methods used.

6. Procedures

    a. Calendar or rhythm method

        1) A woman maintains a calendar recording length of the menstrual cycles over an 8- to 12-month period.

        2) The earliest point in her cycle in which she is likely to conceive is figured by subtracting 18 days from the length of her shortest cycle.

        3) Subtracting 11 days from her longest cycle gives her the last day on which she is likely to be pregnant.

        4) These two numbers represent the beginning and end of the period of time in which she is likely to get pregnant. During this time she abstains from intercourse or uses contraception.

    b. Basal body temperature method

        1) For 3 to 4 months a woman records her body temperature upon awakening and before arising.

        2) A rise in temperature of 0.4 to 0.8°F above normal for 3 days in a row reflects the probable time of ovulation.

        3) Days safe for intercourse are from the beginning of the menstrual cycle or until the temperature has remained elevated for 3 days.

    c. Mucous method: Changes in cervical mucus are observable at the time of ovulation.

        1) Discharge becomes clear and slippery (much like the white of an uncooked egg) during ovulation.

        2) A sample of cervical mucous taken at this time of the cycle and held between the thumb and forefingers will/can be stretched into a thin strand as the fingers are drawn apart.

    d. Symptothermal method: Combination use of the basal body temperature and mucus changes.

OTHER CONTRACEPTIVE METHODS

1. Birth control pills (oral contraceptive pills):

    a. Birth control pills are a combination of synthetic hormones that act on the pituitary to block the secretion of follicle-stimulating hormone

(FSH) and luteinizing hormone (LH), thus preventing ovulation. Also, oral contraceptive pills contain progesterone, which inhibits the development of the lining of the uterus, therefore preventing implantation. In combination, these two hormones also alter the cervical mucosa and affect tubal transport.

b. Advantages:
  1) Taking the pill every day provides 24-hour protection.
  2) Easy to use.
  3) There is no need for preparation prior to intercourse.
  4) A decrease in the amount of premenstrual tension and cramping may occur.
  5) The menstrual cycle is usually more regular, shorter, and less bleeding occurs.

c. Disadvantages:
  1) Expensive.
  2) Side effects include weight gain, breakthrough bleeding, nausea and vomiting, breast tenderness, headache, facial pigmentation changes, nervousness, depression, changes in sexual function. Severe complications include stroke, deep vein thrombosis, embolism.

d. Efficacy: Instruct patient that: Theoretically, if 100 women used this form of birth control perfectly for 1 year, statistically, less than one will get pregnant. If 100 women used this method less than perfectly for 1 year, two will get pregnant. Failures are due to irregular or incorrect use.

e. Dosing schedule:
  1) The woman should take the pill the same time every day to maintain a constant blood level of estrogen and progesterone.
  2) If one pill is missed, the woman should take it as soon as she remembers.
  3) If she missed two pills, she should take both pills as soon as she remembers and use a barrier method of contraception for the remainder of that cycle.
  4) If she forgets three pills, she should contact her health care provider.

f. Problems associated with oral contraceptives:
  1) Break-through bleeding: If it occurs during the midpart of the cycle, continue to take pills and use another method of contraception while experiencing bleeding.
  2) Breast tenderness/fatigue may persist for 3 months, then usually disappears.
  3) Nausea is a short-term side effect. Some women experience relief by taking pills at night.
  4) Weight/appetite change: Some women may experience a weight gain up to 5 pounds because the pill may cause salt and water retention. Instruct the patient to reduce salt intake and reduce high-caloric foods.

    5) Mood change and minor headaches may also be noted. If they persist over 3 months, notify health care provider because an adjustment of the pill may be required. A drop in Vitamin B_6 in the blood may increase nervous tension; therefore, foods high in vitamin B_6 (poultry, grain, cereals, meat), might be beneficial.

  g. In the presence of hemoptysis, restlessness, shortness of breath, pain, Homan's sign, severe headache, dizziness, blurred vision; calf redness, tenderness, swelling, warmth, stop oral contraceptives immediately and seek medical emergency attention immediately.

2. Intrauterine device (IUD):
   a. Description: A device implanted into the uterus through the cervix that secretes progesterone, which prevents implantation of an ovum.
   b. Advantages:
      1) It does not interfere with sexual activity.
      2) It is very effective in the prevention of pregnancy.
      3) No preparation required.
   c. Disadvantages:
      1) The IUD can result in heavy menstrual flow, cramps, and headaches.
      2) Insertion and removal may be painful.
      3) May be costly.
      4) Must be replaced on a regular basis.
   d. Effectiveness: Theoretically, if 100 women use this method for 1 year fewer than two will get pregnant. However, if 100 women use this method, but not perfectly for 1 year, then four will get pregnant. Failure is usually related to undetected expulsion of the IUD.
   e. Contraindications/danger signs:
      1) IUDs are contraindicated in the presence of pregnancy or active infection.
      2) Danger signs include:
         a) Missed or late period.
         b) Severe abdominal pain.
         c) Heavy bleeding during menses, passing clots.
         d) Foul-smelling, purulent discharge.
   f. Patient information:
      1) Instruct patients to notify physician immediately if:
         a) Extreme tenderness.
         b) Heavy bleeding and/or severe cramping.
         c) Unexplained fever or chills.
         d) Severe abdominal pain, usually in the lower region.
         e) Unusual vaginal discharge.
      2) Instruct client to check for string protruding from vagina to ensure that device was not expelled.

3. Diaphragm:
   a. The diaphragm is a curved/rounded rubber dome enclosed by a flexible metal ring. When inserted into the vagina, the diaphragm covers the opening to the cervix to prevent sperm from entering. One edge

of the diaphragm fits closely under the symphysis bone, and the bottom rim rests in the posterior vagina. The diaphragm may be used with spermicidal jelly or cream which adds the additional protection of a second contraceptive method.

b. Advantages:

1) After the diaphragm is properly fitted it requires no medical intervention.
2) It is used only when needed.
3) It is inexpensive.

c. Disadvantages:

1) May affect spontaneity.
2) Can sometimes be felt by partner.
3) Requires comfort with touching oneself and some skill to insert and remove.
4) Must be fitted by health professional and replaced and fit checked at regular intervals.

d. Efficacy: Theoretically, if 100 women use this method perfectly for 1 year two will get pregnant. If used less than perfectly, 19 of 100 will get pregnant. The effectiveness will also depend on whether the diaphragm is used in combination with a spermicide. Failure is usually related to improper fitting or placement of device.

e. Contraindications:

1) Allergy to rubber.
2) Repeated urinary tract infections.
3) Abnormality of pelvic structure.

f. Patient information:

1) Teach patient about insertion:

a) Wash hands.
b) Place approximately 1 tablespoon of spermicide in the dome of the diaphragm and a small amount around the entire rim of the diaphragm.
c) When the edges of the diaphragm are squeezed it forms a wedge shape which is easily, gently inserted into the vagina.
d) When the diaphragm is released the cup spreads out and covers the cervix, which is the opening to the uterus.
e) Instruct patient that:

1) The diaphragm can be inserted up to 2 hours before intercourse.
2) Sexual intercourse should take place within 1 hour following insertion. If not, an applicator of spermicide must be inserted into the vagina.
3) The diaphragm must be left in place for 8 hours after intercourse. If intercourse is repeated within that time, an additional applicator of spermicide should be inserted into the vagina (do not remove diaphragm).
4) Tell patient that removal is easier if woman is sitting on the toilet or squatting while bearing down.

g. Inform patient that:
  1) The diaphragm must be refitted if there is a weight gain or weight loss of 10 pounds or more.
  2) The diaphragm must be refitted 6 to 8 weeks following a pregnancy.
h. Inform patient on care of diaphragm:
  1) After the diaphragm is removed it must be cleansed with warm water and mild soap and gently patted dry.
  2) Replace diaphragm properly in storage container for next use.
  3) Do not use petroleum jelly on the diaphragm because it will cause deterioration of this latex product.
  4) Annual gynecological examination is always recommended.
i. Contraindications: Allergies to spermicide or polyurethane sponge.

4. Condoms:
  a. The condom is a thin rubber device that covers the penis; it prevents sperm from entering the vagina.
  b. Advantages:
    1) Protection against sexually transmitted diseases (STDs).
    2) May be purchased over the counter.
    3) Easily portable.
    4) Inexpensive.
    5) Male participates in contraception.
  c. Disadvantages:
    1) Male may experience dissatisfaction with sensitivity.
    2) May affect spontaneity.
    3) Contraindications: allergies to latex, spermicide.
  d. Efficacy: Theoretically, fewer than one woman will get pregnant out of 100 if this barrier method is used correctly all of the time. Four out of 100 will get pregnant if used correctly most of the time.
  e. Patient information: Instruct patient that:
    1) The condom is placed on the penis before entering the vagina, leaving space at the tip to collect sperm.
    2) Before insertion of the penis into the vagina, spermicide may be inserted to increase protection against pregnancy.
    3) The penis must be protected at all times during foreplay, which includes manipulation of the genital area.
    4) Condoms must be undamaged prior to usage, applied correctly, correctly removed after intercourse, and properly disposed of.
    5) Latex has a shelf life of 2 years; after that latex will deteriorate.

5. Vaginal sponge:
  a. A disposable cup-shaped sponge, which is saturated with a spermicide. This device provides a mechanical and chemical barrier that traps, kills, and absorbs sperm.
  b. Advantages:
    1) Can be purchased over the counter without prescription.
    2) Easy to use.
    3) Provides 24-hour protection.
  c. Disadvantages:

1) Client must be comfortable touching herself and locating cervix.

2) Can be expensive.

   d. Efficacy: It is 89% to 90% effective. Failures are related to improper placement.

6. Spermicide (foam, jelly, suppository preparations):

   a. Spermicides are types of vaginal chemicals that act to kill sperm and may act as a barrier to prevent sperm from entering the cervix.

   b. Advantages:

1) No prescription necessary.

2) May be purchased over the counter.

3) Portable.

4) Inexpensive.

5) May provide some protection against sexually transmitted diseases.

   c. Disadvantages/contraindications:

1) May disrupt spontaneity.

2) Taste may be disagreeable.

3) Application must proceed each act of intercourse.

4) May be perceived as messy.

5) Woman must be comfortable with insertion procedure.

6) Contraindicated if allergies to spermicide exist.

   d. Efficacy: If 100 women use this method of birth control perfectly for 1 year, 5 to 15 will get pregnant. If 100 women use this method less than perfectly for 1 year, 15 to 30 will get pregnant. Failure is due to improper introduction of spermicide into vagina.

   e. Patient instructions:

1) Chemical barriers are designed to keep the vaginal pH near 4. Sperm thrive best with an alkaline pH of 8.5 to 9.0.

2) Foams, creams, and suppositories must be inserted into the vagina before sexual intercourse.

3) Whichever method is used, it must remain in the vagina at least 8 hours after the last intercourse. (Read the package instructions for directions on use.)

4) Can be used with condoms to increase effectiveness.

7. Norplant system:

   a. The Norplant consists of six thin capsules made of a soft, flexible material that releases a continuous dose of hormone into the body, inhibiting ovulation so that eggs will not be produced regularly, and by thickening the cervical mucus, making it difficult for the sperm to reach the egg.

   b. Advantages:

1) The Norplant system is one of the most effective methods of birth control.

2) The contraceptive effect begins within 24 hours if the capsules are placed during a period. Therefore, sexual relations may be resumed without fear of pregnancy.

3) The capsules may be placed at other times as long as patient is not pregnant.

  c. Disadvantages:
    1) Many women can expect an altered bleeding pattern to become more regular after 9 to 12 months.
    2) Very costly.
    3) Requires surgical removal of capsules if pregnancy is desired or if reinsertion is necessary.
    4) Must be replaced by a specially trained physician every 5 years.
  d. Efficacy: The average annual pregnancy rate over a 5-year period is less than 0.1%. This is an average of less than 1 pregnancy for every 1000 women using this contraceptive method.
  e. Patient information:
    1) The Norplant system should be inserted within 7 days after the onset of menstrual bleeding or immediately after an abortion.
    2) The Norplant capsules are placed under the skin on the inner surface of the upper arm through a small incision made under sterile conditions at an office visit.
    3) A local anesthetic is used to numb a small area in the upper arm, a small incision less than $\frac{1}{8}$ in. long is made, and the six capsules are placed one at a time just under the skin in a fan shape using a special instrument.
    4) The incision does not require any stitches; it is covered with a small bandage.
    5) The type of bleeding pattern one will have with the Norplant cannot be predicted.
  f. Inform patient to call health care provider immediately if any of these serious effects occur following insertion of the Norplant system: sharp chest pain, coughing of blood, shortness of breath, pain, redness, tenderness, swelling or discoloration at insertion site, fever.
  g. Instruct patient to monitor for the occurrence of any of these minor symptoms: headaches, nervousness, nausea, weight gain/appetite change, dizziness, acne/dermatitis, breast tenderness. If no improvement after 3 months, consult the health care provider.

REFERENCES

Franklin, M. (1990). Reassessment of the metabolic effects of oral contraceptives. *Journal of Nurse-Midwifery. 35*(6), 358–364.

Franklin, M. (1990). Recently approved and experimental methods of contraception. *Journal of Nurse-Midwifery. 35*(6), 365–376.

King, J. (1992). Helping patients choose an appropriate method of birth control. *American Journal of Maternal-Child Nursing. 17*(2), 91–95.

Lethbridge, D. (1991). Coitus interruptus: Considerations as a method of birth control. *Journal of Obstetric, Gynecologic, and Neonatal Nursing, 20*(1), 80–85.

$\mathcal{M}$AMMOGRAM

Patrice Perez, RN, MSN
Deidra Gradishar, RNC, BS

1. Assess patient's previous experience or awareness of mammography.
2. Explain benefits and risks:
   a. Benefits:
      1) Some cancers can be detected as long as 2 years before they are felt during self-breast examination.
      2. Cancers can be treated early once they are identified. Often, early treatment is less radical than later treatment.
   b. Risks:
      1) Not 100% effective in identifying cancers.
      2) Radiation risk is cumulative. Consequently, even though x-ray exposure is quite low, women who have had many x-rays for other diagnostic purposes might be at greater risk for side effects from x-ray exposure.
3. Explain who should be tested:
   a. Any woman who identifies an irregularity or lump.
   b. Women with strong family history of breast cancer.
   c. Every 3 years for women before the age of 40 and yearly thereafter.
4. Explain the procedure for mammogram:
   a. Each breast is firmly compressed against the x-ray plate.
   b. The technician will manipulate the patient's breast until proper positioning has been achieved.
   c. Several x-ray views of the breast are taken.
   d. Compression of the breast can be quite uncomfortable, but procedure lasts only minutes.
5. Describe measures to be taken if results are abnormal:
   a. Ultrasound examination to determine whether the mass is fluid-filled or solid. [Fluid-filled masses are rarely cancerous, but may be drained by needle aspiration.]
   b. Solid masses may require periodic reevaluation and/or immediate biopsy.
6. Instruct on need for ongoing self-breast examination.

REFERENCES

Doogan, R. A. (1991). The role of mammography in the early detection of breast cancer. *Nurse Practitioner Forum.* 2(4), 217–224.

Elsenhans, V. D. & Vivio, D. (1991). Preventing slippage: assuring follow-up of abnormal test results . . . mammograms. *Nursing Economics.* 9(5), 344–347.

Gram, I. T. & Slenker, S. E. (1992). Cancer anxiety and attitudes toward mammography among screening attenders, nonattenders, and women never invited. *American Journal of Public Health.* 82(2), 249–251.

PELVIC EXAMINATION AND THE PAPANICOLAOU TEST (PAP SMEAR)

Patrice Perez, RN, MSN
Deidra Gradishar, RNC, BS

1. Provide information on purpose of Pap test:
   a. To obtain cells from the surface of the cervix for cancer screening.
2. Discuss candidates for yearly Pap test:
   a. All sexually active women.
   b. Women with risk factors for cervical cancer:
      1) First intercourse/pregnancy before age 18.
      2) Diethylstibestrol (DES) daughter.
      3) History of sexually transmitted disease, especially human papillomvirus and herpes.
      4) Cigarette smoker.
      5) Taking oral contraceptives.
3. Describe the procedure for performing a pelvic examination/Pap test:
   a. After emptying bladder, the woman is placed in lithotomy position.
   b. Examiner performs visual inspection of vulva and perineum, observing for signs of infection, any lesions, or unusual vaginal discharge.
   c. Examiner places gloved finger in the vagina; the Bartholin glands are evaluated for swelling and the Shene glands are inspected for purulent discharge.
   d. Using the fingers, the examiner depresses the lower portion of the vaginal opening while inserting a speculum. The woman is instructed to relax her legs and breathe slowly to relax her pelvic muscles, facilitating the insertion.
   e. The speculum is opened and locked in position so the cervix and vagina can be visualized.
   f. A spatula or a tiny brush is used to obtain cells from the cervix surface. The smear is placed on a microscope slide for laboratory examination.
   g. Samples of secretions may likewise be obtained to test for chlamydia or gonorrhea.

   h. After the speculum is removed, two fingers are again placed in the vagina. The examiner places the other hand on the abdomen and compresses the vagina and the ovaries down toward the fingers in the vagina so the surface and size of the uterus and cervix can be assessed.

   i. Prepare the patient that compression of the ovaries may cause temporary discomfort.

   j. A rectal examination may be included, which involves inserting a finger into the rectum. This allows further assessment of the uterus and ovaries through the thin rectal-vaginal wall.

4. Explain the expected turn-around time and routine for obtaining test results.

REFERENCES

Clay, L. S. (1990). Midwifery assessment of the well woman: the Pap smear. *Journal of Nurse-Midwifery, 35*(6), 341–350.

Ginsberg, C. K. (1991). Exfoliative cytologic screening: The Papanicolaou test. *Journal of Obstetric, Gynecologic, and Neonatal Nursing, 20*(1), 39–46.

Harlan, L., Bernstein, A., & Kessler, L. (1991). Cervical cancer screening: Who is not screened and why? *American Journal of Public Health, 81*(7), 885–890.

$\mathcal{B}$REAST SELF-EXAMINATION (BSE)

Catherine Folker-Maglaya, RN, MSN, IBCLC

1. Assess patient's knowledge/skill with performing breast self-examination.
2. Explain reasons for performing breast self-examination.
   a. The breast is the major site for carcinoma in women.
   b. Until the disease can be prevented, the best means of protection is through early detection and treatment.
   c. Most lumps are found by women themselves.
   d. Most lumps found are not cancerous.
   e. Breast cancer is primarily a disease of women and every woman is at-risk as she grows older. Some factors that increase risk include:
      1) Age (35 and older).
      2) History of breast cancer in close family (mother, grandmother, sister, or aunt).
      3) Onset of menstruation prior to age 12.
      4) Late onset of menopause.
      5) Nullipara (never having given birth).
      6) Birth of first child at age over 30.
      7) Obesity: 40% above ideal weight.
3. Discuss integral components for breast health. In addition to breast self-examination, they include:
   a. Clinical breast examination by health care provider, which consists of a visual inspection with palpation of breasts, chest, and axilla. *Annual examination is recommended for women without breast symptoms.* Encourage the patient to note how the examination is performed and to pay close attention to the amount of pressure applied to the breasts during the examination. *This can serve as guide for the patient when doing self-examination.*
   b. Mammogram (breast x-ray) for women 35 years and older. Refer to Teaching Guide on Mammogram.
4. Instruct regarding performance of breast self-examination:
   a. Self-examination should be performed by women over the age of 20.
   b. Examination should be performed when the breasts will be the least lumpy. If the woman has regular menses, the breasts should be ex-

amined at the end of the menstrual period. If no menses, the examination should be performed on the same day each month. If breast feeding, in addition to above, perform breast examination after breast feeding, when the breasts have been well emptied.

   c. Stress the importance of becoming familiar with one's breast. After learning how normal breast tissue feels, recognition of changes can be made more readily. Confidence will be gained by regular performance of the examination.

5. Instruct the patient in the how-to's of breast self-examination

   a. Lie down and flatten the right breast by placing a pillow under the shoulder of the same breast. If large-breasted, the breast should be supported by the right hand while performing the examination with the left hand.

   b. Use the pads of the index, middle, and ring fingers on the left hand. With a rubbing motion, feel for lumps or thickening, pressing firmly enough to feel the various breast tissues.

   c. Thoroughly feel the entire breast and chest, making certain to examine the breast tissue extending toward the shoulder.

   d. Provide ample time for a complete examination. Small breasts will require a few minutes, while larger breasts will require more time.

   e. Use the same method for feeling every part of the breast (the easiest method should be chosen). Figure 66.1 illustrates the three breast self-examinations methods most commonly preferred by women: circular, vertical strip, and wedge.

   f. After completing the examination of the right breast, examine the left breast in the same manner.

   g. Also examine the breasts while showering or bathing. Lumps can be felt more easily when the skin is wet.

   h. Also examine the breasts before a mirror, checking for noticeable changes in size or contour, a swelling or dimpling of the skin. Squeeze the nipples to check or discharge.

   i. If any changes are noted, contact a physician without delay.

6. Following step-by-step instruction, have patient provide return demonstration. Offer comments for improvement of skills. *This allows the nurse an opportunity to assess and improve patient's ability to perform BSE.*

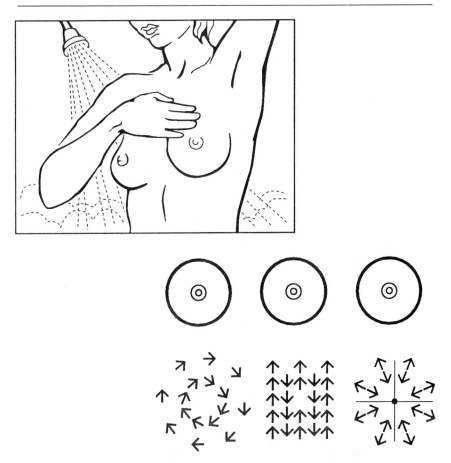

Figure 66.1 Three methods for breast self-examination: circular, vertical strip, and wedge. Reprinted with permission from the American Cancer Society.

REFERENCES

American Cancer Society. (1987). *Special Touch: A Personal Plan of Action for Breast Health Brochure.* Washington, D.C.

Champion, V. (1992). Breast self-examination in women 65 and older. *Journal of Gerontology. 47,* 75–79.

Liff, J., Sung, J., Chow, W., Greenberg, R., & Flanders, W. (1991). Does increased detection account for the rising incidence of breast cancer? *American Journal of Public Health. 81*(4), 462–465.

Stefanek, M. E. & Wilcox, P. (1991). First-degree relatives of breast cancer patients: Screening practices and provision of risk information. *Cancer Detection and Prevention. 15*(5), 379–384.

INDEX

Note: Page numbers followed by t indicate tables; numbers followed by f indicate figures.

DATE DUE	
MAY 0 6 1998	
DEC 0 3 2004	
DEC 0 6 2004	

GAYLORD   PRINTED IN U.S.A.